MEAT SCIENCE
An Introductory Text

P.D. WARRISS

School of Veterinary Science
University of Bristol
Bristol
UK

CABI *Publishing*

CABI *Publishing* is a division of CAB *International*

CABI Publishing
CAB International
Wallingford
Oxon OX10 8DE
UK

Tel: +44 (0)1491 832111
Fax: +44 (0)1491 833508
Email: cabi@cabi.org
Web site: http://www.cabi.org

CABI Publishing
10 E 40th Street
Suite 3203
New York, NY 10016
USA

Tel: +1 (212) 481 7018
Fax: +1 212 686 7993
Email: cabi-nao@cabi.org

A catalogue record for this book is available from the British Library, London, UK

Library of Congress Cataloging-in-Publication Data
Warriss, P. D.
Meat science : an introductory text / P.D. Warriss.
p. cm.
Includes bibliographical references and index.
ISBN 0–85199–424–5 (alk. paper)
1. Meat. I. Title.

TX373.W37 2000
664′.9--dc21

99–048373

ISBN 0 85199 424 5

Typeset in 10/12pt Melior by Columns Design Ltd, Reading.
Printed and bound in the UK by Biddles Ltd, Guildford and King's Lynn.

MEAT SCIENCE
An Introductory Text

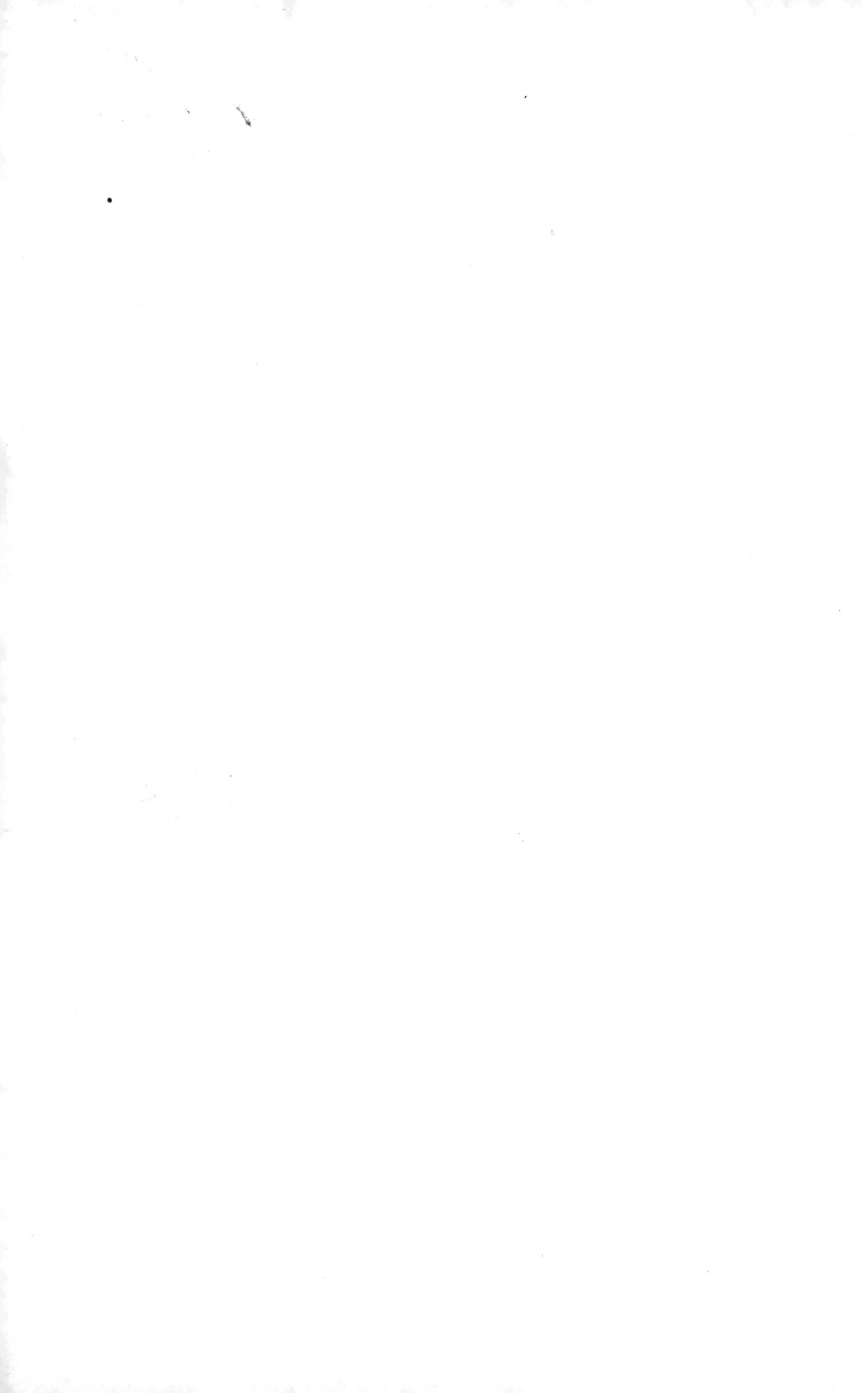

Contents

Preface

The standard reference work in meat science for many years has undoubtedly been R.A. Lawrie's *Meat Science*, first published in 1966. More recently, a number of other works have provided good overviews of the subject but from slightly different perspectives. H.J. Swatland's *Structure and Development of Meat Animals and Poultry* has given us an authoritative work based on a structural approach to meat science. N.G. Gregory has given us a different perspective in his *Animal Welfare and Meat Science* and the technology of meat and meat products is well covered in A.H. Varnum and J.P. Sutherlands' *Meat and Meat Products*. However, for many readers who require a simple overview of the subject, these books may perhaps be too detailed in their treatment and an introductory text would be more useful. The present work is therefore aimed at undergraduate and postgraduate students in food science and technology, animal and veterinary science, and technical staff in the meat industry. It may also be of interest to veterinarians and meat inspectors.

In such a book it is impossible to cover all relevant topics in depth and therefore the object has not been to be comprehensive. Rather, it seemed better to outline the general principles and to provide sufficient references to allow readers to access further, detailed information if required.

I would like to acknowledge the help of many of my colleagues in giving advice and reading through sections of text. Steve Brown helped with production of many of the graphs, Kath McDonnell and Carol Hole typed the manuscript, and John Conibear produced the final text figures from my original sketches. To these people I am especially grateful.

Chapter 1

Producing and Eating Meat

Humans appear to be adapted to an omnivorous diet, based on the shape of their teeth and their unspecialized gut, and it is likely that quite early in human evolution meat began to play a part in our diet. Originally this would have been scavenged from the kills of more effective predators, such as the large cats, until hunting techniques developed. The domestication of animals and the development of animal husbandry ensured a more reliable source of meat and coincidentally reduced the number of species from which it was obtained to about two dozen or so, of which half are now significant sources of meat. These include not only mammals such as cattle, sheep, goats, pigs, buffaloes, camels, yaks, llamas, deer and rabbits but also birds, especially domestic fowls and turkeys, geese and ducks, reptiles such as alligators, fish and various invertebrates. Currently there is also considerable interest in using various new species for meat production (Kyle, 1994) including several antelopes, the American bison and the ostrich.

Despite this range, the important meat-producing species remain domestic cattle, sheep, pigs and poultry. Cattle, sheep and pigs are often referred to as 'red meat' species and poultry as a 'white meat'. The importance of the three red meat species in supplying meat protein differs in different parts of the world. Beef is most important in North and South America, Africa and Europe while sheep are most important in the Near East and pigs in the Far East.

Meat Production and Consumption

World meat production

The total world production of the four main types of meat in 1995 was 197 Mt (GIRA, 1997). The largest amount was pig meat (83.2 Mt) followed by poultry (53.9 Mt), beef (53.2 Mt) and sheep meat (7.0 Mt). Between 1984 and 1994 total meat production increased by an average of 3.8% per year (Table 1.1). The size of the increase differed in the four meats. Over the 10 years, beef production increased by 16% and sheep meat production by 17%. In contrast, pig meat production rose by 41% and poultry meat by 72%. These differences in production reflect differences in preference by consumers. Pig and poultry meat are becoming relatively more popular. This is because of several factors. Pork and poultry are cheaper to produce than beef and sheep meat and they are also generally thought by consumers in the developed world to be healthier to eat. This perceived greater healthiness is partly because of the concern about eating animal fats. The redder meats (beef and sheep meat) tend to be associated in consumers' minds with larger amounts of fat. In contrast, there is little if any visible fat in *skinless* poultry meat and the same is true for pork. This often has inherently relatively little fat now, or the fat has been closely trimmed, and generally has less apparent 'marbling' – the fine strings of fat within the body of the muscle – than beef or sheep meat.

Another factor is the growth of population in parts of the world where pork and poultry are traditionally the preferred meats. For example, the production of pork increased by 122% between 1984 and 1994 in China, compared with 45% in the countries of the European Union (EU) and only 20% in the USA. The geographical variation in the production of the different meats is illustrated in Table 1.2. In Asia and the Far East nearly two-thirds of the total meat production is from pigs. In South America, and Australia and New Zealand, beef production accounts for about half of the total meat produced. In Australia and New Zealand, a quarter of meat production is sheep meat. In Africa and the Middle East nearly a fifth of meat is produced from sheep and over 40% from poultry. These differences probably reflect both preferences of the populations for different sorts of meat and the suitability of the environment for growing the different species. In particular, cattle thrive in extensive grassland regions. Table 1.3 lists the major producers of beef, sheep, pig and poultry meat by country in

Table 1.1. Changes in the world production of meat (Mt) between 1984 and 1994 (based on data from GIRA, 1997).

	1984	1989	1994	Change over 10 years
Beef	45.6	51.0	52.7	+16%
Sheep meat	6.1	6.7	7.2	+17%
Pig meat	55.8	67.9	78.5	+41%
Poultry meat	29.7	38.1	51.2	+72%

Table 1.2. The production of meat in 1995 (Mt) (based on data from GIRA, 1997).

	Total meat	Beef	Sheep meat	Pig meat	Poultry meat
Asia and Far East	68.6	7.4	2.7[a]	43.7	14.8
North America	41.6	14.4	0.2	10.4	16.6
EU[b]	33.0	7.8	1.2	16.0	7.9
South America	18.7	9.3	0.3	2.4	6.6
Former Soviet Union	18.7	7.0	0.9	7.8	3.0
Africa and Middle East	9.6	3.4	1.8	0.5	3.9
Australia and NZ	4.4	2.3	1.1	0.4	0.6

[a] Includes goat meat.
[b] Fifteen member states.

1995. The USA produced 22% of all beef and 26% of all poultry meat. China produced 44% of all pig meat and an estimated 14% of sheep meat.

In many western societies in particular, there have been changes in the relative consumption of the different types of meat. This is illustrated by the situation in the UK (Table 1.4). The consumption of beef and lamb has progressively fallen, that of pork and bacon has remained steady and that of poultry has increased substantially. Poultry meat is now the major meat eaten in the UK and, together with pork, forms nearly two-thirds of overall consumption (Table 1.5). Small amounts of offal, chiefly liver and kidneys, are eaten. The overall consumption of meat in the UK is about 20% below the average for the EU. UK consumers eat only three-quarters of the beef and half the pig meat of the average European, but slightly more lamb and poultry. The discrepancy is even greater between the UK and North American consumers. North Americans eat approximately double the amounts of beef and poultry as are eaten in the UK.

Table 1.3. The major producers of each type of meat in 1995 (data from GIRA, 1997).

Beef		Sheep meat		Pig meat		Poultry meat	
USA	22%	China	14%[a]	China	44%	USA	26%
FSU	11%	FSU	10%	USA	9%	China	17%
Brazil	10%	Australia	9%	FSU	4%	Brazil	8%
China	8%	New Zealand	7%	Germany	4%	France	4%
Argentina	5%	UK	6%	Spain	3%	FSU	3%
Mexico	4%	Turkey	4%	France	3%	Japan	2%

[a] Estimated.
FSU, Former Soviet Union.

Table 1.4. Recent per capita meat consumption (kg) in the UK (source: MLC, 1997).

Year	Beef and veal	Mutton and lamb	Pork and bacon	Poultry	Total meat
1985	19.0	7.1	20.8	15.6	62.5
1987	20.1	6.3	21.2	18.6	66.2
1989	18.5	7.2	21.2	21.4	68.2
1991	17.5	7.3	20.8	23.0	68.8
1993	15.5	5.8	20.9	25.5	67.7
1995	15.3	6.1	20.2	27.0	68.6

Table 1.5. Consumption of different meats in the UK in 1995 (source: MLC, 1997).

	Percentage of total meat consumption
Poultry	37.5
Pork and bacon	28.1
Beef and veal	21.2
Mutton and lamb	8.5
Offal	4.6

The sources of meat

Meat can come from both specialist systems, such as broiler chicken units, beef suckler herds and pig units, and as a by-product of other agricultural enterprises whose main function is not the production of meat. For example, in the UK about a quarter of all cattle slaughtered are culled cows, mostly from the dairy herd. Of the remaining three-quarters of beef, coming from steers, heifers and young bulls, just over half is also from the dairy herd. This contrasts with the situation in the USA where 80% of beef is from beef breeds. Culled laying hens are used for the production of low-value poultry meat products. Even in pig production, where the only product is meat, this can come from culled sows as well as 'clean pigs', that is, animals that have not formed part of the breeding herd.

Concerns about Eating Meat

The nutritional value of meat

Red meat and poultry contribute about a sixth of all protein consumed by humans and, if fish, milk and eggs are included, animal products supply a third. Not only is meat a very concentrated source of protein but this has a high biological value because its composition matches closely that of our own proteins. It contains all the amino acids essential for human health. Meat is also an important source of the B vitamins, particularly B1 (thiamine), niacin (nicotinic acid), B2 (riboflavin), B6 and B12 (cyanocobalamin), and vitamin A (retinol). It is a major source of iron, copper, zinc and selenium. Iron in meat has high bioavailability, the main reservoir being as a component of the haem protein myoglobin. Iron deficiency is the most common nutritional deficiency in the world (Neale, 1992). Haem iron is more easily absorbed from the gut than non-haem iron, for example that in plant materials. What meat does not provide in the diet is carbohydrate, and particularly fibre, and vitamins K and C (ascorbic acid). The nutritional value of meat is further considered in Chapter 6.

Meat as purchased by the consumer often contains a relatively high fat content. Steaks or joints in the UK may contain between 15 and 30% separable fat (Enser *et al.*, 1996). There is still 1 or 2% fat in closely trimmed lean. The white (breast) meat of poultry contains about 1% fat and this rises to 3% in the dark (leg) meat, but, if the skin is included, the fat levels in poultry meat are much higher. Poultry skin contains 33% fat, and the subdermal layers even higher amounts. Fat is an excellent energy source. A high fat content equates to a high energy (calorific) content. To early hunter–gatherer populations this was a very valuable attribute of meat. It may be less beneficial today, with a much-reduced demand for calories in most modern human populations, and consequently there has been a general trend to reduce the amount of carcass fat in animals. Indeed, from the point of view of human health, a high-fat diet is now thought undesirable. However, this statement needs to be qualified. It is not just the amount of fat that is important, but the type. Also, it presupposes that people have the fairly sedentary lifestyle with low dietary energy requirements that is characteristic of a large proportion of the population of developed countries.

Health concerns

The dietary intake of fat varies widely in different cultures. In developing countries much more dietary energy (80%) comes from carbohydrates than in developed countries (55%). The difference in energy from carbohydrates is made up by increased fat consumption. The diets of developing countries are therefore a lot less energy-dense with much higher levels of fibre. Energy-dense diets that are low in fibre tend to be associated with various chronic diseases amongst which are coronary heart disease, cerebrovascular disease and various cancers. An additional factor is that high levels of total fat in the diet are often, but not always, associated with high levels of saturated fat. Coronary heart disease is one of the major causes of death of adults in

North America and Europe. Two factors which are associated with higher risk – high blood cholesterol and high blood pressure – are both seemingly affected adversely by diets high in fat, particularly saturated fat (see Chapter 3), although there seems to be an important genetic component to a person's susceptibility.

In the UK in the last 20 years, two committees have considered the implications for health of fat in the national diet. The National Advisory Committee on Nutrition Education (NACNE), formed in 1979, recommended that fat intake should be reduced by 25% and should provide not more than 30% of the total energy intake. Moreover, saturated fatty acids should not make up more than 10% of the total energy intake. Subsequently, the Committee on Medical Aspects of Food and Nutrition Policy (COMA) published a report in 1984 that focused on the relation between diet and cardiovascular disease. This recommended that total fat consumption should be reduced to 35% of the total energy consumed and that not more than 15% should come from saturated and *trans* fatty acids. *Trans* fatty acids are unsaturated fatty acids (which are characteristic of plant oils) that have been chemically modified (hydrogenated) during food processing so they behave in many ways like saturated fatty acids.

Although the recommendations from the two committees were seemingly slightly different, this is not really so, since the differences can mostly be explained by small differences in definition. The important message was that dietary fat should be reduced and it should be less saturated. Because the proportion of saturated to unsaturated fats is rather higher in animal products, particularly meat and dairy produce, the implications were that consumption of these should ideally be reduced. Inevitably this will influence health-conscious consumers. Their concern about meat eating could well be reinforced by other information. In developed countries a quarter of all deaths are attributed to cancers and about half of these are thought to be related to dietary factors. It has been suggested that eating meat is linked to a higher prevalence of colon cancer. There seems to be little or no conclusive evidence for this except that colon cancer is linked to diets containing low amounts of fibre but high amounts of fat, and therefore energy, and that these diets are likely to be largely dependent on animal products like meat. However, when meat is cooked at high temperatures, and particularly when it is exposed to naked flames or barbecued over hot charcoal, various pyrolysis products may be formed on the surface or derived from the smoked residues. Examples are the polycyclic aromatic hydrocarbons (PAHs) such as benzo(a)pyrene. Although formed in very low amounts, some of these compounds can cause tumours in laboratory animals. They are therefore potentially causes of human cancers but their actual importance is unclear. There is also legitimate concern about the nitrites used in producing cured meats like bacon and ham. Nitrite has been identified as a potential carcinogen, either directly or through the formation of nitrosamines when it reacts with amines. There is therefore considerable interest in reducing the nitrite levels in cured meat products to a minimum.

Food hygiene

Recently there have also been concerns about the healthiness of meat in regard to other aspects of food safety. Animal products are a major potential source of serious food poisoning in man such as that caused by *Salmonella* and *Campylobacter*. In Europe, probably at least 80% of food poisoning occurs through consumption of meat contaminated with these organisms. In the USA, consumption of meat or poultry was implicated in 54% of all reported outbreaks of food-borne illness in which the cause was ascertained between 1968 and 1977 (Bryan, 1980). A concern is that we do not know the real prevalence of the problem. It is thought that only of the order of 10% of cases are actually reported, even in developed countries, and the figure may be as little as 1% in developing countries. Official statistics are therefore likely to underestimate the seriousness of the problem. Nevertheless, it is apparent that the frequency of infection is increasing (Fig. 1.1) and campylobacteriosis is now probably the main food-borne disease in the UK. Where *Campylobacter* is a food contaminant it has almost invariably come from animals. Certain strains of *Escherichia coli*, especially *E. coli* O157:H7, which has been found in the intestine of cattle, have caused serious outbreaks of gastroenteritis. *E. coli* O157:H7 is one of the serotypes of the bacterium that produce verocytotoxins. These enable the organism to penetrate and damage the cells of the gut lining and cause it to be infective and virulent in even small numbers. The O157:H7 serotype is of particular concern when very young children or old people are infected since these groups seem especially at risk of developing severe symptoms. Bacterial contamination of meat can be minimized by careful hygiene practices during carcass dressing and the effects on humans prevented by effective cooking. But modern life styles, and food production and preparation systems, have resulted in greater chances of contamination with correspondingly increased infection rates.

A problem much more difficult to address has been the emergence of bovine spongiform encephalopathy (BSE) in cattle in the UK in the late 1980s. BSE was first reported in Great Britain in November 1986 (Bradley, 1993). This is a neuropathological disease similar to scrapie that has been known in sheep for many decades. Scrapie does not apparently infect humans but there is now strong evidence that the causative agent of BSE (a prion) has crossed species to produce a new

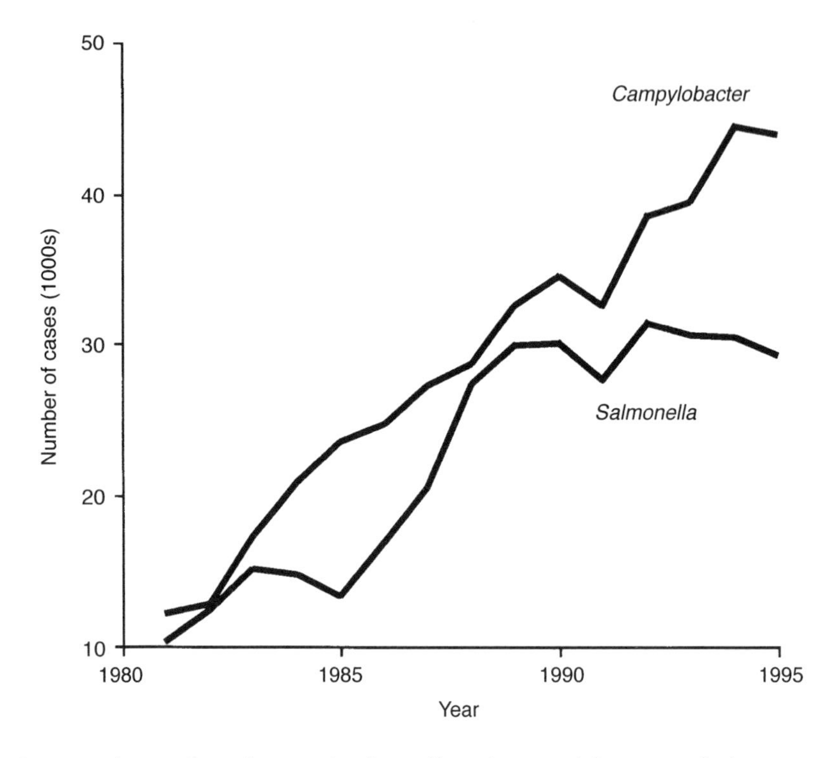

Fig. 1.1. The number of cases of *Salmonella* and *Campylobacter* notified as causes of food-borne disease in England and Wales between 1981 and 1995 (data supplied by the Communicable Disease Surveillance Centre of the UK Public Health Laboratory Service).

strain of Creutzfeldt–Jakob disease (CJD). BSE was probably spread through the UK dairy and beef herds by feeding protein supplements derived from the waste material produced as a by-product of the slaughtering industry. This material is 'rendered' to sterilize it and extract usable fats. It is thought that changes in procedures led to inadequacies in the rendering process allowing survival of the extremely resilient infective prions.

Because encephalopathies may have very long incubation periods before symptoms of the disease are manifested (in cattle this is typically 3–5 years), it is still unclear how many people were infected before effective steps were taken to minimize the risk. These included slaughtering potentially infected animals, removing potentially infective parts of the carcass (particularly the brain and spinal cord) at slaughter and disposing of them so they could not enter the food chain, and changing rendering procedures. The feeding of protein derived from ruminants back to cattle and other ruminants was prohibited in 1988. From 1996 it was prohibited for all animals. These measures have led to a progressive, large reduction in the number of BSE cases. The disease is thought to have reached its peak in 1992 and the incidence began to decline in 1993. It is likely that the disease will eventually be virtually eliminated.

The number of people possibly exposed to infection by consuming potentially infected beef prior to recognition of the problem and implementation of effective preventative measures was large. However, the fact that beef muscle does not appear to be infective, and that eating infected material seems to be an inefficient way of becoming infected *across* species, suggests that the risks to humans of contracting CJD from beef are very small. CJD is an extremely rare disease. Normally less than 20 cases a year are reported in the UK population of more than 50 million people. Nevertheless, the fear of catching such a dreadful disease, albeit with apparently such a small risk, from consuming potentially infected meat had enormous effects on sales. Home beef consumption slumped and there were bans on the export of UK beef. This illustrates how important is the consumer's perceived risk associated with a particular product even though the relation between this perceived risk and the actual risk may be rather weak. This can be because the consumer's assessment of the risk is based on irrational arguments sometimes encouraged by the way information is reported by the media. An interesting discussion of the concept of risk in animal agriculture is given in Kunkel *et al.* (1998).

Bacterial resistance to antibiotics

There is some concern about the development of bacterial resistance to antibiotics (Taylor, 1997). When populations of bacteria are exposed to the appropriate antibiotics, the vast majority of cells will be killed. However, it is possible that, through random mutations, a very small number of cells may survive through having developed resistance. These cells will therefore be selected for and the genetic mutation conferring resistance will be passed to their daughter cells. In this manner, antibiotic resistance can develop and the resistance may be passed on to other bacterial cells through various mechanisms. Of particular concern is the selection of resistant food-borne pathogens (Threlfall, 1992). The development of resistance will be encouraged by inappropriate or unnecessary use of antibiotics. One such use is as growth promoters in animal feeds and there is a body of opinion that suggests that this use should be phased out. About half of all the antibiotics used in the UK are for agricultural purposes and most of these are for growth promotion rather than for treating sick animals. Sweden has banned the use of antibiotic growth promoters for all livestock (Tronstad, 1997) and Denmark has banned virginiamycin, the most widely used growth promoter in pig production. In 1999, authorization for the use of virginiamycin and three other antibiotics as feed additives was withdrawn throughout the EU.

Agricultural sustainability and animal welfare

As if these concerns about the wholesomeness of meat, even if sometimes misinformed or exaggerated, and the consequences of some husbandry practices, were not enough, there are other factors which may result in future reductions in the consumption of meat. Meat production is often associated with a concept of agriculture that is linked to lack of sustainability and long-term damage to the environment. The production of animals from plants is relatively inefficient. Only about a tenth of the energy of one trophic level is passed to the next, the remaining 90% being lost as heat. More food can therefore be produced from an area of suitable land by growing plants and harvesting them directly than by feeding the plants to animals to produce meat. This is of concern in a world where there are still people with not enough to eat.

There is disquiet about the degree of intensification of some modern animal production systems, particularly for non-ruminants like pigs and poultry. These systems, while efficient at producing animal protein, sometimes appear to be doing so at the expense of both damaging the environment, for example by the production of slurry (animal waste) and the build-up of nitrogen, phosphorus and potassium in soils and ground water, and the welfare of animals. In the future, environmental considerations, particularly the disposal of animal wastes, may become one of the major limiting factors in the production of food animals. A major concern with many people is our dependency on naturally occurring animal protein and fat sources to supplement the diets of farm animals. Nearly a third of all fish caught in the world are processed into meal and oil rather than being eaten directly as a protein source by humans. Three-quarters of the fishmeal is used to feed pigs and poultry. A further sixth of the meal and over a quarter of the oil is fed back to farmed fish. Whether this is a sustainable and acceptable way of using a diminishing natural resource is questionable.

To some, this exploitation of the environment and natural resources is linked to an unacceptable exploitation of farm animals generally. Many people are concerned that the meat they eat should come from animals that have been bred, reared, and slaughtered in ways which are sympathetic to the animals' welfare. This is reflected in a move away from more extreme forms of intensive farming, for example the use of veal crates to rear small calves in, and farrowing crates to house parturient sows. A similar related concern is the housing of hens in battery cages and attempts to find welfare-friendly alternatives, but there are people for whom concessions to animal welfare such as these are not sufficient and who turn away from eating meat as a consequence.

A balanced view

These rather negative concerns about meat production and consumption need to be balanced by positive considerations. Certain areas and soils are unsuitable for growing crops useful to man, and animals can be used to exploit these areas indirectly. Sheep can be reared on the hills of northern Britain under conditions unsuitable for cultivating crops, and many natural grasslands can only be effectively exploited by grazing cattle. The production of meat is associated with a large range of other valuable by-products, for example skin and leather, wool, pharmaceuticals and fats. It may itself be linked to the use of the animal for other reasons. A large part of the beef eaten in Europe comes directly or indirectly from the dairy herd, the main object of which is to provide milk. Surplus calves are reared for beef and meat from culled cows forms a sizeable proportion of overall beef production.

Generally, as the wealth of groups of people has increased, so has their consumption of meat implying a preference or natural appetite for meat over a largely vegetarian diet, despite its current somewhat unhealthy image. The reason most people eat meat is that they enjoy eating it, but, perhaps like most things we enjoy eating, the ideal is to consume it in moderation and as part of a well-balanced diet. On the positive side there are major benefits from including meat in the diet. In contrast, there are major health concerns with eating too much fat, and too much saturated fat in particular. Animal products like meat can be a major source of these but the same is true for dairy foods. The dairy industry has addressed the problem by developing low-fat alternatives to its traditional products. The meat industry needs to do the same, both in learning how to produce low-fat fresh meat that tastes good and also in developing more convenient forms of low-fat product for the consumer. Additionally, there will be a need to address consumer concerns about the ethical questions surrounding meat production, in particular the requirements for sustainability of agricultural systems and the need to ensure high welfare standards for the animals reared in them.

Chapter 2

The Growth and Body Composition of Animals

Growth commonly refers to an increase in size or weight of an animal. There is a need to differentiate true growth caused by increase in the amount of living material (an increase in cell mass) from the increase in weight caused, for example, by ingestion of water or food. Sometimes the term growth has therefore been restricted to an increase in size of those parts of an animal which are subsequently capable of growing more. Another aspect of growth is that it involves change in shape and perhaps composition. This is attributable to cellular differentiation and is the main reason why it is of interest in meat science. Generally we want to eat some parts of an animal but not others, or at least we prefer some parts to others. It is therefore important to know how the yield of the desirable parts can be maximized. For example, we might well want to maximize the yield of lean meat and reduce the proportion of fat in the carcass.

Growth in Animals

The growth curve

If the weight of an animal is plotted against its age, an S-shaped or sigmoid curve is produced (Fig. 2.1). The weight increases slowly at first, the rate of increase reaches a maximum and then decreases so the increase in live weight with age in old animals is small. This shape of growth curve can be derived for most animals. The point of inflexion, where the curve changes from concave to convex, occurs at the maximum growth rate and is therefore referred to as the maximum point of growth. Food consumed by the animal is used for two processes: the

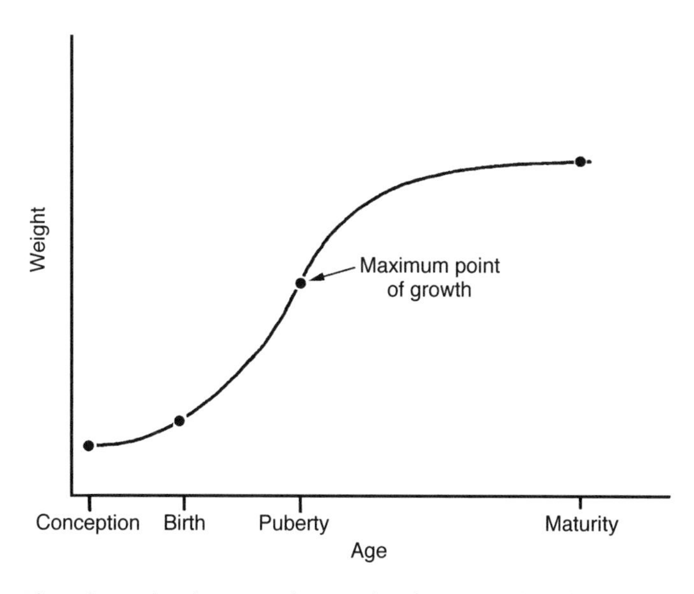

Fig. 2.1. The relationship between the weight of an animal and its age.

maintenance of existing tissues and the growth of new tissue. As growth is fastest at the maximum point of growth it is also most efficient because the proportion of the total energy available to the animal that is used for maintenance of its body is relatively least. At any time, growth is determined by the balance between accelerating and retarding forces. An example of an accelerating force is the increase in the mass of cells making up the body. Examples of retarding forces are the decrease in available space for a tissue to grow, or lack of nutrients. The maximum point of growth is where the two forces balance. This occurs at puberty in mammals. Normally this is at about 30% of mature weight. Human beings are unusual in that the growth curve is distorted by a disproportionately long period as infants and juveniles and that puberty occurs at 60 to 70% of mature weight.

Describing growth

The rate of growth can be described in different ways. The *average growth rate* over a period of time is calculated by dividing the increase in weight over a particular time period by the length of that period:

$$\text{average growth rate} = w_2 - w_1/t_2 - t_1,$$

where w_1 is the weight at the start of the period (t_1) and w_2 is the weight at the end (t_2). This method gives the growth rate in terms of g day^{-1} or kg week^{-1} for example. The *relative growth rate* is calculated as the increase in weight over a period of time divided by the initial weight:

$$\text{relative growth rate} = w_2 - w_1/w_1.$$

This gives the growth rate expressed as a proportional increase, for example a percentage, over the defined time period. The sigmoid curve derived by plotting absolute weight against age is only one way of showing growth. Plotting the average growth rate or the relative growth rate against age produces different types of curve (Fig. 2.2). The plot of average growth rate shows that the animal grows fastest in the period in the middle of its life. However, relative growth rate decreases progressively throughout life, reflecting the fact that the increase in body mass, expressed as a proportion of that already existing, reduces with time.

In many husbandry systems, growth rates are directly influenced by the feeding system. For example, beef animals may be maintained

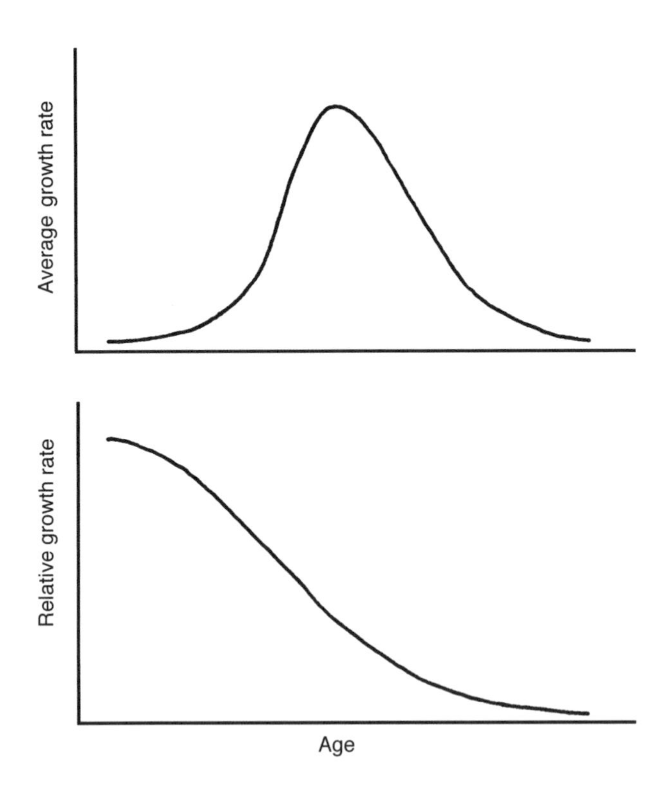

Fig. 2.2. The relationships between average and relative growth rates and age.

over winter on relatively small amounts of poor quality food when their growth slows or stops altogether. During the following spring this 'store' period is replaced by a 'finishing' period when the availability of new, highly nutritious pasture allows rapid 'compensatory' growth to occur.

The process of growth

As indicated above, growth consists of the combination of increase in the total body cell mass and differentiation of these cells. The differentiation makes certain tissues, organs or parts of the body grow at different rates from that of the whole body and leads to a change in shape as well as size. It is a point of common observation that human babies have relatively big heads compared with adults. The same is true for other young mammals including meat species. These often also have relatively long thin legs. The change in shape of meat animals as they matured was first carefully documented by John Hammond at the School of Agriculture of the University of Cambridge in the 1930s (Fig. 2.3).

Because they grow at different rates, different parts of the body mature at different times. This applies whether regions of the body, different types of tissues or different examples of a particular tissue are considered. The head develops faster and matures earlier than the thorax, which in turn matures before the loin. Central nervous tissue matures before bone, which matures before muscle. The last tissue to mature is fat and, within this tissue, different depots mature earlier or later. The first to mature is the fat surrounding the kidneys (perinephric), followed by that between different muscles (intermuscular), that just under the skin (subcutaneous) and finally the fat within the muscles (intramuscular).

There are obvious biological reasons for these sequences of maturity. They also have implications for the production of animals with desirable carcass characteristics. For example, as fat is the last tissue to be laid down, leaner carcasses can be produced by killing animals after the majority of muscle growth has occurred but before much fat has been deposited. However, this objective might have to be balanced against a requirement for larger carcass size and some minimal amount of fat in it. Similarly, a balance has to be struck between wanting a minimal level of intramuscular fat to maintain eating quality of the lean (see Chapter 6) while wanting to reduce overall fat levels in the carcass for economic and health reasons. A concise overview of the growth and development of meat animals is that of Trenkle and Marple (1983).

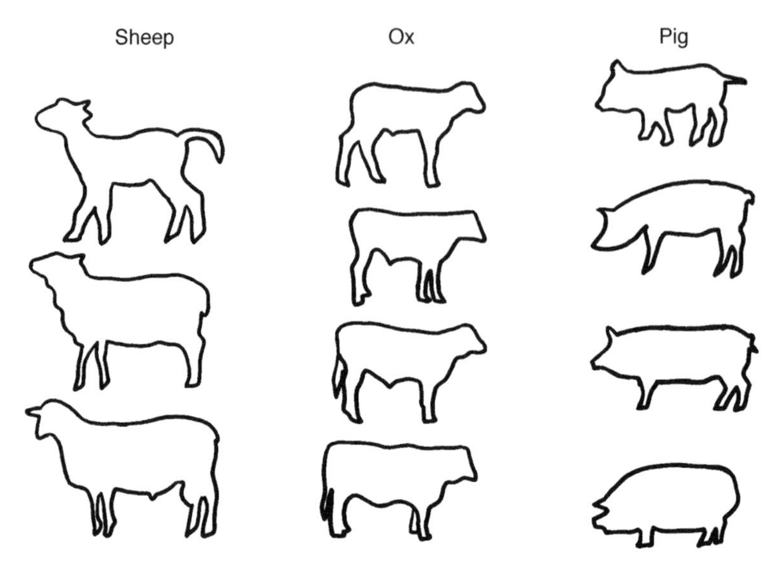

Fig. 2.3. Tracings from photographs of sheep, cattle and pigs at different stages of maturity (the tracings are from photographs reproduced in Pálsson (1955) and based on those originally published by Sir John Hammond in the 1930s).

Describing different relative growth

Changes in the proportion and composition of an animal as it grows are caused by differences in growth rates of the different body parts. A very useful way of describing this relative growth is by expressing the size of the particular part of interest (y) in relation to the size of the whole body (x) in terms of an equation originally developed by J.S. Huxley in the 1930s. This is:

$$y = bx^k,$$

where b and k are constants. The value of k describes the relative growth rate. If $k > 1$ the part becomes proportionally larger in bigger animals. If $k < 1$, the part becomes proportionally smaller in bigger animals. In the former case the part is said to be positively allometric and in the latter negatively allometric. An example of positive allometry is the size of antlers in red deer (*Cervus elaphus*). These are *relatively* larger in older, larger stags as well as being larger in *absolute* terms. The concept of allometry has also been referred to as heterogony. The equation seems to fit many actual examples well and therefore can be very useful in summarizing growth data. However, its real biological significance is not completely clear.

The equation can also be used to compare the growth of different parts of the body to one another, rather than the growth of one part to the whole. In this case, when $k = 1$ the two components grow at the same rate. By taking logarithms of both sides the equation becomes much more convenient to use because the relationship is transformed into a linear one:

$$\log y = \log b + k \log x.$$

Tulloh (1964) gave equations in this form which described the growth of bone, muscle and fat as functions of carcass weight in sheep. The equations were:

log *bone* weight = −0.474 + 0.678 log carcass weight;

log *muscle* weight = −0.239 + 0.978 log carcass weight;

log *fat* weight = −1.136 + 1.594 log carcass weight.

These relationships are plotted in Fig. 2.4. Note that, with an increase in carcass weight, the percentage bone decreases ($k<1(0.678)$), the percentage fat increases ($k>1(1.594)$) and the percentage muscle changes only slightly ($k\sim1(0.978)$). This means that increasing carcass weight from about 15 to 20 kg reduces the proportion of bone in the carcass by 10%, increases that of the fat by 16% and reduces the relative muscle content by 4% (Table 2.1). Doubling the carcass weight from 15 to 30 kg reduces the proportion of bone by 26% and muscle by 9%, but increases that of fat by 40%.

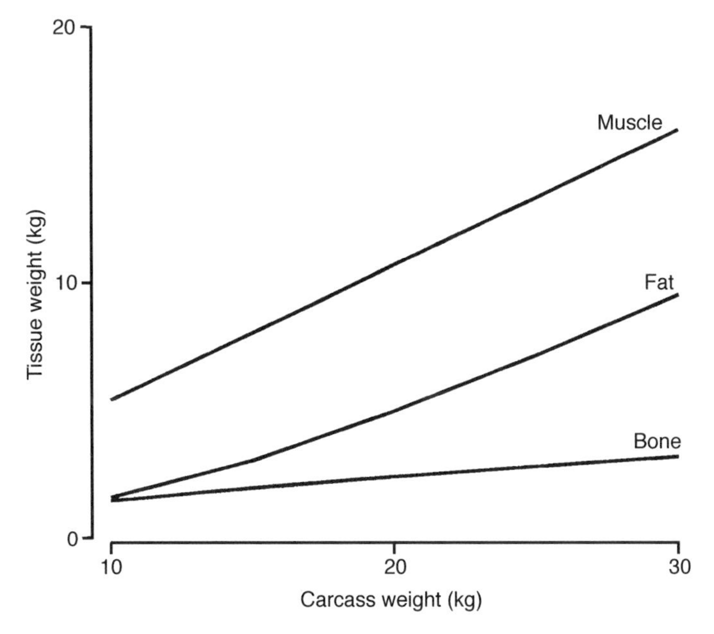

Fig. 2.4. The weights of bone, muscle and fat in sheep carcasses based on Tulloh's (1964) equations.

Table 2.1. Percentages of bone, muscle and fat in different sized sheep carcasses (based on data in Tulloh, 1964).

Carcass weight	Bone (%)	Muscle (%)	Fat (%)
15	16	61	24
20	14	58	28
30	12	55	33

Strictly speaking, when using the allometric equation to examine the relation of one part of the carcass to the whole, the whole should *not* include the part. However, in practice this requirement is often ignored with little apparent harm. Thus, whole carcass weight is used in Tulloh's (1964) equations, rather than carcass weight minus the tissue of interest (e.g. fat).

Growth of muscle and fat

The growth of tissues consists of two processes. First, the number of cells increases by cell division. This is referred to as hyperplasia. Second, the cells increase in size. This is referred to as hypertrophy. Most of the hyperplasia occurs before birth. About 30–40 cell divisions take place during gestation compared with only two to four post-natally. After birth the cells hypertrophy so tissue mass increases with little change in the number of cells.

Muscle growth

The cells that will form muscle fibres are called myoblasts. Each has a single nucleus. The myoblasts fuse into muscle 'straps' which subsequently lose their separate cell membranes to form multinucleated myotubes. These are immature muscle fibres. They elongate into mature fibres. Only a few cells, called satellite cells, retain the capacity to replicate after birth. These act as a reserve for the development of new myoblasts. The functional units of contraction within the fibres are sarcomeres. As muscle fibres grow in length, new sarcomeres are added at the ends. There are contractile organelles within fibres called myofibrils. Myofibril numbers increase by splitting longitudinally. Larger species of animal have more muscle fibres in their muscles but the size of the fibres is similar. So-called 'double-muscled' animals (Arthur, 1995), which occur in certain beef breeds, have a larger number of fibres in their muscles than normal animals, hence the pronounced 'muscling' when mature. Having a larger number of fibres present at birth leads to more rapid growth than in animals having smaller numbers. In any case, muscle growth in the first few days after birth is very rapid because of the onset of hypertrophy.

Fat growth

Fat occurs in a specialized connective tissue called adipose tissue. Fat cells are referred to as adipocytes. Their size differs in different fat depots and at different stages of growth. They are larger in depots that are laid down earlier and can reach 100 μm in diameter. Four major depots can be recognized: subcutaneous, perinephric, omental and that around and within the muscles (inter- and intramuscular). The omentum is the fold of peritoneum connecting the stomach and other abdominal viscera. It is sometimes referred to as the caul. About 98–99% of mature fat cells consist of actual fat (triglyceride).

The proportion of the total body fat in each fat depot varies between species. For example, cattle and sheep have proportionally more abdominal fat and less subcutaneous fat than pigs (Wood and Butler-Hogg, 1982). At the same overall level of body fat, pigs had 68% of the dissectable fat in their bodies subcutaneously, compared with 43% in sheep and 24% in dairy cattle. The corresponding figures for the abdominal fat found around the kidneys and in the pelvic cavity (perirenal–retroperitoneal fat) were 6, 10 and 17%. There is also variation within species. Beef cattle tend to have proportionally more subcutaneous fat and less in the abdomen.

Control of growth

A very large number of hormones and growth factors have been implicated in the control of various aspects of growth. These may operate by promoting or inhibiting the proliferation or differentiation of cells. They often have different effects in different sorts of cell. Important examples are insulin, growth hormone (somatotrophin), insulin-like growth factors and epidermal growth factor. Growth hormone, produced by the pituitary gland at the base of the brain, appears to promote growth through peptide hormones called somatomedins.

Insulin inhibits protein degradation in the fed state; cortisol promotes degradation of protein in the fasting state. The sex hormones, oestrogens and androgens, influence the growth of male and female animals to produce the obvious differences in size and fatness of the sexes. Insulin-like growth factor appears to influence the growth of all muscles in the body. That is, it acts systemically; but local growth promoting factors are also present which have a limited sphere of influence. For example, immobilizing a muscle in a stretched state leads to its rapid growth by stimulating the muscle fibres to produce 'mechanical growth factor'. At a general level, the growth of bones determines the growth in length of muscles.

Carcass Yield and Composition

Carcass yield

There are many parts of a living animal that we do not want to eat. Examples are the hide or fleece and the contents of the gastrointestinal tract. Of the weight of the live animal therefore, only a proportion is useful as saleable meat. The most important is the carcass but the liver, kidneys and, to a limited extent, various other visceral components also have value as food items. For illustrative purposes, the approximate composition of a slaughtered steer is given in Table 2.2. The definition of the carcass varies somewhat in the different species, and in different dressing specifications and methods of preparation for sale. For example, the carcasses from sheep and cattle have the head removed immediately after slaughter but in pigs this may be delayed until after chilling and further butchery. In beef carcasses, abdominal fat may be removed but not in those from pigs and sheep. In pigs the skin is included. However, in general terms the carcass consists of all those parts of the animal that will eventually be sold as joints or steaks of meat. The weight of the carcass in relation to the weight of the live animal is therefore an important measurement of meat yield. It is normally expressed as killing-out percentage. Particularly in North America the term 'dressing percent' is preferred. In both, the carcass weight is expressed as a percentage of the weight of the live animal just before slaughter:

$$\text{killing-out percentage} = (\text{carcass weight}/\text{live weight}) \times 100.$$

Live weight varies depending on gut fill and so the time of weighing should be standardized in regard to time of feeding. The carcass is usually weighed immediately after preparation – removal of the hide or fleece and viscera – and before cooling in a refrigerated chill room. During cooling, water, and therefore weight, is lost by evaporation. This might amount to 1.5–2% of the initial carcass weight. For example, in the UK, to predict cold weight for a pig carcass weighing between 56.5 and 74.5 kg, 1.5 kg is deducted from the hot carcass weight if the interval between bleeding and weighing is less than 46 min; between 46 and 180 min the rebate is 1.0 kg. It is therefore important to know whether the killing-out percentage is based on the hot or cold carcass

Table 2.2. The components of the body of a slaughtered steer and their approximate proportion of the live weight.

Component	Weight (kg)	Percentage of live weight
Carcass	265	53
Gut contents	64	13
Hide	49	10
Gut	41	8
Head, lungs, trachea, diaphragm	31	6
Blood lost at slaughter	20	4
Liver and kidneys	11	2
Gut fat	8	2
Other small components	11	2
	500	100

weight since hot killing-out percentages will always be higher. In cattle particularly, the weight of the fat associated with the kidneys (referred to as kidney knob and channel fat – KKCF) can be significant. Whether KKCF has been included in the carcass weight is therefore also important to know. Excluding the KKCF can reduce the measured killing-out percentage by two percentage points.

The average killing-out percentage differs in the different species (Table 2.3). Sheep and cattle have proportionately bigger guts while pig carcasses include the skin, feet and head. These values are for illustrative purposes only. Killing-out percentages can vary widely between breeds, at different levels of fatness, between sexes and in animals reared in different husbandry systems. A major effect is that due to selection for improved carcass muscularity. This is illustrated by the improvement in killing-out percentage seen with more modern, highly selected breeds of pigs. The Pietrain and Hampshire breeds, which have values of above 79%, compare with more traditional breeds such as the Gloucester Old Spots and Tamworth, with values of below 75% (Warriss *et al.*, 1996). In cattle the trend is for killing-out percentage to increase with better 'conformation'. Thus, it is higher in beef breeds or beef crosses. It is also higher in bulls compared with steers. This is illustrated by the information in Table 2.4.

Carcass conformation

Conformation describes the shape of the carcass and is a reflection of the proportion of muscle to bone in it. Carcasses with good conformation have the appearance of thicker, more defined muscles. At the same level of fatness these carcasses yield more lean meat, and joints and steaks of better appearance. They are therefore preferred by butchers

Table 2.3. Approximate killing-out percentages for different species.

Species	Killing-out percentage
Sheep	~50
Cattle	~53
Pigs	~75
Broiler chickens	~72

Table 2.4. Killing-out percentages in steers and bulls of dairy (Friesian) and beef cross (Charolais × Friesian) breeds reared on a cereal based diet (based on data abstracted from the MLC Beef Yearbook, February 1993).

	Friesian		Charolais × Friesian	
	Steers	Bulls	Steers	Bulls
Live weight (kg)	405	448	446	495
Killing-out percentage	52.6	53.4	53.1	53.9

and command a higher price. For this reason modern breeds of animal have been selected for better carcass conformation. The effect of this selection is illustrated by the carcasses from eight breeds of pig shown in Fig. 2.5. The modern meat breeds such as the Pietrain, Hampshire and Duroc have noticeably much better developed, rounded hams than the traditional unselected breeds like the Saddleback, Oxford Sandy and Black and Gloucester Old Spots.

This difference is also seen in the muscle development in other parts of the carcass. Table 2.5 shows the carcass composition of pigs from three breeds killed at the same live weight. The Tamworth is an unimproved breed and contrasts with the Pietrain which has been highly selected for carcass quality. The Large White is intermediate. With greater selection, the weights of shoulder, loin and ham joints have all progressively increased. The cross-sectional area of the important muscle in the back, the musculus longissimus dorsi (see Chapter 3) has also increased dramatically. This improvement in area is mainly attributable to an increase in the depth of the muscle, rather than its width, illustrating the way selection has led to 'plumper' muscles.

As mentioned above, the improvement in muscularity can be measured in terms of the muscle:bone ratio. Animals with high muscle:bone ratio show good carcass conformation. This relation between conformation, muscle size and muscle:bone ratio is illustrated for cattle by data from Kempster *et al.* (1988) and shown in Table 2.6. The beef breeds had better conformation, larger muscles and higher muscle:bone ratios. They also had a greater percentage of the lean meat in the high-value parts of the carcass. A discussion of the relation between conformation and the yield and distribution of lean meat in carcasses can be found in Kempster *et al.* (1982a).

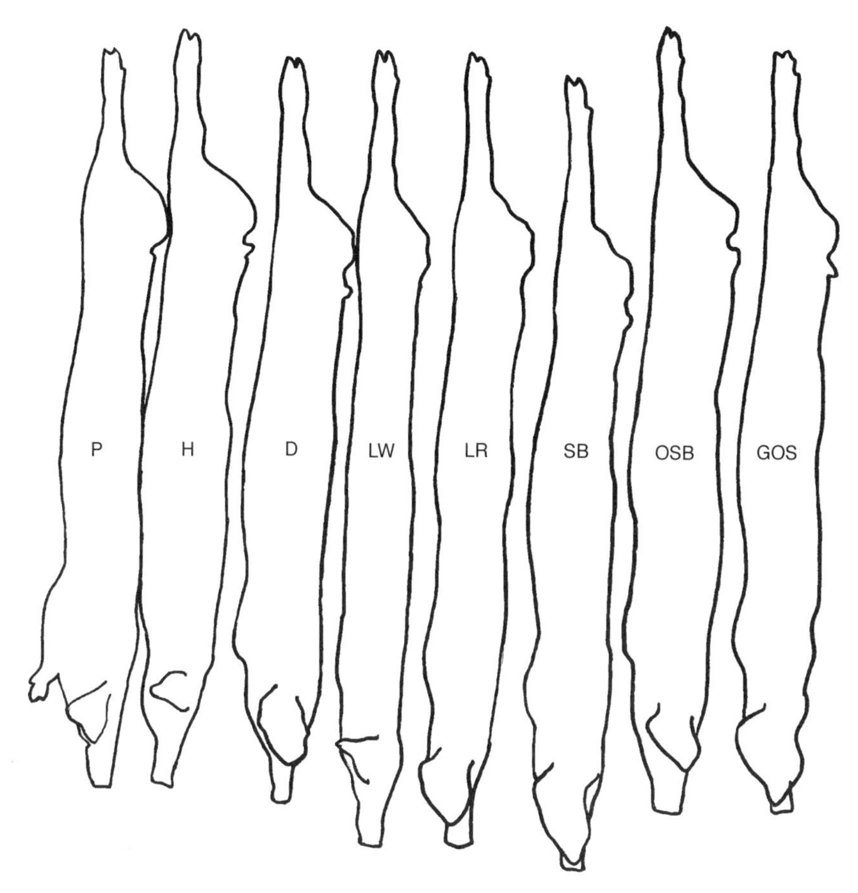

Fig. 2.5. Tracings of photographs of carcass sides from eight breeds of pig showing improved development of the ham in the selected breeds on the left compared with traditional breeds on the right (P, Pietrain; H, Hampshire; D, Duroc; LW, Large White; LR, Landrace; SB, Saddleback; OSB, Oxford Sandy and Black; GOS, Gloucester Old Spots).

The relative growth of muscle and fat tissues

Because fat, particularly subcutaneous fat, is the last tissue to mature, older animals tend to be fatter. Fat is deposited mainly from the onset of puberty. Therefore, at the same carcass weight, so-called late-maturing cattle breeds, such as the Limousin, Simmental and Charolais, in which puberty is relatively delayed, tend to be leaner than early-maturing breeds such as the Angus and Hereford. Dairy breeds of cattle have carcasses with more muscle and less fat than beef breeds. Male animals are leaner than females and grow to a larger mature size. Castration removes this anabolic effect of the male sex

Table 2.5. The carcass composition of pigs from three breeds. The Tamworth represents an unimproved breed, the Pietrain extreme selection for carcass quality.

	Tamworth	Large White	Pietrain
Killing-out percentage	73.9	76.7	80.0
Backfat thickness (mm)	18.6	12.3	11.0
Shoulder weight (kg)	11.6	13.0	13.4
Loin weight (kg)	9.6	9.8	10.2
Belly weight (kg)	4.4	4.4	4.4
Ham weight (kg)	11.4	12.6	14.0
Area of cross-section of m. longissimus dorsi (LD) (cm^2)	36	43	55
Width of LD (mm)	93	93	95
Depth of LD (mm)	39	46	59

Values corrected to the same live weight (63 kg).

Table 2.6. Conformation, muscle development and muscle:bone ratios in steers from five breed-types of cattle slaughtered at 24 months of age at the same fatness (based on Kempster *et al.*, 1988).

Breed	Conformation score[a]	Cross sectional area of LD muscle (cm^2)	Muscle:bone ratio	Percentage lean in high value parts of carcass
Canadian Holstein[b]	2.7	61	3.5	44.0
Friesian[b]	4.5	62	3.7	44.2
Hereford	6.2	60	3.9	44.3
Simmental	6.6	69	3.9	45.3
Charolais	7.8	72	3.9	45.2
Limousin	8.1	74	4.3	45.3

[a] Fifteen-point scale, higher is better.
[b] Purebred, all other breeds represent the Sire breed which was crossed with Friesian dams.

hormones and castrated males are as fat as females (Table 2.7). A very useful review of much of the early work on the growth and development of the different tissues of meat animals, and the methods used to estimate them, is given in Berg and Walters (1983).

The energy required for growth

The two main edible components of an animal's carcass, muscle (lean) and adipose tissue (fat), require different amounts of energy to lay down. Energy is measured in joules (J). The temperature of 1 g of water is raised by 1°C by 4.2 J of energy in the form of heat. One gram of

Table 2.7. Estimates of the average percentage fat levels in the carcasses from male, female and castrated animals in the UK.

	Ox	Pig	Sheep
Entire males	19	17	23
Females	23	22	27
Castrated males	22	23	26

protein has an energy content of about 17 kJ; 1 g of chemical fat has a higher energy content (about 38 kJ). The fat also requires more energy to synthesize. In the tissues of animals, protein and chemical fat are associated with water. Muscle contains about 75% water and 20% protein. Adipose tissue contains only about 30% water, although this is rather more variable. The difference in their water contents increases further the difference in the energy content of the lean and adipose tissues. The energy content of 1 g of muscle is about 4 kJ while that of 1 g of adipose tissue is around 26 kJ. Adding 1 g of adipose tissue to an animal's body therefore increases its energy content more than six times that of adding the same weight of muscle.

The greater energy associated with laying down fat means that animals must consume proportionately more food to gain the same amount of weight when they are in the later stages of growth in which fat deposition is occurring. As animals grow fatter therefore, they become less efficient in terms of body weight gain for each unit of food eaten. Food energy is used for both the maintenance of existing tissues and the growth of new tissue. The maintenance requirement for energy is minimized with fast growth and thus maximum food intake, but maximum food intake may produce over-fat carcasses. It may therefore be necessary to maximize growth rate at some (early) stages of development but reduce it at other (later) stages to produce a compromise between efficiency of growth and desirable carcass fatness. In practical terms, the situation is complicated by differences over the growth period in the efficiency with which animals convert the energy and protein in food into the energy retained in their own bodies. A review of the energetic efficiency of growth is given by Webster (1980).

Variation in carcass composition

As animals get older and heavier the proportion of fat in their carcasses increases and the proportion of muscle and bone decreases. This is illustrated for sheep in Table 2.1 and it is shown for cattle in Fig. 2.6. This shows that while the *absolute* weights of all tissues increased in older, heavier carcasses, only the *percentage* fat increased, the *percentages* of

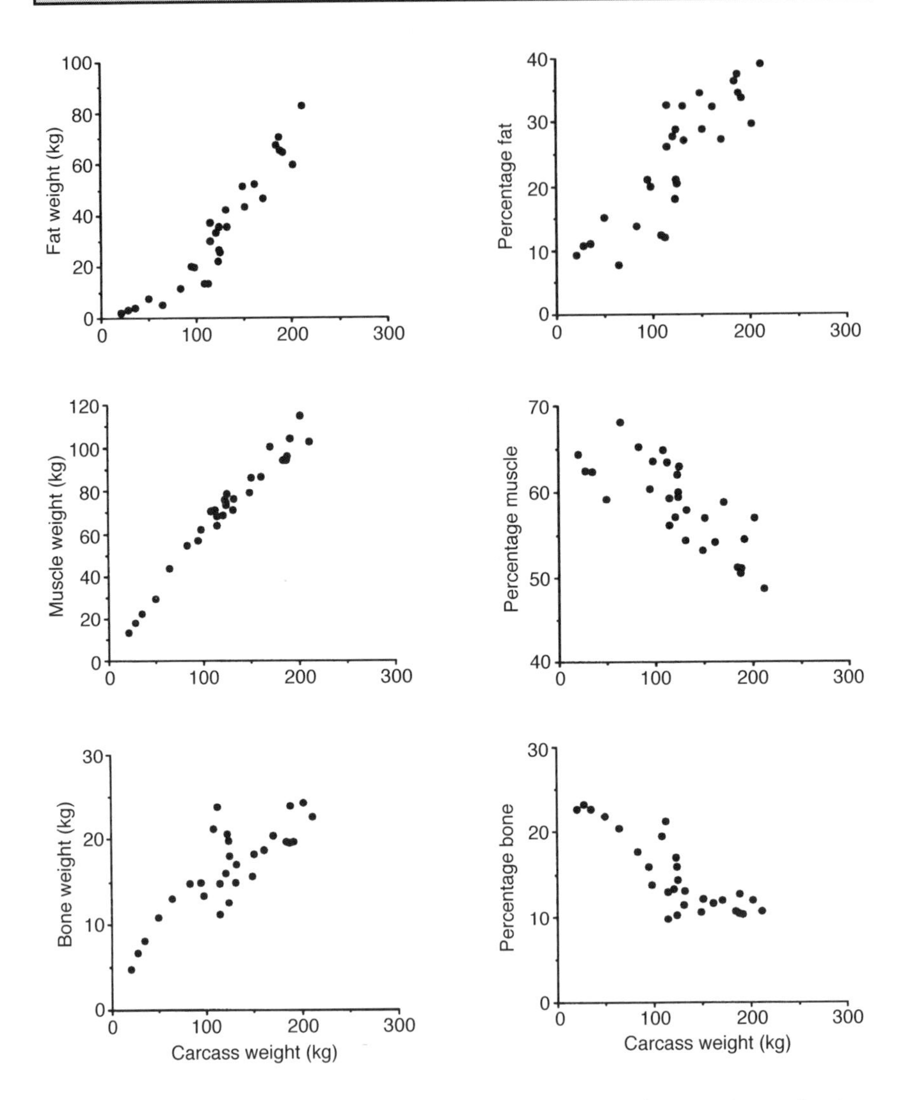

Fig. 2.6. The amounts of fat, muscle and bone in carcasses from cattle ranging in age from 10 days to 12 years (based on data in Callow, 1948).

muscle and bone decreasing progressively. A good account of much of the early work on determining the distribution of tissues in, and the chemical composition of, carcasses can be found in the papers in Tribe (1964).

Entire males produce carcasses with more muscle than do castrated males. Dairy cattle such as the Friesian have carcasses with more muscle and less fat than beef breeds such as the Hereford or Limousin. The Texel and Southdown breeds of sheep have more muscle than

Suffolk or Oxford breeds. At a particular fat level the value of a carcass is influenced by the muscle:bone ratio. A higher ratio is obviously better since it equates to more saleable lean meat as well as better carcass conformation. Beef breeds have a higher ratio than dairy breeds and entire males have a higher ratio than castrates.

Sex has a major influence on fatness and conformation in cattle. Young bulls produce the leanest carcasses, followed by culled cows and steers, with heifers on average producing the fattest. Table 2.8 illustrates this with the frequency distribution of fat class scores for cattle killed in the UK in 1994. Table 2.9 gives the corresponding distributions for conformation class. Young bulls also produce carcasses with the best conformation, followed by steers and then heifers. Although they are very lean, cow carcasses have very poor conformation. Excluding these cow carcasses, fatness and conformation are inversely related in the other three sex classes.

The 'target' levels for beef are 4L or leaner for fatness and R or better for conformation. In 1994 in the UK, 33% of heifers, 43% of steers and 60% of young bulls fell into the target sector, the remaining animals having too much fat, or poor conformation, or both. The increasing use of young bulls, rather than steers, in the UK may have

Table 2.8. Fat class distribution (%) in cattle killed in the UK in 1994 (data abstracted from *MLC Year Book* statistics).

	Fat class		
	Leaner than 4L	4L	Fatter than 4L
Heifers	19.8	50.3	30.0
Steers	23.5	53.8	22.7
Cows	35.8	34.0	30.2
Bulls	63.0	32.9	4.1

There are five main classes according to fat cover but with classes 4 and 5 subdivided into low (L) and high (H) subgroups.

Table 2.9. Conformation class distribution (%) in cattle killed in the UK in 1994 (data abstracted from *MLC Year Book* statistics).

	Conformation		
	Better than R	R	Worse than R
Heifers	8.2	41.2	50.7
Steers	15.0	43.0	42.0
Cows	0.8	3.6	95.6
Bulls	29.6	33.4	37.1

There are five main conformation classes (E, U, R, O, P) based on the shape of the carcass profiles. Classes U, O and P are each divided into an upper and lower band.

led to an overall reduction in fatness in beef carcasses. However, despite apparent preferences for leaner meat in the 1980s and 1990s there was little or no evidence of reduced fat in UK carcasses up to 1985 except for pigs. Between about 1975 and 1985, while the separable fat content of the average pig carcass fell from 27.4% to 22.8%, the composition of beef and lamb carcasses did not change appreciably (Kempster *et al.*, 1986). In 1985 the average beef carcass contained 22.2% separable fat (equivalent to 20.2% chemical fat) and the average lamb carcass 25.6% (equivalent to 23.5% chemical fat). The corresponding chemical fat in the pig carcass was 19.4%.

Growth-promoting Agents

Growth-promoting steroids

The importance of the sex hormones, both androgens and oestrogens, in controlling fatness and growth is illustrated by the use of synthetic growth-promoting substances (anabolic steroids) based on them. Androgens have actions like the male sex hormone testosterone. Oestrogens have actions like the female sex hormone oestradiol. Progestagens act like the female hormone progesterone, the main physiological function of which is to suppress oestrus, and have been used to enhance the effects of the other sex hormones. Trenbolone acetate is a synthetic androgen that promotes growth by decreasing protein degradation in muscle. Similarly, the synthetic oestrogen zeranol also promotes growth by decreasing protein degradation. Both hormones therefore work by reducing protein *turnover* rather than by increasing protein synthesis. As might be expected, the effects of synthetic sex hormones depend to a degree on the sex of the animal to which they are administered since it is the balance of male and female hormones which is important. Females tend to respond better to androgens and males to oestrogens. Castrates tend to respond best to a combination of androgens and oestrogens.

The use of anabolic sex steroids, usually as implants, was widespread in cattle in Europe until banned in the EU (EU Directive 88/146/EEC). There was concern about the potential effects of steroid residues on humans who consumed the meat and offal from treated animals particularly if the recommended dose rates had not been adhered to. Nevertheless, the compounds are still in use in many countries outside the EU, including North America. Examples of anabolic sex hormone products are given in Table 2.10. Anabolic sex steroids are usually administered as compressed tablets implanted into the tissues of the ear (a non-edible part of the animal). Other growth promoting steroids that have been used are the stilbenes (diethyl

Table 2.10. Examples of products containing anabolic sex hormones.

Product name	Hormone	Manufacturer
Finaplix®	Trenbolone acetate	Hoechst
Ralgro®	Zeranol	Crown Chemicals
Compudose®	Oestradiol	Elanco
Synovex S®	Oestradiol + progesterone	Syntex
Synovex H®	Testosterone + oestradiol	Syntex

stilboestrol, hexoestrol) which were banned in the EU in 1981 and also North America, because of concerns, possibly unfounded, that they could cause cancer in people eating meat.

β-Adrenergic agonists

A class of pharmacological compounds that has shown enormous potential to alter the muscularity and ratio of lean to fat in meat animals is the β-adrenergic agonists. These have chemical structures similar to the naturally occurring catecholamines, adrenaline (epinephrine) and noradrenaline (norepinephrine). Adrenaline and noradrenaline are hormones that are secreted in response to stressful situations (see Chapter 10). Noradrenaline is also the neurotransmitter found in the sympathetic nervous system (equivalent to the acetylcholine of the parasympathetic system). Examples of β-adrenergic agonists are clenbuterol, cimaterol, salbutamol and ractopamine. Figure 2.7 shows how their chemical structures relate to that of adrenaline.

β-Adrenergic agonists are so called because they act on cells via β-receptors on the cell membrane. The β-receptors can be subdivided into two types. β_1 receptors are characteristic of cardiac and intestinal muscle; β_2 receptors are characteristic of bronchial and uterine smooth muscle. However, both β_1 and β_2 receptors occur in many tissues including skeletal muscle and fat. The β-adrenergic agonists of interest in animal production mainly affect β_2 receptors but the classification into β_1 and β_2 is not clear-cut and some β_1 activity is also evident.

The potential value of β-adrenergic agonists in meat animals lies in their so-called repartitioning effects. They reduce the amount of fat in the body and increase protein accretion so promoting muscular development. They appear to do this by both reducing the production of fat (lipogenesis) and increasing fat breakdown (lipolysis; Cardoso and Stock, 1998). Their action on protein accretion seems to be through reducing breakdown, so favouring the synthesis component of the normal protein turnover. Some muscles, particularly those with a high proportion of type II, glycolytic, fast contracting fibres (see Chapter 3), are more affected than others. Although they influence circulating

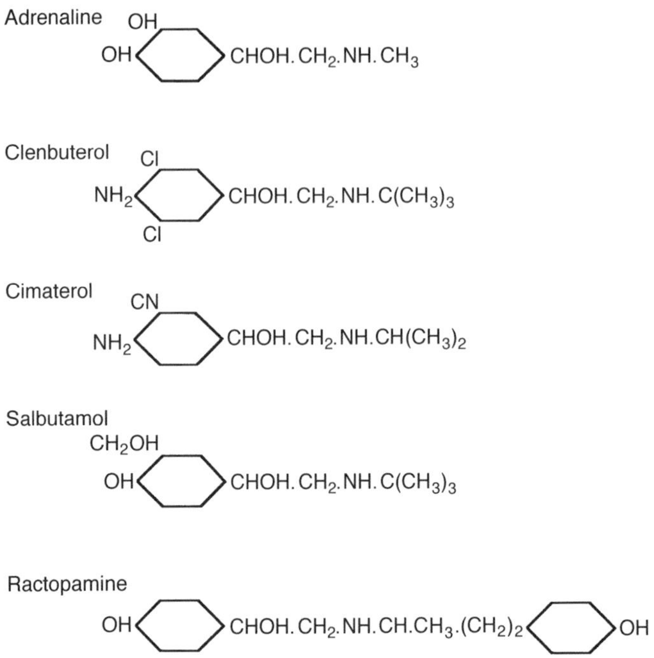

Adrenaline OH
OH CHOH.CH_2.NH.CH_3

Clenbuterol Cl
NH_2 CHOH.CH_2.NH.$C(CH_3)_3$
Cl

Cimaterol CN
NH_2 CHOH.CH_2.NH.$CH(CH_3)_2$

Salbutamol
CH_2OH
OH CHOH.CH_2.NH.$C(CH_3)_3$

Ractopamine
OH CHOH.CH_2.NH.CH.CH_3.$(CH_2)_2$ OH

Fig. 2.7. The chemical structures of adrenaline and four β-adrenergic agonists.

levels of insulin, growth hormone and the thyroid hormones, it is not thought that the effects of β-adrenergic agonists are mediated through these.

Unlike anabolic steroid hormones, β-adrenergic agonists are effective in all sexes to the same extent. They are orally active and so can be administered in the feed, usually at levels of between 1 and 10 ppm. They are therefore effective at very low doses. Although they may show small effects on growth rate this is not a consistent effect and is generally more apparent in ruminants than in non-ruminants. Carcass yield is improved by around 1–2% in pigs and poultry and by up to 5–6% in cattle and sheep. There is evidence that this is due to both an increase in carcass weight and a decrease in the size of the viscera. The carcasses have better conformation. The increases in muscle development are accompanied by reductions in subcutaneous, intermuscular and intramuscular fat. The effects of administration of a β-adrenergic agonist to pigs are illustrated in Table 2.11. A comparison of the effects of treatment with β-adrenergic agonists on pigs and sheep is shown in Table 2.12. These figures illustrate the potential gains to be had from administration of β-adrenergic agonists. However, the gains are offset by potentially poorer meat quality. Some β-adrenergic agonists may produce meat that

Table 2.11. The effect of a β-adrenergic agonist on carcass composition in pigs.

	Control animals	Pigs treated with β-adrenergic agonist	Change in relation to control group
Killing-out percentage	77.6	78.8	↑
Backfat thickness (mm)	12.6	11.0	↓
Cross-sectional area of the m. longissimus dorsi (cm^2)	50.4	55.9	↑
Percentage muscle in foreloin joint	50.3	55.0	↑
Percentage fat in foreloin joint	35.7	31.6	↓
Percentage bone in foreloin joint	14.1	13.4	↓

Based on data published in Warriss *et al.* (1990a, b).

Table 2.12. Comparative effects of β-adrenergic agonists in pigs and sheep (data for pigs as in Table 2.11; data for sheep from Warriss *et al.*, 1989c).

	Percentage change over control animals	
	Pigs	Sheep
Killing-out percentage	+1.5	+7.6
Backfat thickness	−13	−36
Cross sectional area of m. longissimus dorsi	+11	+28
Proportion of muscle in foreloin	+9	+15
Proportion of fat in foreloin	−11	−10
Proportion of bone in foreloin	−5	−26

is darker and duller in colour, and tougher after cooking. The darker colour is caused by reduced glycogen levels in the muscles at slaughter leading to a higher ultimate pH in the muscles. Toughness may result from a lower activity of proteolytic enzyme systems *post mortem* (see Chapter 5). By reducing intramuscular fat, β-adrenergic agonists may also reduce other eating quality characteristics.

Porcine and bovine somatotrophin (PST and BST)

Giving frequent injections of growth hormone (somatotrophin) to pigs reduces carcass fat and increases muscle development. Some studies have shown increases in lean tissue growth rate and reductions of fat deposition of up to 20%. Food conversion is also more efficient. It is unclear whether there are any major deleterious effects on muscle quality but marbling fat tends to be reduced in line with overall carcass fat and this might influence tenderness. Similar effects on fat and muscle development have been seen with administration of BST to ruminants. Somatotrophins can be produced in relatively large quantities by bacteria using recombinant DNA techniques to insert the appropriate genes. However, because they also occur naturally, they may be more acceptable to consumers than β-adrenergic agonists even though not currently permitted in the EU.

Describing and Predicting Composition

Carcass classification and grading

Tables 2.8 and 2.9 are derived from information summarizing the classification of beef carcasses in the UK. Classification schemes are used to describe carcasses and allocate them to categories based on criteria such as fatness and conformation. They provide a common point of reference between producers of animals, and wholesalers and retailers of meat. Strictly, classification schemes should be differentiated from grading schemes. Grading schemes put different values on the carcasses placed in each of these uniform classes. The value is dependent on how useful the carcass is for a particular purpose and therefore how much someone will be willing to pay for it. The description of carcasses in classification schemes enables people to buy and sell them unseen. It also facilitates carcasses going to the appropriate use. For example, the requirements for carcasses destined to be butchered into meat sold in a retail supermarket will be different from those going for processing. Classification schemes also aid marketing since they lead automatically to product uniformity. In contrast, grading schemes may produce uniform top grades but variation in the poorer grades. This is because the poorer grade carcasses can be poor for different reasons. They might be too fat, or too poorly muscled, but both sorts of carcasses are included together.

Another potential problem with some systems is that the terms used to describe the grades tend to be emotive. Thus, using words like 'poor', while possibly correct, is likely to prejudice people against buying the carcass. Even the worst grades therefore are likely to be called 'good' and the really good grades indicated as better by calling them 'prime' or 'choice'. To avoid this kind of problem, classification schemes may use code letters. The European beef classification scheme for conformation uses E, U, R, O and P, with the U, O and P classes subdivided into upper and lower bands.

By combining fatness and conformation, a matrix or grid is produced. At its extremes this has four types of carcass: lean with small muscles, fat with small muscles, fat but well-muscled and lean and well-muscled. For illustration, the percentage distribution of carcasses in 1994 in the UK in the matrix system used in the EU for beef classification is shown in Table 2.13. The EU beef classification scheme also requires recording of cold carcass weight and sex. Other characteristics that may be included in classification and grading schemes, especially for beef, are breed/type, age, muscle colour and graininess, the amount of intramuscular fat (marbling), and colour and texture of the subcutaneous fat. In the USA, marbling in beef is considered to be very important because larger amounts tend to be associated with more tender, juicy meat. Beef with large amounts of evenly distributed marbling therefore receives a higher quality grade in the United States Department of Agriculture (USDA) system.

The ideal classification system is one that is absolutely precise and where the classes can be exactly related to commercial value. Because of the importance of the relative amounts of fat and lean in determining this value, the EU pig scheme predicts percentage lean in the carcass from measurements of fat and/or muscle depth. For example, the equation used to predict percentage of lean meat in a pig carcass from the backfat thickness (P_2) alone is:

$$\text{lean meat} = 65.5 - [1.15 - \times P_2\ (\text{mm})] + [0.077 \times \text{cold carcass weight (kg)}].$$

The P_2 value is the backfat thickness measured in millimetres at the level of the head of the last rib and 6.5 cm from the mid-line of the carcass. The EU class is based on this calculated percentage lean (Table 2.14). If the precise amounts of lean and fat in a carcass can be predicted, 'component' pricing can be used. In this, the value of the whole carcass is determined exactly by the sum of the values of lean and fat components separately.

Much of the grading of beef and lamb carcasses is done subjectively by trained graders because of the difficulty of finding appropriate instrumental methods. Grading of pig carcasses is inherently easier due

Table 2.13. Percentage distribution of carcasses from steers, heifers and young bulls in the UK in 1994 (based on data in the *MLC Beef Yearbook* 1995).

Conformation class (increasing muscularity)	Fat class (increasing fatness) → 1	2	3	4L	4H	5L	5H
E		0.1	0.1	0.1			
U+		0.2	0.8	1.1	0.4		
U−		0.5	2.9	6.0	2.5	0.2	
R	0.1	1.2	8.3	21.3	9.1	0.7	0.1
O+	0.1	1.1	7.1	14.8	5.8	0.7	0.1
O−	0.1	0.9	3.7	5.3	1.7	0.3	0.1
P+		0.3	0.6	0.6	0.2		
P−	0.1	0.1	0.1				

Table 2.14. The percentage lean in pig carcasses given different EU grades.

EU grade	Lean meat percentage
S	60+
E	55–59
U	50–54
R	45–49
O	40–44
P	<40

to the much greater proportion of fat in the subcutaneous depot. The thickness of this can be measured directly. However, there is much interest in looking for instrumental methods for the ruminant species, for example, using such techniques as video-image analysis (Allen, 1984).

Methods of predicting body and carcass composition

Because of the importance of carcass composition, particularly the proportion of lean to fat, many methods have been devised to estimate it from simple measurements or using more sophisticated procedures. Subcutaneous fat depth in pig carcasses can be measured using a ruler or an optical probe. Optical probes are pushed through the skin and fat. The boundary between fat and lean is seen in an illuminated window and the fat depth is read from a scale. In the 1980s electronic grading probes, such as the Fat-o-Meater from Denmark and the Hennessy Grading Probe from New Zealand, were developed. These detected the boundary between fat and lean by the change in light absorbance as the probe tip passed through. A major advantage over the optical probe was that by pushing the probe through the underlying muscle tissue the depth of this could be measured as well. The combination of fat and lean measurements potentially produces much more accurate estimates of lean content (Fortin *et al.*, 1984; Kempster *et al.*, 1985).

Traditionally, carcass grading in pigs has been based on single measurements of fat thickness made over the m. longissimus dorsi (see Chapter 3) at the level of the last rib (for example, in the UK the P_2 value is made 6.5 cm from the dorsal mid-line). However, this tends to underestimate the leanness of more muscular carcasses. This can be important in assessing carcasses from pigs from a diverse genetic background with relatively large differences in conformation and fatness. Improved prediction comes from the use of a larger number of sampling sites as has been pioneered in Denmark with the use of automatic multiple-probe grading systems. Better predictive measurements are always being sought, more modern approaches using combinations of measurements or sophisticated electronic scanning devices, for example using total body electrical conductivity (Hicks *et al.*, 1998).

For research purposes a wide range of often very complex techniques has been used to measure body composition in both the live animal and the carcass. In live animals the methods have included dilution techniques, combinations of linear measurements, magnetic resonance imaging, computer-assisted tomography and dual energy X-ray absorptiometry (Lister, 1984; Mitchell *et al.*, 1996). The composition of whole carcasses has been predicted either by dissection into fat, lean and bone, or by chemical analysis of lipid, protein, ash and water, of sample or 'indicator' joints. Often part of the loin joint is chosen (Planella and Cook, 1991; Nour and Thonney, 1994; Swensen *et al.*, 1998). A very thorough review of carcass evaluation techniques is that of Kempster *et al.* (1982b).

A particular technique that has been used to assess the composition of both live animals and their carcasses is measuring the velocity of ultrasound through the body tissues. Ultrasound has a frequency above 20 kHz, the upper limit of human hearing. Measurements are usually made at frequencies of 1–5 MHz. When a pulse of ultrasound is passed through an animal's body a small proportion (2%) is reflected back as 'echoes' from the boundaries between different tissues. The characteristics of these echoes can be used to generate a picture of the relative positions of these tissues. This is the principle used in machines such as the Scanogram (Ithaco Incorporated, USA) and the Vetscan (BSC, UK) which produce two-dimensional displays of the tissues below the scanning head. From these the thickness of fat layers or the cross-sectional areas of muscles can be deduced.

As well as recording these echoes to estimate body composition, the speed at which the ultrasound passes through the tissues can be used. This is because the speed is different in muscle and fat. It is about 1.6 km s^{-1} in muscle and 1.4 km s^{-1} in fat (Miles and Fursey, 1974). By measuring the speed through a part of the animal's body consisting of soft tissues the proportions of muscle and fat can be calculated. It is important that the pathway of the sound is not deflected by bone and, if used in the live animal for predicting lean and fat in the carcass, that it does not pass through organs or body cavities. Additionally, the speed is influenced by temperature and, importantly, the effect is different for lean and fat. This is a slight limitation to the value of the technique for assessing the composition of carcasses. It can therefore be used for large carcasses, for example from adult cattle, when measured reasonably soon after slaughter but is less useful for rapidly cooling lamb carcasses.

A comparison of the use of various ultrasonic techniques for measuring beef carcass composition in the live animal was made by Porter *et al.* (1990) and a good review of the use of the speed of ultrasound to measure composition is that of Fisher (1997). There can be significant between-operator variation in the interpretation of images from pulse echo techniques (McLaren *et al.*, 1991). Measuring the speed of ultrasound through muscles has also been used to estimate the amount of intramuscular fat present in beef (Park *et al.*, 1994).

Chapter 3

The Chemical Composition and Structure of Meat

Considering its complexity, an animal's body consists of relatively few kinds of chemical substances. About 55–60% is water. This, and the 3–4% or so of minerals, make up the inorganic component. The remaining 35–40% consists of organic substances. These are complex compounds of carbon (C), hydrogen (H) and oxygen (O), sometimes together with nitrogen (N), sulphur (S) or other elements, which are in general found only in living organisms. Three major categories of organic compound are of importance to us: proteins, fats and carbohydrates. The approximate composition of an animal in terms of these components is given in Table 3.1. These figures are given only as an illustration. As we have seen in Chapter 2, the proportions of some components, especially fat, can vary greatly. Muscle tissue consists of about 75% water and 20% protein. A large part of the remaining 5% is fat with very small amounts of carbohydrate (principally glycogen), free amino acids, dipeptides and nucleotides.

The Chemical Composition of Meat

Proteins

Proteins have a very wide range of functions. They may be structural (e.g. the collagen of connective tissues like tendon), contractile (e.g. the actin and myosin that make up the major part of muscle), or enzymes which catalyse chemical reactions (e.g. creatine kinase, which catalyses the regeneration of adenosine triphosphate from adenosine diphosphate; see Chapter 5). They may be hormones (e.g. insulin, which regulates the level of glucose in the blood) or antibodies

Table 3.1. The approximate chemical composition of an animal like a pig.

Substance	Percentage
Inorganic	
Water	60
Minerals	4
Organic	
Proteins	20
Fats (lipids)	15
Carbohydrates	1

involved in immunological responses. They may have transport functions (e.g. the haemoglobin of blood and the myoglobin of muscle, which carry oxygen) or osmotic functions (e.g. blood plasma albumin). Proteins principally contain carbon, hydrogen, oxygen, nitrogen and sometimes sulphur. They are made up of chains of amino acids, of which there are 20 common ones. Animals cannot synthesize the amino group ($-NH_2$) which characterizes amino acids so must have protein in their diet. However, given a protein source, many amino acids can be synthesized by the animal. These are therefore sometimes referred to as *non-essential* amino acids to differentiate them from the *essential* amino acids, which cannot be synthesized. Essential amino acids may be essential for particular types of animal, but not others, or may only be essential at particular stages of life. The amino acid proline is essential for chicks but not adult birds. Lysine is an essential amino acid for pigs and the content of lysine in a particular diet may therefore be the limiting component in terms of how fast the pig can grow. Amino acids have the general formula:

$$\begin{array}{c} R \\ | \\ H - C - COOH \\ | \\ NH_2 \end{array}$$

A carbon atom has a carboxyl or carboxylic acid ($-COOH$) group and an amino group ($-NH_2$) attached to it. R represents a side chain that differs in the different amino acids. In the simplest case R is a hydrogen atom and this produces glycine; in alanine it is a methyl group (CH_3; Fig. 3.1). In lysine it is $NH_2(CH_2)_4$. In cysteine a sulphur atom is incorporated ($HS.CH_2$). When two molecules of cysteine are reduced and linked by an –S–S– bond, cystine is produced. Disulphide bonds between cysteine molecules (Fig. 3.2) are important in contributing to the overall structure of proteins. Various carbon ring structures may also be incorporated as in tyrosine (containing a benzene ring) and proline (containing a pyrrole ring). The amino group from one amino acid can condense with the

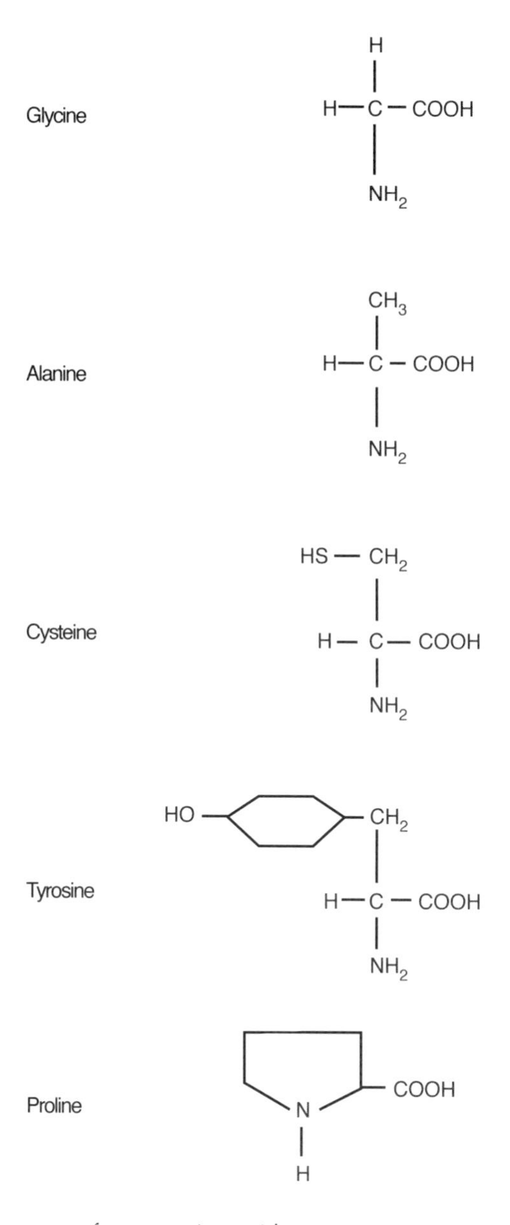

Fig. 3.1. The structures of some amino acids.

carboxyl group of any other to form a peptide linkage or bond (Fig. 3.3). Condensation reactions are those in which a water molecule is produced.

In this way chains of amino acids can be formed with a backbone of alternating pairs of carbon atoms and a nitrogen atom (–CCNCCN,

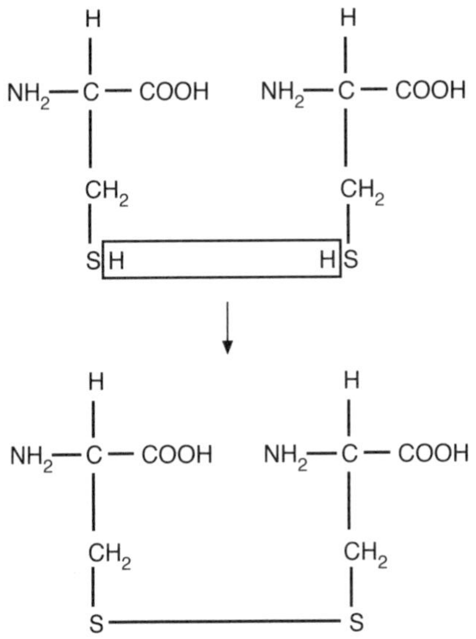

2 × cysteine

Cystine

Fig. 3.2. The formation of a disulphide bond between two amino acids.

etc.). Short, isolated chains are referred to as peptides, or polypeptides if longer. The –CCNCCN– backbone of the chain of amino acids forms a helical coil with the R groups sticking outwards from it. This is known as the alpha helix and produces the 'secondary' structure of the protein. The 'tertiary' structure is formed by the alpha helix being bent into a more complex shape. The structure is maintained by forces generated by the component amino acids, and held by hydrogen bonds and various other mechanisms. Hydrogen bonds form between the nitrogen of the amino group and the oxygen of the carboxyl group of different amino acids. Some proteins may be extremely large molecules. The bluish pigment haemocyanin, found in the blood of some crustaceans and snails, can have a molecular weight of 5 million. A protein may consist of more than one polypeptide chain. For example, haemoglobin, the oxygen carrying pigment of mammalian blood, has four chains, each with a molecular weight of 17,000. Myoglobin, the corresponding muscle pigment, has only one such chain. Proteins may be combined with lipids in lipoproteins and with carbohydrates in glycoproteins.

Most proteins are denatured at relatively low temperatures (<60°C) and also on exposure to acid conditions. They are most susceptible to denaturation at their isoelectric point – the point at which the electric charges on their amino and carboxyl groups exactly cancel one another. Denaturation leads to loss of solubility in aqueous solutions and loss of enzymic, immunological or hormonal properties. Because proteins

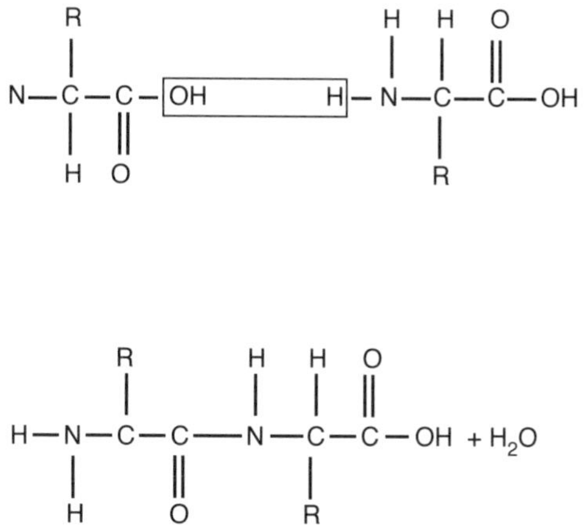

```
     R                    H   H   O
     |                    |   |   ||
 N—C—C—[OH          H]—N—C—C—OH
     |  ||                    |
     H  O                     R
```

```
          R        H   H   O
          |        |   |   ||
 H—N—C—C——N—C—C—OH  + H2O
    |     ||       |
    H     O        R
```

Fig. 3.3. The formation of a peptide bond between two amino acids.

constitute such a large part of muscle, denaturation and changes in their solubility and other functional properties have a major effect on the structure and characteristics of meat, affecting its appearance and ability to hold or bind water. This is especially true in meat products in which the meat is comminuted and mixed with other components to form gels and emulsions.

Collagen

Collagen is one of the commonest proteins in the body forming a major component of connective tissues. Collagen fibres are made up of long, rod-like tropocollagen molecules that form protofibrils. Each tropocollagen molecule consists of three polypeptide chains (alpha chains) twisted together into a coiled triple helix. Each polypeptide is about 1000 amino acids long. The polypeptides have a characteristic order of amino acids with a high content of glycine, which occurs at every third position, then usually but not always, proline and hydroxyproline:

> – glycine – proline – hydroxyproline – glycine – (another amino acid) – etc.

Proline and hydroxyproline together form nearly a quarter of all amino acid residues. The amino acid hydroxyproline is relatively uncommon in proteins. Hence, analysis of the hydroxyproline concentration in meat samples can be used to estimate their connective tissue contents. There are various types of collagen, often referred to using roman numerals (I to XI, etc.) and each characterized by having different constituent polypeptide chains. The epimysium, perimysium and endomysium (see p. 55) are composed of different collagens (Table 3.2).

At the 'amino-group' end of the non-helical part of the tropocollagen molecule are formed intermolecular cross-links that give collagen its strength. Important cross-links form between lysine molecules through production of an aldimine ($CH=N–CH_2$) bond. This occurs by an oxidative deamination reaction catalysed by the enzyme lysyl oxidase to give aldehyde groups that spontaneously condense with those from other lysine residues. The enzyme can be inhibited by substances referred to as lathyrogenic agents, so-called because they are found in the family of plants which includes the sweet pea (*Lathyrus odoratus*) and the chick pea (*Lathyrus sativa*). A potent lathyrogenic agent is the amino acid beta-amino proprionitrile. Because the enzyme is needed for the normal development of all tissues containing collagen (and elastin), inhibition leads to skeletal deformities and weakening of arteries and other tissues. The condition is known as lathyrism. Chick peas contain small amounts of lathyrogens. Normally these are not sufficient to cause problems in animals that eat them. However, eating large quantities, especially if raw, and also eating the leaves of the plants, can cause lathyrism (Bailey, 1972).

Collagen in tendons is more cross-linked than collagen in cartilage from organs like the external ear or nose. The cross-linking makes the tendon collagen more resistant to tensile stress. As animals get older the collagen cross-links are stabilized and the average diameter of the fibrils increases. A study of the role of the different connective tissue structures in determining the texture of beef was made by Light *et al.* (1985). The highest correlation with toughness was with the amounts of heat-stable cross-links in the epi-, peri- and endomysium. After cooking, the cross-links weaken but do not break, so contributing to the toughness of meat from old animals. Cooking collagen from young animals produces gelatin, which is soft and soluble. The gelatin forms a gel on cooling. The collagen from old animals is much less soluble. This is illustrated by results from Goll *et al.* (1964) who cooked muscle from cattle ranging in age from young calves to cows 10 years old (Table 3.3).

The tropocollagen molecules are aligned in a repeating parallel, staggered arrangement so parts of one molecule overlap with parts of

Table 3.2. The collagen composition of the connective tissue sheaths.

Connective tissue sheath	Surrounds	Collagen type
Epimysium	Whole muscle	Type I
Perimysium	Fibre bundles	Types I and III
Endomysium	Fibres	Types IV and V

Table 3.3. Release of protein and hydroxyproline on heating beef biceps femoris muscle at 70°C for 15 min (based on data in Goll *et al.*, 1964).

	Calves (<49 days old)	Steers (409–495 days)	Cows (5 years)	Cows (10 years)
Soluble protein[a]	863	409	171	82
Hydroxyproline[a]	88	36	10	4

[a] As μg ml^{-1} of solution.

others to form fibres. In the perimysium the fibres then form a criss-cross lattice at an angle to the main axis of the muscle fibre so enabling change in its length and shape. Crimping of the collagen fibres also facilitates this, the crimps straightening out when the muscle changes length.

Carnosine, anserine and balenine

These peptides occur in small but varying amounts in meat; carnosine and anserine in all species, but anserine especially in the muscles of some birds, and balenine in muscles of pigs and the baleen whales. They are found in higher concentrations in muscles with low oxidative capacity – usually paler-coloured muscles. They are dipeptides, consisting of β-alanine and histidine (in carnosine), 1-methylhistidine (in anserine) or 3-methylhistidine (in balenine). Their physiological role is unclear but they may act as buffers to prevent large changes in acidity (pH) which otherwise could occur during anaerobic muscle activity which produces lactic acid. They therefore maintain the pH of the living muscle in the physiological range of 6.8–7.4 and will obviously also contribute to the buffering capacity of meat *post mortem*. Their occurrence in high concentrations (2%) in the muscles of whales may be an adaptation to the importance of anaerobic metabolism during diving and the need to protect the tissues from the effects of a build-up of lactic acid.

Fats

Fats, or more correctly lipids, form essential parts of cell membranes and also act as a vehicle for energy storage. They also form the basis of steroid hormones. Fats are a very concentrated energy source. The energy value of fat is almost double that of carbohydrate or protein. Animals that are able to accumulate large amounts of fat can survive long periods without sufficient food, for example over winter, and lose relatively little body weight. Hibernating animals have large fat depots. Lipids are a very diverse group of substances chemically but are characterized by their relative insolubility in water and high solubility in organic solvents such as ethyl ether and chloroform. They all contain principally carbon, hydrogen and oxygen. The commonest forms are fats and oils (hence the use of the collective term 'fat'). These are triglycerides in which three fatty acid molecules are linked to (typically) glycerol, or more rarely other higher alcohols, by ester linkages. The fatty acids are therefore referred to as 'esterified'. The nature of the individual fatty acids making up the triglyceride determine its melting point, potential for oxidation and, to a degree, its nutritional value. The general formula for a fatty acid is:

$$\begin{array}{l} CH_3 \\ | \\ (CH_2)_n \\ | \\ COOH \end{array}$$

The simplest fatty acid is acetic acid (CH_3 COOH) with two carbon atoms. In naturally occurring fatty acids the length of the carbon chain varies from about 4 to 22 and is, for reasons not fully understood, usually an even number. There are two general types based on whether or not they contain double bonds (C=C) between the carbon atoms. Saturated fatty acids do not whereas unsaturated fatty acids do. The unsaturated fatty acids can have a single double bond (monounsaturated) or two or more (polyunsaturated). Fatty acids with two or more double bonds are therefore known as polyunsaturated fatty acids (PUFAs).

Examples of saturated fatty acids are butyric acid, palmitic acid and stearic acid. An example of a monounsaturated acid is oleic acid, and examples of polyunsaturated acids are linoleic and linolenic acids. The structures of palmitic and oleic acids are:

Palmitic acid: $CH_3 - (CH_2)_{14} - COOH$

Oleic acid: $CH_3 - (CH_2)_7 - CH = CH - (CH_2)_7 - COOH$

A shorthand way of designating fatty acids is commonly used. It gives the number of carbon atoms in the chain (the chain length) followed by the number of double bonds (Box 3.1).

Oleic, palmitic and stearic acids are some of the commonest naturally occurring fatty acids. Fatty acids containing double bonds can exist as *cis* or *trans* isomers. Isomers are molecules that have the same molecular formulae but either a different structure or a different arrangement of the atoms in space. *Cis* and *trans* isomers have the latter. The majority of naturally occurring fatty acids in animal fats are

Box 3.1. Examples of the designation of fatty acids.

Butyric acid	C4:0 (4 carbons, no double bonds)
Palmitic acid	C16:0 (16 carbons, no double bonds)
Stearic acid	C18:0 (18 carbons, no double bonds)
Linoleic acid	C18:2 (18 carbons, 2 double bonds)
Linolenic acid	C18:3 (18 carbons, 3 double bonds)

the *cis* forms. Three fatty acids: linoleic, linolenic and arachidonic acids, cannot be synthesized by animals (although arachidonic acid can be synthesized from linoleic acid) and are therefore referred to as essential fatty acids and must be obtained from the diet. They are abundant in the oils found in plant seeds.

An important characteristic of polyunsaturated fatty acids is where the first double bond occurs from the methyl (CH_3) end of the molecule. In linolenic acid this is three carbon atoms away. It is therefore referred to as an $n-3$ fatty acid. In linoleic acid the first double bond is six carbons away and it is referred to as an $n-6$ fatty acid. Sometimes the terms 'omega 3' and 'omega 6' are used. The $n-3$ and $n-6$ fatty acids are not interconvertible by animals and result in two functionally distinct groups of polyunsaturated fatty acids. Important examples of these groups are eicosapentaenoic ($n-3$) and docosahexaenoic ($n-3$) acids, and arachidonic acid ($n-6$) referred to previously. Both groups have important metabolic functions but there is evidence that, for man, a dietary ratio of 4 or 5:1 for $n-6$: $n-3$ polyunsaturated acids is desirable. Higher ratios, common in western diets, are less desirable. The proportion is especially important in relation to the incidence of cardiovascular disease. For instance, the $n-3$ fatty acids reduce blood clotting while the $n-6$ acids counteract this effect.

Plant oils are rich sources of linoleic acid and, to a lesser degree, linolenic acid. Linseed oil is the only common plant oil to contain high levels of linolenic acid. Linoleic acid can be used by the animal to synthesize arachidonic acid, and linolenic acid can be used in the synthesis of eicosapentaenoic (EPA) and docosahexaenoic (DHA) acids (Box 3.2). However, to a degree the synthetic pathways compete with one another such that a diet rich in linoleic acid (for example those which are characteristic of many developed countries) can lead to a deficiency of EPA and DHA. Consuming EPA and DHA directly in the diet can compensate for this. Even small increases in consumption appear to reduce significantly the incidence of disease. This explains the early observation, and apparent paradox, that the lowest levels of coronary heart disease were seen in Greenland Eskimos and Japanese fishermen, populations with very high fat diets normally thought prejudicial to cardiovascular health. However, these diets were based

Box 3.2. Important members of the $n-3$ and $n-6$ series of fatty acids.

$n-3$	$n-6$
Linolenic acid (C18:3)	Linoleic acid (C18:2)
↓	↓
Eicosapentaenoic acid (C20:5) (EPA)	Arachidonic acid (C20:4) (AA)
↓	
Docosahexaenoic acid (C22:6) (DHA)	

on fish. These, especially oily fish like mackerel, are a rich source of EPA and DHA. This is because their own diet is based directly, or indirectly through the food chain, on micro-algae (particularly diatoms and dinoflagellates) which are major synthesizers of them. Red meat also contains long chain $n-3$ polyunsaturated fatty acids, but at low levels. There is therefore considerable interest in finding ways of increasing the levels to make a greater contribution to the diet and so promote health.

The general formula for a triglyceride is:

$$\begin{array}{l} CH_2\ COO - R_1 \\ | \\ CH\ COO - R_2 \\ | \\ CH_2\ COO - R_3 \end{array}$$

where R_1, R_2 and R_3 may be the same or different fatty acids. Thus, the formula for tristearin, or the triglyceride of stearic acid and the major triglyceride in beef fat, is:

$$\begin{array}{l} CH_2\ COO\ C_{17}\ H_{35} \\ | \\ CH\ COO\ C_{17}\ H_{35} \\ | \\ CH_2\ COO\ C_{17}\ H_{35} \end{array}$$

Triglycerides that contain mainly saturated fatty acids are solid at room temperature (20°C) and are often referred to as fats. Those containing a large proportion of unsaturated fatty acids are, by contrast, usually liquid. They therefore form oils. The triglyceride composition of animal fats is consequently very significant in determining their softness or hardness. Most animal fats are solids at room temperature. Most plant fats are not; hence groundnut (peanut), corn, rapeseed (canola) and olive oils. Lard is the fat of pigs; suet is the fat from around the kidneys of cattle and sheep. Beef fat contains up to 25% stearic acid, which is why it is harder than pork fat containing only about half this amount. The fats from fish and marine mammals tend to be polyunsaturated, containing up to six double bonds, and therefore are oils (cod liver oil, whale oil) at room temperature or above. Obviously, because fish are cold blooded it is important that their fats do not solidify at low temperatures and hence they must contain more unsaturated fatty acids. Within the body of warm-blooded animals, different fat depots may have different degrees of saturation. The fat from around the kidneys is very saturated (and hard at room temperature) compared with the subcutaneous fat. This is probably a reflection of the fact that the temperature of the body just under the skin is slightly cooler than that in the deep parts such as inside the abdomen. This temperature effect probably accounts for the softness of whale blubber fat. The proportions of saturated and unsaturated fatty acids in some fats and oils are shown in Table 3.4.

The differing proportions of the constituent saturated and unsaturated fatty acids illustrate their importance in determining the hardness or softness of the fat. The saturation of lamb or mutton fat is notable and may account for the 'greasy' mouth feel associated with eating it since it often has a melting point above that of the mouth temperature. The fatty acid composition of meat in the UK has been surveyed recently (Enser *et al.*, 1996).

For reasons of human health there is interest in trying to increase the proportion of polyunsaturated fatty acids to saturated fatty acids (the P:S ratio) in meat. It is not difficult to increase the proportion of unsaturated fatty acids in non-ruminants like pigs and poultry because the fat laid down in their bodies closely reflects the characteristics of the dietary fat. So, feeding pigs diets high in linseed, rapeseed or fish oils results in softer, more unsaturated carcass fat. The process is more difficult in ruminants. Unsaturated fats in the diet are hydrogenated by the rumen microorganisms to much more saturated fats. This is why the carcass fat of cattle and sheep is hard, despite the fact that the grass they eat contains mainly unsaturated fatty acids. However, about a

Table 3.4. Fatty acid composition of some fats and oils (as a percentage of the total fatty acids; based on data in Pearson, 1981).

	Lamb	Beef	Pork	Chicken	Salmon	Corn oil
Saturated fatty acids	53	45	40	35	21	13
Unsaturated fatty acids	47	55	60	65	79	87
Ratio (saturated/ unsaturated acids)	1.1	0.8	0.7	0.6	0.3	0.2
Hardness of fat	Hard →					Soft

tenth of the ingested unsaturated fatty acids do seem to pass through the rumen unchanged and feeding ruminants diets very rich in them can make the carcass fat softer, although the effect is relatively small (Enser *et al.*, 1998). A major problem with unsaturated fats is their sensitivity to oxidation and this may limit the degree to which production of meat with more unsaturated fats, and more desirable P:S ratios, can be achieved.

Other important lipids

Phospholipids are found as a major structural component of cell membranes but include the lecithins also found in blood plasma. Phospholipids are esters of glycerophosphoric acid. The fatty aids they contain are unsaturated. Sphingomyelins are an important constituent of nerves and glycolipids are also found in cell membranes. Steroids have a characteristic ring structure. The commonest is cholesterol, found in cell membranes and as a precursor of steroid hormones such as oestrogens and corticosteroids. Beef fat contains about 0.1% cholesterol. As well as being esterified with glycerol in triglycerides fatty acids can exist in the un-esterified form [non-esterified (NEFA) or free fatty acids (FFA)] and are the principal way in which body fat stores are mobilized and carried in the blood.

Lipid oxidation

Unsaturated fatty acids are very prone to oxidation. This is why linseed oil was so useful in the manufacture of paints: the oil oxidized in air to hard waterproof substances. Even in meat in which most of the fat is saturated the cell membranes contain phospholipids. The polyunsaturated fatty acids present in these can react with oxygen to form fatty acid hydroperoxides. These are unstable and break down into various compounds including aldehydes, ketones and carboxyl compounds, which can produce off-flavours. The process is relatively rapid, often occurring within 1–2 days in meat that has been cooked then kept refrigerated. This leads to the rather stale, rancid flavour referred to as 'warmed-over flavour' or WOF (Sato and Hegarty, 1971; Kerler and Grosch, 1996). However, off-flavours caused by lipid oxidation can also occur in uncooked meat. Generally, the propensity of meats to show the problem is directly related to their content of unsaturated fat. Therefore fish is more prone than poultry meat which in turn is more susceptible than the red meats. Of these, pork is the worst, followed by beef then lamb. The process of lipid oxidation is autocatalytic. The products of the reaction catalyse further reactions so that once started the reaction rate increases rapidly. Three stages can be recognized. In the *initiation* stage a fatty acid molecule (RH) breaks down to produce a free radical (R°). Free radicals are unstable and very reactive molecules. The fatty acid may also react with oxygen to produce a lipid peroxy radical (ROO°).

$$RH \rightarrow R^\circ + H^\circ$$

$$RH + O_2 \rightarrow ROO^\circ + H^\circ.$$

The H of the RH is the hydrogen of the methylene group (CH_2) adjacent to a double bond. Therefore, the more double bonds in the fatty acid molecule, the more prone it is to oxidation. In the second, *propagation* stage the free radical reacts with oxygen to produce a lipid peroxy radical. This then reacts with another fatty acid molecule to give a lipid hydroperoxide (ROOH) and another free radical.

$$R^\circ + O_2 \rightarrow ROO^\circ$$

$$ROO^\circ + RH \rightarrow ROOH + R^\circ.$$

Hydroperoxides can decompose to give various alcohols, aldehydes and ketones and it is these, particularly the aldehydes, which produce the off-odours and flavours associated with lipid oxidation. In the third, *termination*, stage, two free radicals may react together and a free radical may react with a lipid peroxy radical. Thus, free radicals are destroyed. They may also be destroyed by reaction with antioxidant or other molecules.

The initiation stage can be catalysed by a number of factors. Amongst these are light and heat, metal ions like iron and copper, and the iron-containing haem pigments like myoglobin and cytochromes. Free iron and haem pigments also catalyse the breakdown of the hydroperoxides formed in the propagation stage. Of the two forms of iron – the free iron and that in the haem molecule – the latter is thought to be the more important catalyst. Degradation of haem can release free iron. Ferrous iron can react with oxygen to give superoxide anion which then converts to hydrogen peroxide. This can produce hydroxyl radicals, which then react with fatty acids to initiate oxidation.

Lipid oxidation is promoted by processes that damage the muscle structure, such as mincing or comminuting. This exposes the fatty acids to oxygen and catalysing factors such as iron and haem.

Oxidation is also promoted by sodium chloride. The processes used to make products such as sausages, which contain minced meat and salt, therefore provide ideal conditions for oxidation. However, nitrite, often also added in cured products, and chelating agents such as citrates and phosphates, which sequester, or mop up, free metal ions, inhibit it. Other factors that affect the propensity of fat to undergo oxidation in meat are the haem pigment concentration, the storage temperature and availability of oxygen. Redder muscles, containing higher concentrations of haem pigments, are oxidation prone. Storage at high temperatures increases the rate of oxidation while freezing reduces it. Reducing the availability of oxygen by packing meat in, for example, nitrogen, or by vacuum packing it, will inhibit oxidation. So, to a degree, will keeping it in larger pieces where the ratio of the surface area to volume is minimized. Although all unsaturated fatty acids are susceptible to oxidation, the problem is greater the larger the number of double bonds since this is where breakdown of the molecule is initiated. Thus, both linoleic and linolenic acids have the same chain length (18 carbon atoms), but linolenic acid has three double bonds, compared with the two of linoleic acid. Its rate of oxidation is correspondingly much greater.

In the living animal, natural antioxidants reduce the level of lipid oxidation, so also limiting the production of dangerous free radicals which could damage other molecules. Several enzymes (glutathione peroxidase, catalase and superoxide dismutase) act to prevent oxidation. Natural antioxidants include vitamin C (ascorbic acid), β-carotene and vitamin E (α-tocopherol). Vitamin E is especially important. This can be taken advantage of by supplementing animal diets with the vitamin so the levels present in the meat *post mortem* are enhanced, sometimes up to eightfold those of unsupplemented animals. Vitamin E is lipid soluble and so accumulates in fats, particularly in cell membranes where it is most effective. The use of vitamins C and E as antioxidants is further dicussed in Chapter 8. An account of lipid oxidation and its effects on flavour in meat is given in Gray and Crackel (1992).

Measuring lipid oxidation

The most useful technique for following lipid oxidation in meat, rather than in just pure fat, is to measure the production of the aldehydes and ketones. This is done by heating the meat with thiobarbituric acid (TBA) when a pink coloured product is formed. This colour is measured after extraction into an organic solvent. To improve the specificity of the method the heating is usually combined with steam distillation. This separates the aldehydes and ketones, which are allowed to react with the TBA. Because the main oxidation product is malonaldehyde the degree of lipid oxidation is usually expressed in parts per million (ppm) of malonaldehyde. This figure is often referred to as the TBA number or value. Values above 0.5 indicate some oxidation and values above 1 possibly unacceptable levels.

Carbohydrates

In terms of overall composition these form a relatively minor component of animals but in muscles a particularly important one. Carbohydrates are composed of carbon, hydrogen and oxygen with the ratio of hydrogen to oxygen always 2:1. There are two main classes: sugars include monosaccharides such as glucose ($C_6H_{12}O_6$), also known as dextrose, and disaccharides such as sucrose ($C_{12}H_{22}O_{11}$) – the 'sugar' of common parlance that we use in our tea and coffee. Polysaccharides include glycogen $(C_6H_{10}O_5)_n$ which is a polymer of glucose. Polymers are large molecules made up of chains of repeated units sometimes with branches to the chains. Glycogen consists of up to 50,000 glucose or glucosyl units. It is comparable in function to the starch of plants in that it acts as an energy store, and especially as a readily available source of glucose. It is found particularly in the muscles and the liver. Although it occurs at a much lower concentration in the muscles (10–20 mg g^{-1}) the much greater muscle bulk means that the overall weight of glycogen stored is a lot larger (perhaps double) than in the liver. The liver nevertheless contains a higher concentration (50 mg g^{-1}), at least in well-fed animals. In the initial stages of fasting in animals, the liver glycogen is mobilized to maintain blood glucose concentrations at a constant level. Muscle glycogen can be used to produce energy for contraction under anaerobic conditions (where oxygen is absent), eventually being broken down into lactic acid.

Nucleotides

Nucleotides are complex molecules made up of three constituent parts, phosphoric acid (H_3PO_4), a sugar molecule containing five carbon atoms (a pentose) and a purine or pyrimidine molecule. Purines and pyrimidines are characterized by having rings containing both carbon and nitrogen atoms. Nucleotides form the basis of the nucleic acids, RNA and DNA. The purine-containing nucleotide, adenylic acid, is also known as adenosine monophosphate (AMP). AMP can have one or two extra phosphate molecules added to it to produce adenosine diphosphate (ADP) and adenosine triphosphate (ATP) respectively.

The importance of these extra phosphates is that they are joined to the AMP molecule by what are referred to as energy-rich bonds. These bonds, particularly that of the third phosphate in ATP, act as stores of chemical energy. Thus, when ATP is hydrolysed to ADP:

$$ATP + H_2O \rightleftharpoons ADP + H_3PO_4$$

the energy in the bond becomes available to fuel other processes in the animal's body. One of these is muscle contraction.

Examples of pyridine nucleotides are nicotine adenine dinucleotide (NAD) and nicotine adenine dinucleotide phosphate (NADP). These are important as coenzymes – compounds necessary for the activity of particular enzymes – because they act as hydrogen carriers. They are also important in the development of meat flavour, acting as flavour enhancers.

The Structure of Meat

Carcass meat consists of lean, fat and bone, together with connective tissue. The fat can be subcutaneous (lying under the skin of the animal), intermuscular (lying between individual muscles) or intramuscular (occurring within the body of the muscle). Subcutaneous fat is relatively easy to trim to produce leaner-looking meat; intermuscular fat is more difficult to remove simply. Intramuscular fat is also referred to as marbling fat because when abundant it gives a marbled appearance to the lean.

Muscles and their structure

The most important component of meat is the muscle. Indeed, when people think of meat they often only consider the muscle and the terms meat and muscle are sometimes used interchangeably. Muscles removed from a carcass frequently have a complex shape resulting from the complexity of their operation in the live animal and their attachment to the skeleton. The way the carcass is handled *post mortem*, allowing some parts of the musculature to contract while others are stretched, adds to this complexity. Nevertheless, all muscles have the same basic structure, consisting of muscle cells (fibres) bound together into bundles which are themselves often arranged in larger groupings. This arrangement is defined by connective tissue sheaths that eventually transmit the force developed by contractions of the individual fibres to the skeleton. The muscle fibres usually run in a direction parallel to the long axis of the muscle but can run obliquely. The muscles are attached to the skeleton through the tendons. Note that while *tendons* join muscle and bone, *ligaments* join different bones together.

Because muscles can only contract, they are only able to pull on the skeleton, not push. Hence they are effectively arranged in opposing pairs or groups. A simple example is that of the biceps and triceps muscles of the human upper arm. The biceps contracts to bend or raise the forearm and is referred to as a flexor muscle. The triceps contracts to straighten the forearm and is known as an extensor muscle. As their names suggest, the biceps has two heads each with a tendon attaching it to the shoulder blade, the triceps three heads and three tendons attaching it to the shoulder blade and long bone (humerus) of the upper arm. The importance to meat of muscles operating in opposing groups of flexors and extensors is that, in the carcass *post mortem*, muscles that are in a highly contracted state are likely to be balanced by a group of relaxed muscles. The state of contraction can considerably influence meat texture.

The muscle is supplied with blood through an artery and vein and is innervated by nerves. The nerves consist of numerous nerve fibres originating in the central nervous system and ending in specialized end plates called neuromuscular junctions.

Some important muscles

A good account of the anatomy of the muscles and fat depots of the carcasses of meat animals is given in Gerrard (1980). An extremely detailed description of the muscles of the ox is that of Butterfield and May (1966). Muscles are given Latin names which describe their characteristics or position; hence musculus longissimus dorsi. Often the musculus is abbreviated to 'm.' or omitted altogether. The m. longissimus dorsi (LD), sometimes referred to as the m. longissimus thoracis et lumborum, runs the whole length of the back and is the main muscle seen when 'chops' or 'rib-steaks' are cut from the posterior rib region and the loin. It lies dorsal to the transverse process of the vertebrae (Fig. 3.4). Perhaps rather confusingly, it is sometimes referred to as the 'eye' muscle. On beef carcasses it is possible to access it if each side of the carcass is 'quartered' by cutting between, for example, the last and last-but-one ribs so dividing the side into fore and hindquarters. It forms the 'striploin' joint.

The m. psoas major (PM) or psoas muscle forms the 'fillet'. It runs posteriorly under the transverse processes of the vertebrae in the loin region from the level of the head of the last rib. It is therefore easily accessible on the inside of the dressed carcass. The m. supraspinatus (SS) and m. infraspinatus (IS) are the muscles of the shoulder blade or scapula. The SS runs dorsal to the spine on the scapula; the IS runs ventral to the spine. Because the spine can be felt from the outside of

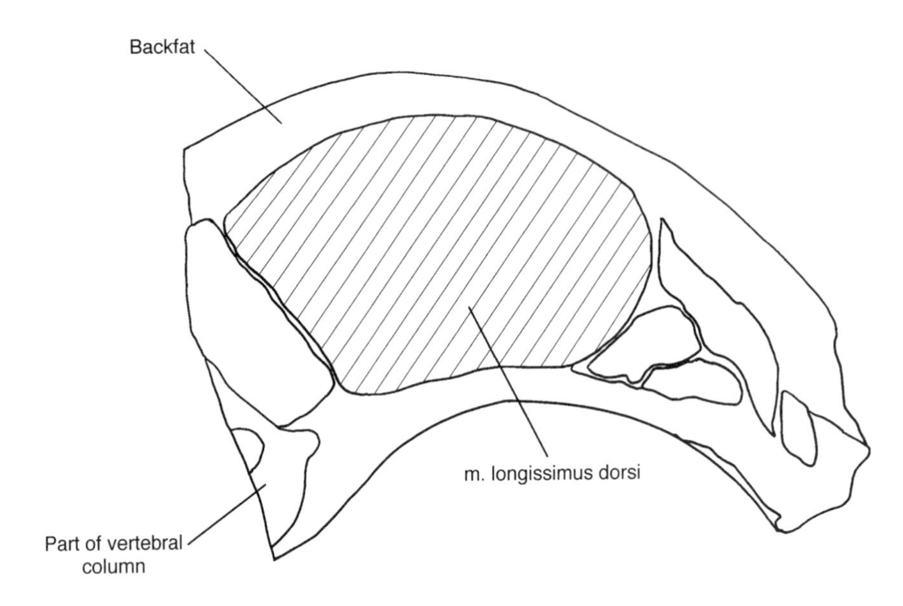

Fig. 3.4. Tracing of a photograph of a pork chop showing the longissimus dorsi muscle.

the forequarter, the muscles are relatively straightforward to locate. The m. biceps femoris (BF), m. semimembranosus (SM), m. semitendinosus (ST) and m. adductor (AD) are all large muscles of the hind limb. The SM and AD are on the medial (inside) part of the limb, the BF on the lateral (outside) part. In beef the BF forms part of the rump joint. A portion of the SM is often exposed when the tissue around the anus is cut to release the rectum prior to removal of the gut during carcass dressing. It can also be exposed on the cut medial surface when the carcass is split into two sides (Fig. 3.5). The SM forms the topside joint in beef. The AD is also cut during splitting.

The most important muscle in poultry is the breast muscle (m. pectoralis). Modern strains of broiler chicken and turkey have been selected to have very large breast muscles even though their major role – to flap the bird's wings in flight – is not required. The m. pectoralis is attached to the sternum, or keel, and the humerus. Pulling down on the humerus pulls the wing down. The wing is raised by a smaller muscle, the m. supracoracoideus, that lies behind the m. pectoralis. This is also attached to the keel and humerus. However, the tendon to the humerus is inserted on the opposite side of the bone and runs over a smooth, rounded surface in the bone of the shoulder girdle. It operates like a rope through a pulley in effect to change its direction of operation. The articulation of the wing with the body is strongly supported by the 'wishbone' formed of the fused clavicles.

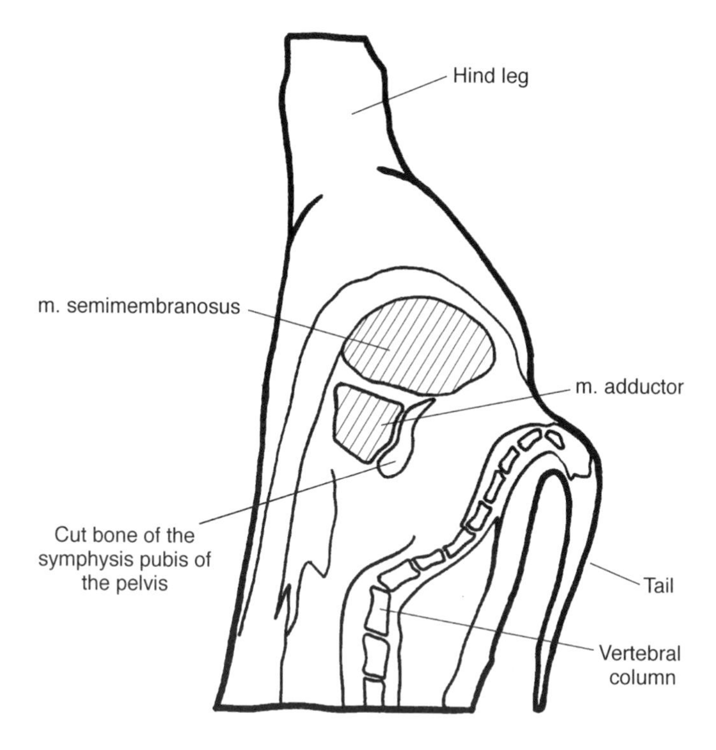

Fig. 3.5. Tracing of a photograph of the medial surface of the hind part of the left side of a pig carcass to show the exposed surfaces of the m. semimembranosus and m. adductor. The m. biceps femoris lies 'behind' these two muscles and would be accessible from the lateral aspect of the carcass by making an incision through the skin of the leg.

The connective tissue sheaths

The structure of the muscles is largely defined by sheaths of connective tissue. There are three levels of organization (Fig. 3.6). Individual muscle fibres are surrounded by a fine network of connective tissue, the endomysium. Bundles of fibres are surrounded by the perimysium, and the whole muscle is contained within the epimysium. In some cases the epimysium may appear to extend into the body of the muscle. This is so with the beef LD where there is an epimysial extension into the dorsal surface of the muscle.

The main component of the connective tissue is collagen, together with the protein elastin. The LD of an ox contains about 0.5% collagen and 0.1% elastin. These form fibres that are embedded in an amorphous ground substance. Collagen fibres are straight, inextensible and non-branching. Elastin fibres are branched and elastic. Elastin

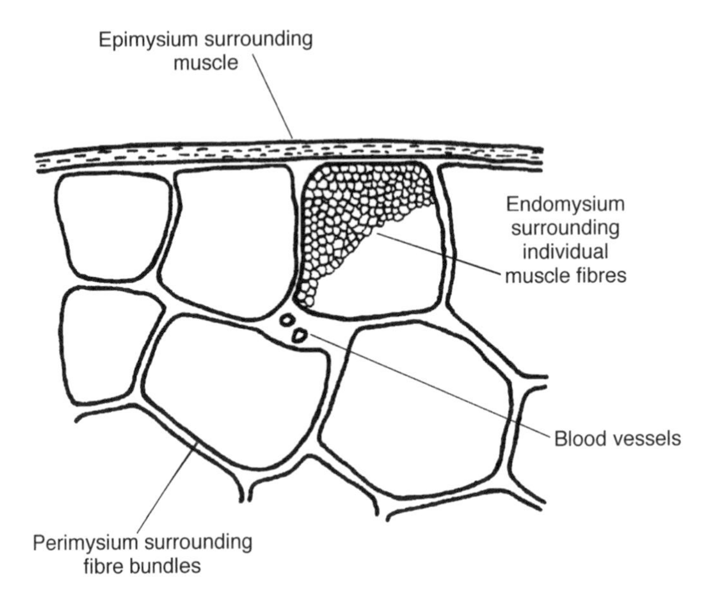

Fig. 3.6. Schematic cross-section of part of a muscle to show the connective tissue sheaths.

occurs especially in the walls of blood vessels and in ligaments. It also contributes to the elasticity of skin. A particularly good source is the neck ligaments of cattle, the ligamentum nuchae. Collagen can form very strong structures. As well as the connective tissue sheaths of the muscles it is a major component of skin, and is the reason why leather, made from tanned skin, is so strong.

The microscopic structure of the muscle fibre

Detailed accounts of the microscopic structure of skeletal muscle are given in many standard physiology textbooks, for example, Reece (1991). Each fibre is functionally equivalent to one cell even though it has been formed by the fusion of several myoblasts (see Chapter 2). The fibre may be several, or even tens of centimetres, long but is usually only about 60–100 μm in diameter. In young animals the diameter may be much less. Fibres contain all the organelles normally found in living cells: nuclei (more than one because each fibre is effectively formed from more than one cell), mitochondria and an extensive sarcoplasmic reticulum (equivalent to the endoplasmic reticulum of other types of cell) all within the sarcoplasm (cytoplasm; Fig. 3.7). The mitochondria contain the enzymes involved in aerobic metabolism. The sarcoplasmic reticulum acts as a store for calcium ions: these are

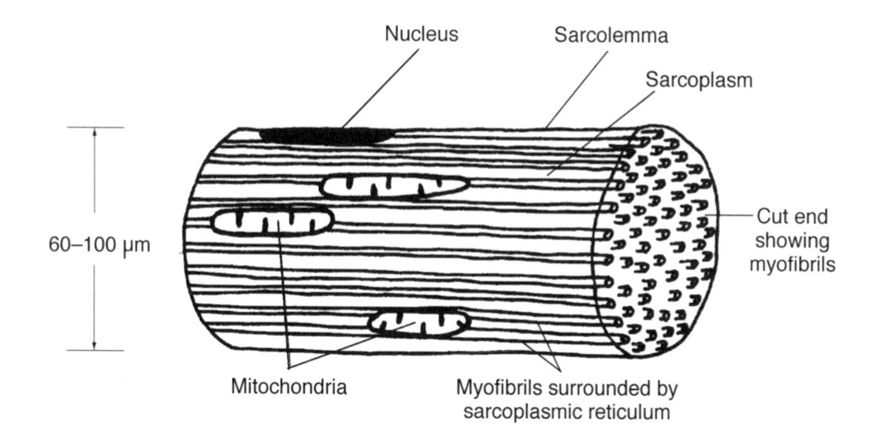

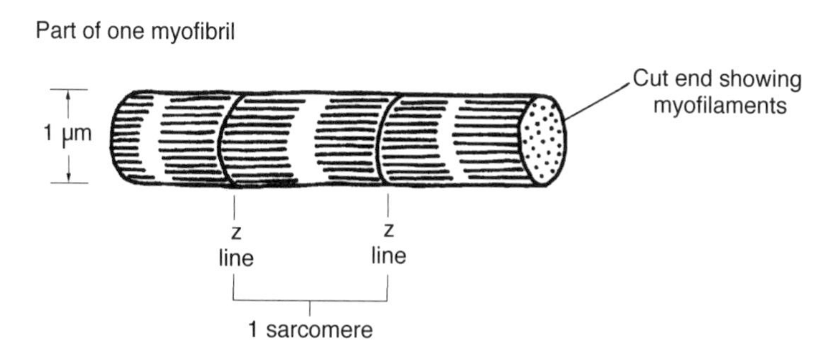

Fig. 3.7. Schematic representations of part of a fibre and one of its constituent fibrils.

released to initiate muscle contraction and reabsorbed (or sequestered) to stop it. The sarcoplasm also contains lysosomes, which act as a reservoir of various proteolytic enzymes, and granules of glycogen. Bounding the cell is a membrane, the sarcolemma (plasmalemma). The sarcolemma folds in to give a system of tubules that form a network through the fibre (the T-tubules) particularly in the region of the Z lines (or Z discs – see later). The system comes into intimate contact with distended regions of the sarcoplasmic reticulum to form 'triads'. The T-tubules and sarcoplasmic reticulum form a functionally continuous system. The nuclei lie just below the sarcolemma.

A unique feature of muscle fibres is that, embedded in the sarcoplasm, are regularly arranged fibrils. In a single fibre there might be between one and two thousand fibrils each about 1 μm in diameter and running longitudinally. Together the fibrils may occupy about 80% of the volume of the fibre. Each fibril is itself made up of smaller elements called filaments. These are of two sorts, thick filaments (about 15 nm in diameter) consisting mainly of the protein myosin and thin filaments (about 7 nm in diameter) consisting mainly of the protein actin. Under certain conditions actin and myosin can react together to produce contraction of the system and therefore the whole muscle. When they are in this state they are sometimes referred to in combination as actomyosin. Fibres, fibrils and filaments are sometimes also given the prefix myo- to indicate their relation to muscle, hence: myofibre, myofibril and myofilament.

Red and white fibres

Based on their complement of enzymes, and the activities of these enzymes, muscle fibres can be categorized into different metabolic types. The essential difference is between fibres with a predominantly oxidative (aerobic) metabolism and those with a mainly glycolytic (anaerobic) metabolism (see Chapter 5). Aerobic metabolism requires the availability of oxygen; anaerobic metabolism can occur in the absence of oxygen. Oxidative fibres have more mitochondria, containing red cytochromes, and a higher concentration of the red pigment myoglobin in their sarcoplasm. Oxidative fibres therefore appear red in colour. Cytochromes are an essential part of the mechanism (oxidative phosphorylation) by which nutrients are oxidized by the cell to liberate energy. Myoglobin transports oxygen within the cell, just as the haemoglobin of the red blood cells transport oxygen from the lungs to the rest of the body. Glycolytic fibres contain relatively small amounts of cytochromes or myoglobin and therefore appear white.

Some fibres have both oxidative and glycolytic metabolic capability. They may appear pink in colour and are sometimes referred to as intermediate fibres. Red, oxidative fibres often contain fat droplets whereas white, glycolytic fibres have a high glycogen content. Red fibres are characterized histochemically by having relatively weak ATP-ase and phosphorylase activity but strong activity of enzymes involved in aerobic metabolism like cytochrome oxidase and succinic dehydrogenase. ATP-ases hydrolyse ATP and phosphorylases are important in the initial stages of glycogen breakdown. White fibres, in contrast, have strong ATP-ase and phosphorylase activity but weak aerobic enzyme activity. Intermediate fibres tend to have strong ATP-ase and glycolytic enzyme activity, but variable activity of the enzymes of aerobic metabolism.

Different muscles contain different proportions of the different fibre types and this determines the macroscopic colour of the muscle.

In poultry and pigs, the differences in colour of different muscles in the carcass are more noticeable than the differences in ruminants. In broiler chickens and turkeys especially, the breast meat (m. pectoralis) is very pale compared with the meat on the legs. In pigs, the LD in the back is pale and the AD in the ham, for example, is dark. Ruusunen and Puolanne (1988) measured the proportions of red, intermediate and white fibres in the LD and AD of Finnish and German pigs (Table 3.5). Both muscles contained all three fibre types. The proportion of red fibres was lower, and the proportion of white fibres higher, in the paler LD, but two-thirds of the fibres in the dark AD were white and both muscles contained about 12% intermediate fibres. The figures for the pigs from the two countries were remarkably consistent. However, the actual designation of the different fibre types can be influenced by the particular histological staining method used to differentiate them, and different proportions of fibres, particularly white and intermediate types, have been reported by other workers.

From a functional point of view, red fibres tend to be 'slow twitch' and white fibres 'fast twitch'. Slow-twitch and fast-twitch refer to the contraction speed. Slow-contracting fibres are characteristic of postural muscles whereas fast-contracting fibres are found especially in muscles whose main role is in rapid but intermittent movement. The relation between contraction speed and the metabolic characteristics of the fibre, as reflected in its categorization as red, white or intermediate, is actually rather more complex than implied here. Two types of fast-twitch fibres are sometimes recognized. Type IIA are fast-twitch red and Type IIB are fast-twitch white fibres. They are differentiated from Type I fibres which are slow-twitch red (Fig. 3.8).

There are morphological differences between fibre types. Generally, white fibres have a greater diameter. Red fibres have a larger number of capillaries associated with them, as might be imagined from their reliance on oxidative metabolism, and therefore a requirement for more oxygen during activity.

Table 3.5. Fibre type composition of two pig muscles (data from Ruusunen and Puolanne, 1988; LD = m. longissimus dorsi, AD = m. adductor).

	Percentage red	Percentage intermediate	Percentage white
LD			
Finnish pigs	6.3	13.9	79.8
German pigs	5.8	10.3	83.9
AD			
Finnish pigs	22.2	11.7	66.1
German pigs	20.5	11.7	67.8

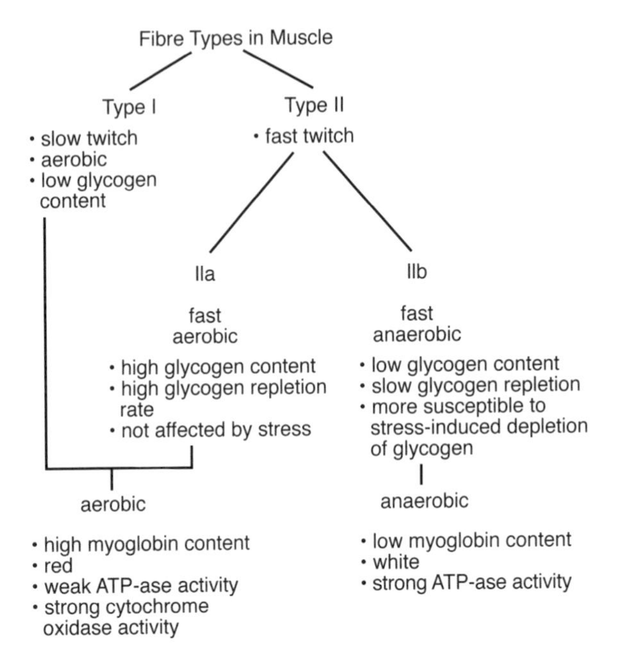

Fig. 3.8. A summary of the main characteristics of the different fibre types in muscle.

The banding pattern seen in muscles

A characteristic feature of photographs of longitudinal sections of skeletal muscles when seen under the microscope is the regular transverse bandings or striations. These have given the name 'striated' as an alternative to 'skeletal' muscle. Unless specially stained with dyes, muscles do not usually appear striated when in correct focus under the ordinary light microscope. However, the striations can be seen by using either a polarizing or a phase contrast microscope. The reason for this is that the striations are caused by alternating bands of protein which have a higher or lower refractive index. The bands with high refractive index are birefringent. Birefringent materials alter the plane of vibration of light passing through them and this can be detected in the polarizing microscope.

Birefringent materials are described as optically anisotropic. Non-birefringent materials are isotropic. The dark bands in muscle seen under the polarizing microscope therefore became known as A-bands (after anisotropic) and the intervening (clear) bands as I-bands (after isotropic). It is now known how these bands relate to the structural relationships of the thick and thin filaments. The A-band is formed by the thick filaments, together with the overlapping thin filaments, and the I-band by mainly just the thin filaments (Fig. 3.9). Because the

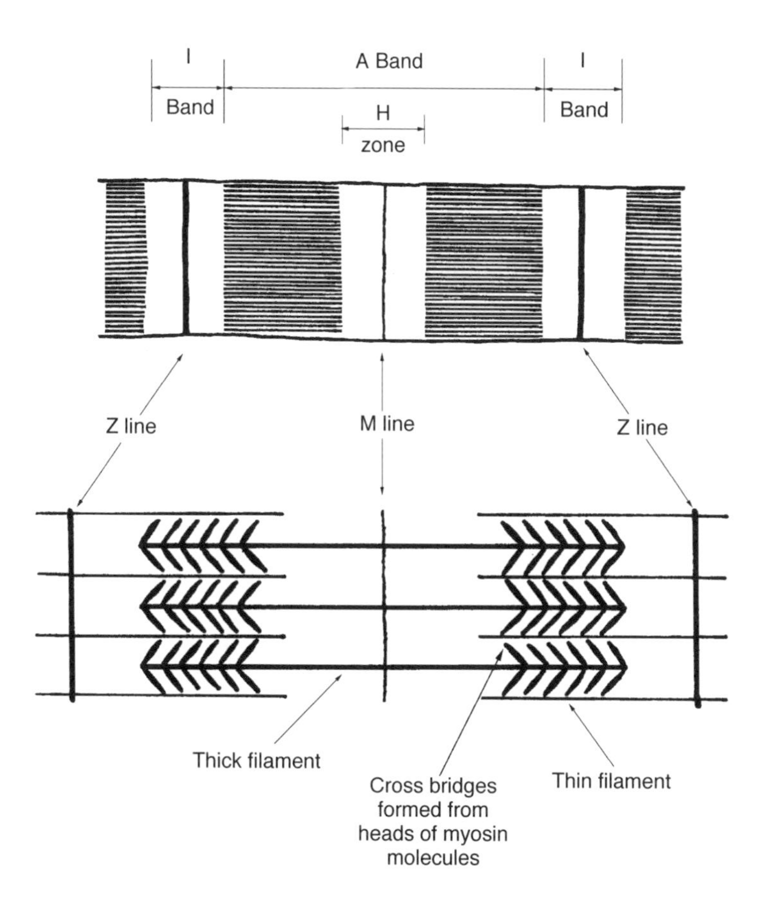

Fig. 3.9. The banding pattern of the muscle fibril and the correspondence with its fine structure shown schematically.

myofibrils are exactly aligned, the banding pattern continues across the fibres.

Early microscopists also identified various other lines and zones, including the H zone, and the M and Z lines. The Z line is of particular functional significance. It is really a disc through which the thin filaments pass (and is often therefore also referred to as the Z disc). Adjacent Z lines delineate the functional unit of the myofibril – referred to as a sarcomere. A myofibril consists of thousands of sarcomeres. The sarcomere length, defined by the distance between Z lines, varies with the state of contraction of the muscle but averages between about 1.5 and 2 μm. Differences in the degree of contraction also lead to variation in the details of the banding pattern observed. These differences are now known to reflect differences in the degree of overlap of the thick and thin filaments.

The arrangement of the thick and thin filaments

The thick and thin filaments interdigitate in a very regular way so that each thick filament is surrounded by six thin ones and each thin filament by three thick ones (Fig. 3.10). The actual pattern seen in transverse section will vary with the position of the cut. Close to the Z line only thin filaments will be visible; in the centre of the sarcomere only thick filaments. Also, in reality the thick and thin filaments are very close together. This is necessary to allow the interaction of myosin and actin molecules during contraction. The 'cross-bridges' visible in some electron micrographs of muscles are formed by part of the myosin molecules – the heads – linking on to the actin molecules. H.E. Huxley (1969), in a classic paper, gave a full explanation of the structural organization of the myofibril in terms of the relationship between thick and thin filaments, the role of the cross bridges in contraction, and the relationship of the ultrastructural details of organization to the structure seen in microscopic preparations.

The Contractile and Other Muscle Proteins

Myosin and actin

Myosin and actin are not restricted to muscle but are found in many mobile cells such as spermatozoa and even in some non-mobile cells. As mentioned previously, in muscle, myosin and actin form the major parts of the thick and thin filaments respectively. The myosin molecule consists of a head region joined via a neck to a tail. Overall it is about 150 nm long with a molecular weight of 520,000. The head itself consists of two pear-shaped parts or lobes and the tail is formed of two long strands wound around one another in a helical fashion (Fig. 3.11). The strands are made up of six subunits, two heavy chains and four light chains. Their composition varies and leads to different types of myosin.

The long ends of the tails of several hundred myosin molecules aggregate to form the thick filament and the heads stick out at regular intervals to form the cross-bridges. When they aggregate, half the myosin molecules have their heads facing one end of the thick filament, the other half the other end. A central bare zone is formed from just the tails of the molecules. The myosin molecules pack together so that the heads forming the cross bridges make a helical repeating pattern around the thick filament. The neck region between head and tail is flexible so allowing the head to move and possibly acting as a lever to amplify any movement. It also seems to introduce an elastic element that may help the generation of force during isometric (fixed

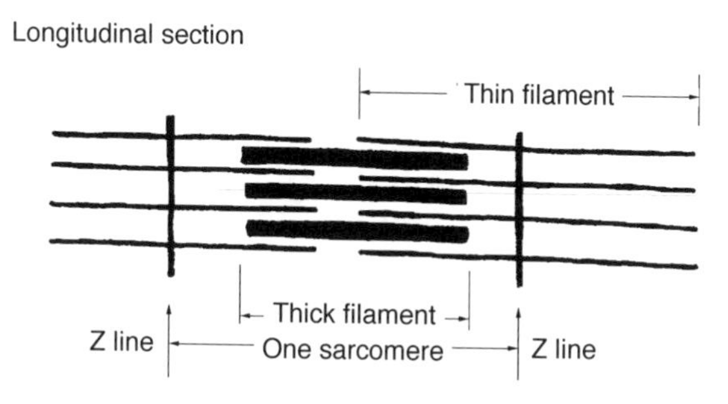

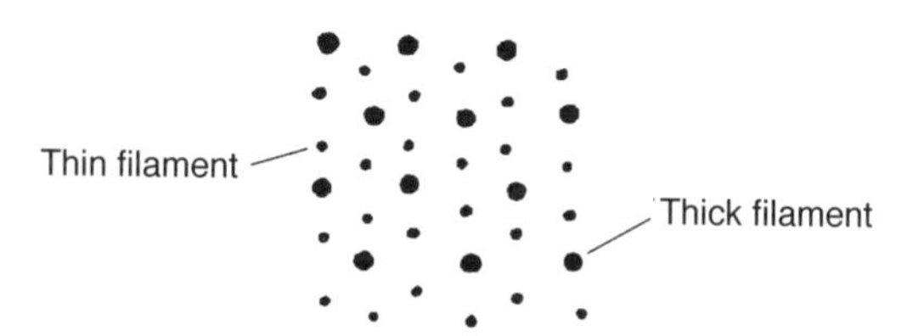

Fig. 3.10. Arrangement of the thick and thin filaments.

length) contraction of the muscle. During contraction the myosin head is thought to undergo a conformational change so it tilts and levers against the actin of the thin filament.

Actin consists of globular molecules (G-actin) with a molecular weight of about 42,000 that, in certain conditions (in relatively concentrated salt solutions), polymerize to form double helical chains (F-actin). These form the basis of the thin filaments together with two other proteins, tropomyosin and troponin, arranged in a regular, repeating pattern (Fig. 3.12). In the figure the G-actin molecules are

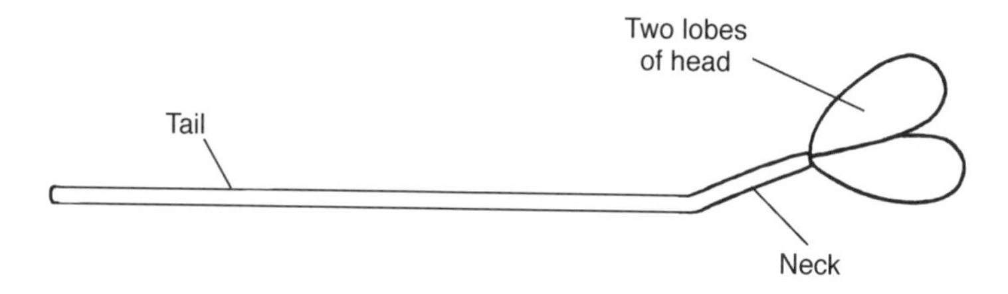

Fig. 3.11. Schematic representation of a myosin molecule.

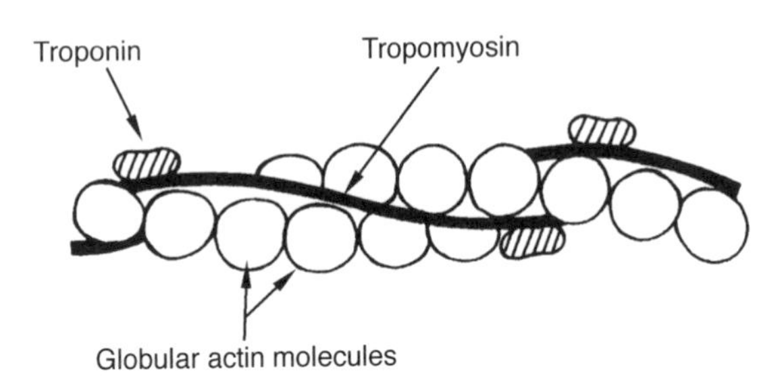

Fig. 3.12. The arrangement of actin, tropomyosin and troponin in the thin filament.

drawn as spherical beads but in reality are not this shape. Tropomyosin and troponin together make up about 10% of the myofibrillar proteins. The rod-like tropomyosin molecules lie between the actin chains, with troponin at the cross-over points. Troponin consists of three subunits (C, I and T). Tropomyosin and troponin are involved in the control of contraction by calcium ions. A summary of the characteristics of the main myofibrillar proteins is given in Table 3.6.

The cytoskeleton

Within the myofibril, the myofilaments are maintained in their relative positions by a cytoskeleton made up of a number of other proteins. Notable amongst these are titin (sometimes called connectin) and nebulin. Titin is an extremely large protein (MW = 3,000,000), which joins the myosin of the thick filament to the Z disc, probably forming what are known as the gap filaments. Nebulin (MW = 500,000) forms a system that probably maintains the orientation of the filaments in the plane transverse to the long direction of the myofibril. It may also prevent over extension or stretching of the sarcomeres. The Z disc contains a number of proteins including α-actinin and desmin. The cytoskeleton also maintains the architecture of the myofibrils within the myofibre. For example, the myofibrils are linked to the sarcolemma by transverse structures called costamers containing the protein

Table 3.6. The characteristics of the main myofibrillar proteins.

Component	Molecular weight	Percentage muscle weight
Myosin	520,000	5–6
Actin	42,000	2–3
Tropomyosin	66,000	0.8
Troponin	80,000	0.2

vinculin. A review of the proteins forming the cytoskeleton is given in Maruyama (1985).

Other proteins of the muscle

The myofibrillar proteins form about 60% of the total muscle protein. The remaining 40% consist mainly of the ordinary cellular proteins, especially the enzymes, normally found in all types of cell and, because they occur in the sarcoplasm, referred to as the sarcoplasmic proteins, and the stroma proteins (Table 3.7). The latter are rather insoluble and consist largely of the connective tissue components (collagen and elastin).

The myofibrillar and sarcoplasmic proteins can be extracted using appropriate-strength salt (e.g. potassium chloride) solutions. Fairly dilute salt solutions (0.04 M) extract the sarcoplasmic proteins. More concentrated solutions (0.4 M) are required to extract myosin. If the solution is then diluted to about 0.1 M the myosin molecules aggregate into 'rods' in which the molecules appear to arrange themselves in a way very similar to that in the thick filament, with the heads sticking out at the ends and a middle part consisting only of tails. Actin can be extracted with 0.6 M potassium iodide. In concentrated salt solutions the molecules polymerize to form chains as in the thin filaments.

Muscle Contraction

The mechanism of muscle contraction

The mechanism of muscle contraction, referred to as the sliding filament hypothesis, was put forward in another classic paper by H.E. Huxley and J. Hanson (1954). During muscle contraction the interdigitating thick and thin filaments of the myofibrils slide over one

Table 3.7. The proportions of myofibrillar, sarcoplasmic and stroma proteins in muscle.

Component	Percentage muscle protein	Percentage wet muscle weight
Myofibrillar proteins	60	10
Sarcoplasmic proteins	20	5
Stroma proteins	20	5
	100%	20%

another. They are linked by the cross-bridges formed by the heads of the myosin molecules. These cross-bridges 'ratchet' along the actin chains of the thin filaments. With different degrees of contraction, different degrees of overlap of thick and thin filaments occur and different amounts of force are developed. The different degrees of overlap are reflected in the sarcomere length and the distance between the visible striations. Maximum force is developed when all the available cross bridges on the thick filament are aligned with the thin filament (at a sarcomere length of about 2.1 μm). The striations therefore move closer together on contraction. A.F. Huxley and R.M. Simmons (1971) suggested an explanation of how the smooth force between the thick and thin filaments could be generated. They proposed the existence of elastic components in the cross bridge structure that would produce the continuous development of contraction actually seen.

Adenosine triphosphate (ATP) and the energy for contraction

Both myosin and actin bind ATP. Each of the lobes of the head of the myosin molecule can bind an ATP molecule and each globular actin molecule also binds a molecule of ATP. However, on polymerization of the actin into chains; this ATP is hydrolysed to ADP. The myosin molecule acts as an ATP-ase but its activity is enhanced greatly by the presence of actin. The hydrolysis of ATP by the actomyosin ATP-ase is the mechanism by which contraction is fuelled. The details of this process by which chemical energy is converted into movement are, however, still unclear.

The sarcoplasmic reticulum and the control of contraction

The sarcoplasmic reticulum forms a complex membrane system surrounding each myofibril and is functionally continuous with the T-tubule system formed by the sarcolemma. It has a fundamental role in controlling the contractile process. Muscles normally contract in response to a nervous stimulation. This causes acetylcholine to be released by the neuromuscular junction. Acetylcholine is a neurotransmitter, interacting with, or binding to, a receptor molecule on the surface of the sarcolemma. The acetylcholine produces a local depolarization of the muscle fibre membrane; in effect the polarity of the membrane reverses. Normally the inside of the cell is maintained at a negative potential (−90 mV) by a differential distribution of potassium (K^+) and sodium (Na^+) ions across the membrane. The concentration of K^+ is high inside the cell and that of Na^+ high outside. During depolarization, K^+ ions move out and Na^+ ions move in.

The local region of depolarization spreads across the membrane surface. Because the sarcolemma is functionally continuous with the sarcoplasmic reticulum, the depolarization is transmitted into the cell and to the individual fibrils. Normally, the sarcoplasmic reticulum maintains the concentration of calcium ions (Ca^{2+}) in the sarcoplasm very low (less than 0.1 μM) by active pumping. Depolarization causes a momentary very large release of Ca^{2+} from the sarcoplasmic reticulum back into the sarcoplasm. The 100-fold increase in Ca^{2+} (to about 10 μM) removes the normal inhibition exerted by tropomyosin and troponin on the attraction between myosin and actin and so causes a contraction. Details of the control of contraction are not fully understood. However, the calcium ions saturate troponin – C, changing the relative positions of the three subunits. This displaces the tropomyosin, exposing the binding site on the actin so allowing it to react with ATP on the head of the myosin molecule. The ATP-ase system is activated, ATP is hydrolysed and the actin and myosin molecules pull together. When the calcium ions are re-sequestered by the sarcoplasmic reticulum, inhibition returns and the contractile force ceases.

Anything that interferes with this chain of events can prevent muscle contraction. Some Indian tribes of South America hunt animals using arrows tipped with a poison called curare, which is made from a plant extract. Curare binds to the acetylcholine receptor on the muscle cell membrane, so blocking the effect of the acetylcholine, and thus paralysing the animal. The animal dies from asphyxiation because the chest muscles are paralysed. Nowadays, derivatives of curare are used as muscle relaxants in people undergoing surgery.

A review of the interaction between myosin and actin, the regulatory roles of tropomyosin and troponin, and the role of calcium in controlling muscle contraction, is given in Weber and Murray (1973). The physiology of the neuromuscular junction and the role of acetylcholine was described by Hubbard (1973).

Chapter 4

The Slaughter of Animals

The methods used to slaughter animals can affect carcass and meat quality, the animals' welfare and the safety of the personnel operating the system. Many methods are influenced by religious beliefs. For example, some Jews and Muslims will not consume the meat from animals unless these have been slaughtered according to a set of religious codes. An important consideration is that in most forms of religious slaughter the animals are not stunned before they are killed by sticking and exsanguination. Stunning refers to rendering the animals unconscious and sticking refers to severing some of the major blood vessels in the neck or thorax so the animal bleeds to death (exsanguination). Stunning prevents any possibility that the animals should feel pain or distress during exsanguination.

Handling and Ante-mortem Inspection

Handling animals up to the point of stunning

Animals awaiting slaughter are often held in special pens or areas in a lairage. The animals in the lairage form a reservoir so that the slaughterline can be maintained full and can therefore be operated efficiently. The lairage also allows the animals to rest and calm down if they are fatigued or stressed by transport or by unloading from vehicles. This can make them easier to handle in the confines of the stunning pen and may improve meat quality.

While in lairage animals need to be handled considerately. This includes provision of bedding, water to drink and, if appropriate, food. Conditions should be such that the animals can rest adequately in unmixed groups. When they are moved this should be done in such a manner that the animals do not become stressed. Use of sticks and goads should be avoided. Stressed animals are more likely to be fractious and likely to fall or bruise themselves, as well as being a danger to the personnel handling them. Poultry are transported and held in plastic crates. This makes it impossible to provide them with food and water and the time they spend in lairage therefore needs to be minimized. The ante-mortem handling of animals is discussed in greater detail in Chapter 7.

Ante-mortem inspection

Animals are inspected before they are slaughtered. This may enable identification of clinical signs of diseases which could either be transmitted to humans (zoonoses) or other animals, or make the meat unfit for human consumption. It may also enable identification of animals which have had medicines or other pharmacological agents given to them, or which are injured and should therefore be handled separately and possibly slaughtered immediately to prevent further suffering.

Some symptoms of disease, such as in tetanus, rabies or poisoning, may be more obvious in a live animal than in the carcass. It is important to detect some serious diseases at the earliest opportunity to prevent further infection and contamination. Examples are anthrax, and foot and mouth disease. Anthrax is a highly contagious disease caused by a bacterium *Bacillus anthracis*, which produces infective spores. It affects animals and humans and is rapidly fatal. Anthrax was once commonly referred to as woolsorter's disease because of its prevalence in people handling sheeps' wool. In the past this was not infrequently contaminated with the anthrax spores. Infected animals are listless and sometimes have bloodshot eyes and respiratory problems. Foot-and-mouth disease is caused by a virus and is highly infectious, although rarely fatal to animals. The disease gets its name from the blisters that form in the mouth and on the feet (although other areas of the body, like the udder, can be affected). The mouth blisters cause characteristic drooling from the mouth and lip smacking. Although mortality is low, the reduced productivity associated with the disease makes it economically very serious.

In the UK and many other countries, anthrax and foot-and-mouth disease are notifiable. That is, immediately on detection the relevant government authorities must be informed so that appropriate measures can be taken to restrict the spread of the disease. There are various other notifiable diseases. Examples are swine fever, African swine fever, brucellosis, rabies and tuberculosis.

Stunning

Stunning methods

Particularly with large animals, stunning is important to immobilize the animal to facilitate severing the blood vessels (sticking) to kill it. Operator safety would be severely compromised by trying to stick a conscious animal unless it was fully restrained. Manual restraint is feasible for small animals like sheep but not for cattle. Restraint in specially designed pens is a feature of Jewish slaughter in high throughput plants in Europe and North America. The value of stunning in preventing the animal feeling pain or distress at exsanguination has been mentioned already. To be effective in this regard the stunning process must render the animal insensible immediately, or, if it is not immediate, the process must be completely pain and stress-free. By relaxing the body, some stunning techniques may also benefit carcass quality.

There are different ways in which animals can be stunned. They fall into three main types. The first is use of a mechanical instrument (captive bolt pistol, percussion stunner or free bullet) which traumatizes the brain so that the animal loses consciousness instantaneously. The second is use of an electrical current passed through the brain. The third is the induction of unconsciousness by immersion in an anaesthetic gas such as carbon dioxide. All methods should be considered to serve *only* to render the animal unconscious. After stunning the animal must be killed by exsanguinating it as soon as possible. This is normally done by severing the blood vessels in the neck (the carotid arteries and jugular veins) or the blood vessels from which they arise where they enter the heart at the base of the throat (chest sticking).

Particularly in the case of the use of a mechanical instrument, or in the application of the current in electrical stunning, it is important that the animal is sufficiently restrained to allow accurate shooting or application of the electrical current. This is another reason for ensuring that the animal is not distressed or fractious at the point of stunning. In the case of pigs, sheep and goats, the animal may be held in a V-shaped or monorail-type restraining conveyor, or may be manoeuvred by the slaughterman himself. For cattle a restrainer can also be used but it is more common to confine the animal in a stunning box. It may still be necessary to restrain the head of the animal. An overview and detailed account of much of the early scientific studies on stunning techniques is given in Leach (1985).

Use of a free bullet

Generally this is only used for large bulls and boars. It is less easy to ensure safety with this method because of the danger of the bullet passing through the animal's body and ricocheting. It may, however, be necessary if the animal has a very thick skull that would preclude effective use of the captive bolt pistol.

Captive bolt and concussion stunning

These methods developed from use of the pole-axe. This was an axe with a hammer at the back and fitted with a long handle (or pole). Later, especially in the early beef packing plants in North America, it was replaced by a small-headed sledge hammer with a long handle. In the captive bolt pistol (Fig. 4.1) the bolt is driven into the animal's brain by either the detonation of an explosive cartridge or by compressed air. Air-operated systems are common in North America.

Different sized cartridges are used for different kinds of animal. For example, a 4–6 grain (1 grain = 0.065 g) cartridge would be effective for a large, heavy bull while 1–2 grains would be sufficient for sheep. All

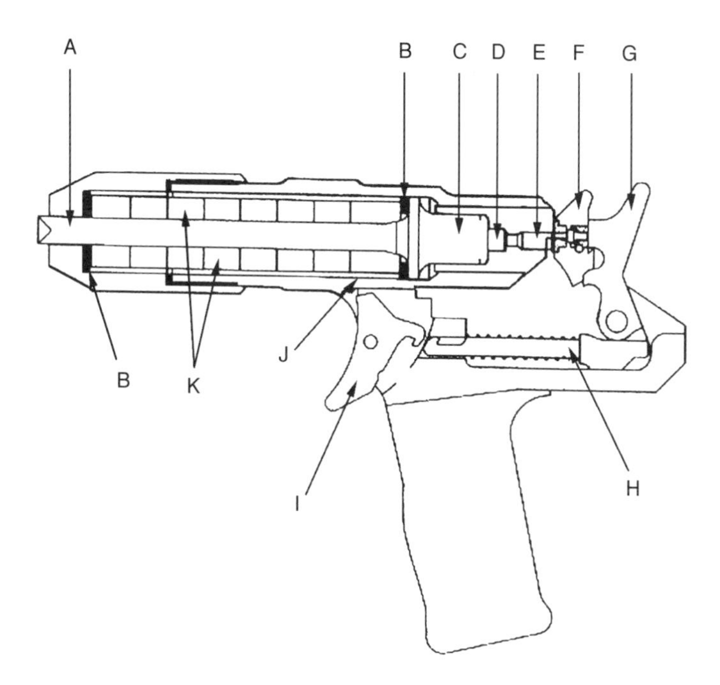

Fig. 4.1. Schematic diagram of one type of captive bolt pistol (reproduced by courtesy of the UK Humane Slaughter Association) (Key: A, bolt; B, stop washers; C, flange and piston; D, expansion chamber; E, breech; F, ejector, housing the firing pin; G, hammer; H, trigger mechanism; I, trigger; J, undercut; K, recuperator sleeves).

current models of captive bolt pistol take 0.22 or 0.25 calibre cartridges.

To stun an animal it is not necessary to penetrate the brain. Concussion alone can be effective and some equipment is designed to give a non-penetrating blow to the head. This is usually through a mushroom-shaped 'bolt'. Concussion stunning is best restricted to mature cattle since it relies on a reasonable thickness of bone over the brain. This is because it is important that the bone does not break. If the bone is broken some of the energy of the impact will be absorbed rather than being transmitted to the brain. The neuropathological changes caused by concussion stunning of cattle have been described (Finnie, 1995).

For effectiveness the important factors in using percussion stunning are positioning of the blow and the energy transmitted. The energy can be calculated from the mass (weight) of the bolt and its velocity. Because the energy is a function of movement it is kinetic energy and can be calculated using the formula:

$$KE = \frac{1}{2} mv^2$$

where: KE = kinetic energy; m = mass of bolt; and v = velocity of bolt. If the mass is in g and the velocity is measured in ms^{-1} the energy is in joules (J). About 200 kJ are required for an effective stun in adult cattle with correct application. Notice that the velocity of the bolt has the major effect on the energy delivered because the velocity term is squared. Things that reduce the velocity of the bolt, like the build up of carbon deposits from the burning explosive, will seriously reduce the energy delivered and compromise an effective stun. The position of shooting should be such that maximum damage is done to the brain. Because the brain is slightly differently positioned in relation to the head shape, different shooting positions are optimal for the different species (Fig. 4.2). Goats and horned sheep need to be shot in the poll position because of the bony mass found on top of the skull, or the tissue associated with the horns, in these animals.

Electrical stunning

Electrical stunning is used mainly for poultry, pigs and sheep, but has been employed for mature cattle in some countries. Usually, a voltage ranging from 150 to 700 V (AC, 50–60 Hz) is used depending on the system. Higher voltages are generally better. It is important that the electric current is passed through the brain, so the positioning of the electrodes through which the current is applied is important. The effectiveness of stunning is determined by the amount of *current* passed through the brain. This can be determined from Ohm's Law:

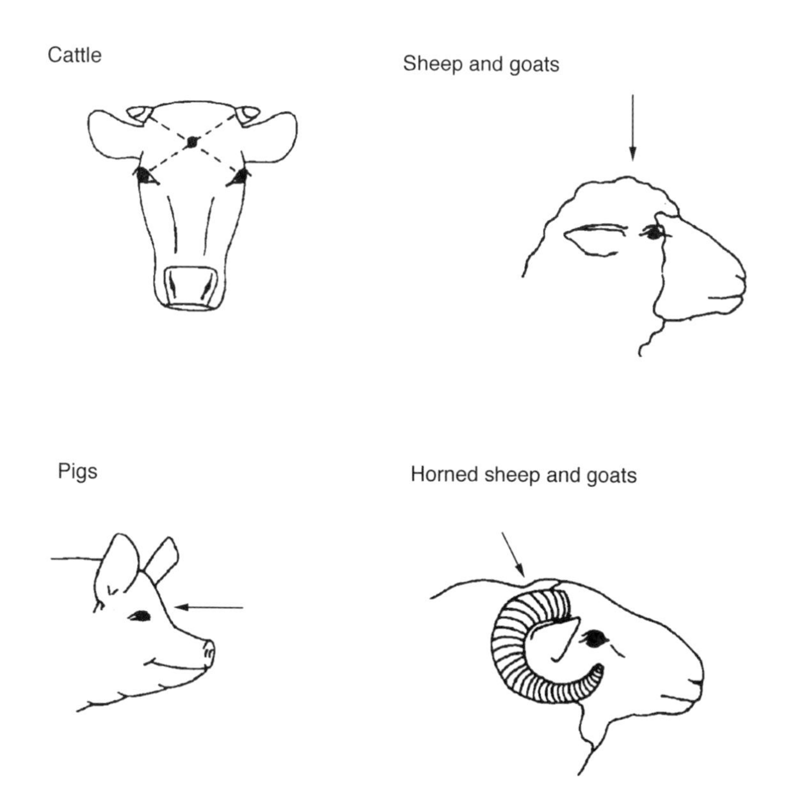

Fig. 4.2. Positions for stunning the different species with a captive bolt pistol as recommended by the UK Humane Slaughter Association (reproduced by courtesy of the HSA).

current = voltage/resistance.

With alternating currents, resistance is more correctly termed impedance. More current is therefore passed with higher voltages and lower resistances of the animal's body tissues. The actual resistance will depend on various factors such as how good the contact with the electrodes is, and whether the skin is wet. Electrode design is also very important and, for pigs, has been excellently reviewed by Sparrey and Wotton (1997). The amount of current required for an effective stun in practical situations in the different species varies (Table 4.1).

The current should be passed for 3 s. Traditionally, in red meat species, the electrodes are applied only across the head using various designs of tongs. These often have a scissor-like operation. The ideal electrode position for pigs and sheep is between the eyes and the bases of the ears on each side of the head. This is referred to as head-only stunning. Newer techniques for red meat species, and conventional

Table 4.1. The amounts of current which have been recommended for stunning different species.

Species	Current (amps)[a]
Chicken	0.105
Rabbit	0.3
Lamb	0.6
Sheep	1.0
Goat	1.0
Calf	1.0
Pig	1.3

[a] For head-only stunning where the electrodes are placed on opposite sides of the head so they span the brain.

poultry stunning, use head-to-body stunning. In this, current flows both through the brain and between the head and the rest of the body through the heart (Wotton *et al.*, 1992). The electrical current flowing through the heart stops it so the animal is killed as well as stunned. The extra electrodes for head-to-body stunning are usually placed on the back, or sometimes on the foreleg or 'brisket' (chest). In poultry stunning, the birds are suspended by their legs from metal shackles. The shackles are connected to ground and their heads dip into a water bath maintained at an electrical potential. Current therefore flows from the water, through the head and body, to the shackles. Head-to-body stunning of cattle with electricity requires 2.5 amps for 3 s through the brain followed by 2.5 to 3 amps for 14 s via neck and brisket electrodes to stop the heart.

The advantage of head-to-body stunning, in which the animal's heart is stopped, is that it is irreversible. It is not possible for the animal to regain consciousness. In head-only stunning, the animal will recover if it is not exsanguinated promptly. It is therefore essential to reduce the time between stunning and exsanguination to the minimum. Normally no more than 15 s should elapse before sticking.

Stunning with gases

Pigs may be stunned by exposure to carbon dioxide gas. A concentration of 80–90% by volume (in air) is used. Because carbon dioxide is heavier than air it can be contained within a pit and the animals lowered into it. There are various designs of apparatus. An example is shown in Fig. 4.3. Under normal conditions the pigs remain in the gas for about 90 s. Prolonging the exposure time kills many of the pigs, rather than just stunning them. Carbon dioxide is acidic (forming carbonic acid with water) so is rather pungent at concentrations greater

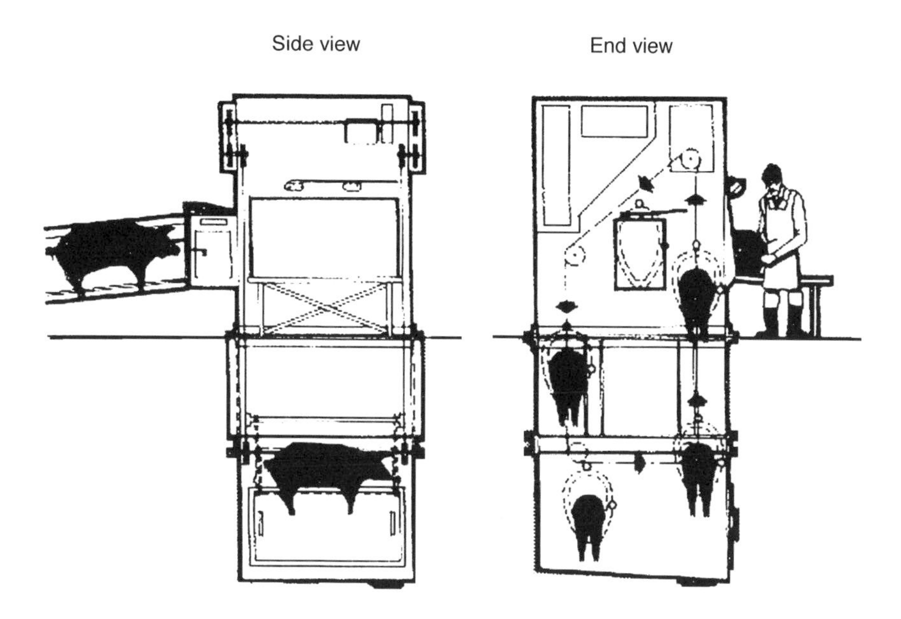

Fig. 4.3. Diagram of the Butina Compact carbon dioxide stunning system for pigs (reproduced from Grandin, 1980, with permission from the author).

than about 30%. Additionally the gas is a potent respiratory stimulant, causing gasping and possible respiratory distress. These characteristics make it aversive to animals and the induction phase of anaesthesia can be stressful. It is therefore important to ensure that the pigs are exposed rapidly to the highest concentrations of the gas very quickly after the initial exposure. Carbon dioxide works because the carbonic acid formed when it dissolves in the blood reduces the pH of the cerebrospinal fluid that surrounds the brain. The acidification disrupts brain function so the animal loses consciousness when the pH falls below about 7.1. The presence of even high concentrations of oxygen does not influence this effect.

Recently the use of stunning by anoxia has been investigated. In this, the stunning occurs through lack of oxygen. Unlike exposure to carbon dioxide, anoxia stunning appears to be completely stress-free. The anoxic conditions are produced by using the inert gas argon. The important thing is to reduce the oxygen concentration in the gas to 2% or less. Because it is tasteless and odourless argon is not detectable by animals and the gas's high density makes it relatively easy to confine in a chamber. Unfortunately, the duration of unconsciousness after removal from the gas is very short, unlike in carbon dioxide stunning. Consequently it is essential to kill the animals by prolonged exposure, rather than simply using the gas to stun. Adding 30% carbon dioxide to the argon (to produce a 70% argon:30% carbon dioxide mixture) has benefits which could outweigh the potential small perception of pungency which might occur at this concentration. The time to insensibility is reduced slightly so the stunning is faster, the anaesthetic properties of the carbon dioxide reduce the severity of the convulsions that occur during anoxia and the amount of argon used is reduced. Because argon is relatively expensive this reduces the cost of the process. So far, commercial use of anoxia stunning has focused on its advantages for slaughtering poultry. Being able to kill birds in their transport crates (see Chapter 7) eliminates the stress associated with manual removal and hanging on the shackles prior to electrical stunning (Mohan Raj, 1993, 1994b). Recently, however, trials have demonstrated the use of the technique for pigs (Mohan Raj, 1999).

Recognizing an effective stun

Effective percussion stunning leads to the animal immediately collapsing, stopping rhythmic breathing and becoming rigid with head extended. The position of the eyeball is fixed. This phase (the *tonic* phase) typically lasts 10–20 s and is followed by a period of involuntary kicking movements of its legs (the *clonic* phase). Gradually the animal relaxes. Electrical stunning causes a disruption of the normal electrical activity in the brain producing an epileptiform (electroplectic) fit. This is similar to the epileptic fit suffered by some unfortunate humans and, by analogy with their experience, the animal is completely unconscious at this time. During electrical stunning there is a large increase in the release of glutamate and aspartate in the sensory cortex of the brain (Cook, 1993; Cook *et al.*, 1995). These act as neurotransmitters, overexciting the neurones and producing the seizure. The epileptiform fit is characterized by an initial tonic phase when the animal becomes rigid and rhythmic breathing ceases with the eyeball fixed. The head is extended or raised and the hind legs flex under the body. After 15–20 s the clonic phase starts in which kicking or paddling movements occur. If the animal is not killed by exsanguination it will recover. Rhythmic breathing will return followed by the resumption of consciousness. The amount of clonic convulsions shown may be reduced by head-to-body stunning. The most reliable, and easiest to recognize, indication of all effective stunning in cattle, sheep and pigs is cessation of rhythmic breathing. However, this is not true for poultry where the brain stem, which controls breathing, recovers very quickly – long before the pain reflex returns and the bird starts to become aware of its surroundings and resumes consciousness.

Effects of stunning methods on carcass and meat quality

Correct percussion stunning tends to reduce the chances of carcass bruising and reduces the prevalence of 'blood splash'. Captive bolt stunning in pigs leads to a lot of convulsions and these tend to promote faster muscle acidification. This may result in PSE (pale, soft, exudative) meat. Similarly, very prolonged application of electrical stunning currents can stimulate the musculature and lead to faster acidification. Electrical stunning can sometimes cause problems of blood splash, haemorrhaging or broken bones, particularly in pigs when very high voltages are used, and if the animals are not suitably restrained and supported. This is because of the violent muscle contractions that sometimes result from passage of the current. In particular, broken backs, with associated haemorrhaging, can occur in pigs stunned using head-to-back electrode placement (Wotton *et al.*, 1992). The meat quality of pigs stunned with carbon dioxide gas is generally considered to be good.

Gas stunning of poultry has certain advantages over conventional electrical systems. These may promote the occurrence of haemorrhaging in the meat and bone breakages under certain conditions (Gregory and Wilkins, 1989a). Haemorrhages downgrade the value of the product and bone breakages may lead to bone fragments being left in filleted muscles. Both these problems are reduced in gas-stunned birds. Additionally, birds killed by anoxia show an increased rate of pH fall in the breast muscle (Mohan Raj, 1994a; Poole and Fletcher, 1995) enabling the carcasses to be held for a shorter time *post mortem* before portioning or filleting, without the danger of muscle shortening and so leading to tougher meat.

Slaughter

Pithing

This is the use in adult cattle of a long flexible rod (a pithing cane), made of plastic or stainless steel, to destroy the parts of the brain and spinal cord that control movement so that reflex muscular contractions do not occur subsequently. These could make dressing difficult and dangerous for the slaughtermen. The pithing cane is inserted into the hole made in the skull by the captive bolt pistol and pushed down the vertebral canal containing the spinal cord. In many modern systems pithing is no longer practised. A major concern is that there is a danger of introducing microbiological contamination into the inside of the vertebral column and thence to other parts of the carcass because the blood circulatory system is still intact. Shackling by the hind legs and hoisting the animal after stunning but before bleeding has reduced the dangers of involuntary carcass movements.

When slaughtering sheep the practice has sometimes been to sever the spinal cord where it enters the skull at the occipito-atlantal junction just after the blood vessels in the neck are cut. This procedure has the same effect as pithing cattle in preventing carcass movements, but it does not affect the sensibility of the animal if this has not been previously stunned. It is not a way of causing insensibility.

A very similar procedure still occasionally used for killing cattle, for example in some South American countries, employs a short-bladed, double-edged knife (a puntilla) which is used to sever the spinal cord by stabbing down dorsally through the neck and into the occipito-atlantal space. This process produces instant paralysis but does not cause unconsciousness and therefore cannot be considered humane.

Sticking

It is important to sever both carotid arteries and both jugular veins, or the blood vessels from which they arise nearer the heart. Chest sticking may have advantages in promoting faster exsanguination. Cutting only one carotid will prolong the time to death. On average, brain death occurs between about 15 and 20 s after correct sticking. By this time around 50% of the total blood which will be lost through exsanguination has been removed (Fig. 4.4). The pattern of blood loss is strikingly similar in the different species implying a common mechanism of loss. Only about 40–60% of the animals' total blood is lost at exsanguination, a weight of blood equivalent to about 4–5% of their live weight. The remaining blood is probably largely retained in the viscera rather than the carcass. A beating heart is not necessary for effective exsanguination and stunning methods that cause cardiac arrest do not affect the amount of blood retained in the meat. The residual blood content of lean meat is between 2 and 9 ml kg^{-1} muscle. There is no evidence that this volume is influenced by different slaughter methods, or that large amounts of residual blood affect the keeping quality of meat. However, different stunning methods, and whether the animal is stuck while lying prone or hanging from a shackle, can slightly affect the volume of blood lost.

So-called back bleeding can occur with poor sticking technique in pigs. Pigs are stuck by inserting the knife at an angle of 45° and about 5 cm anterior to the breastbone (sternum) in the midline. This severs the main arteries and veins entering the heart. In back bleeding the knife is pushed too far forwards into the chest cavity and punctures the pleural membrane lining the thorax. This allows blood to bleed back into the thorax. The blood stains the walls of the rib cage and may form clots.

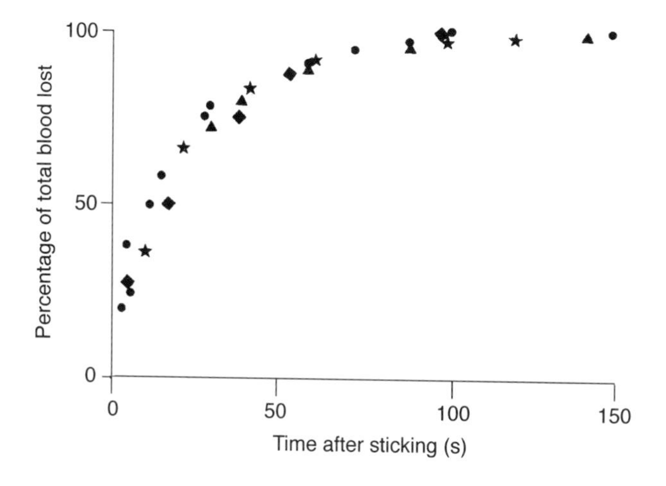

Fig. 4.4. Rate of loss of blood at exsanguination. Modified from Warriss (1984a) (● pigs: Warriss and Wotton, 1981; Swatland, 1983; ▲ calves: Cooper and Morris, 1978; ♦ lambs: Blackmore and Newhook, 1976; ★ broiler chickens).

Sometimes pig and cattle blood is collected for human consumption (for example to make blood sausage). A hollow knife is used. It is connected to a tank kept under a partial vacuum and an anticoagulant like sodium citrate may be used to prevent the blood clotting. Alternatively the blood may be stirred to collect the fibrin and maintain the major part liquid. Obviously it is important to prevent contamination of the blood and to ensure that it comes only from healthy animals.

Religious slaughter

The main religious slaughter methods are *shechita*, used by Jews, the slaughter method used by Muslims to produce *halal* meat, and *jatka* used by Sikhs. In shechita and jatka the animal is not stunned prior to killing it by exsanguination. In general, the religious slaughter methods used to produce halal meat do not use prior stunning, although some forms of stunning may in fact be acceptable to some adherents of the Islamic faith. In shechita and halal slaughter the major vessels of the throat are severed by a transverse cut and in jatka the animal is decapitated with a single stroke using a sword. Legislation in many European countries requires that animals are stunned before exsanguination, but there are usually exemptions for those slaughtered by shechita and halal methods. Neither Jews nor Muslims consume pork so the methods can apply to cattle, sheep, goats and poultry.

Small animals can be restrained manually, for example sheep may be placed on their backs on a cradle, but larger cattle must be held in a special pen. The Cincinnati pen designed for Jewish slaughter employs a chin lift device to extend the neck of the animal while in a normal standing position.

In many western cultures preslaughter stunning is considered important for welfare reasons and there is thus some debate about the ethics of religious slaughter. Useful descriptions of the procedures and equipment used in religious slaughter, together with discussions of the ethical questions associated with the practices, have been given by Anil and Sheard (1994) and Grandin and Regenstein (1994). In regard to animal welfare, three important questions were raised. Was the preslaughter handling and restraint unduly stressful, was the incision used to cut the throat painful, and was insensibility or unconsciousness achieved soon enough after the incision? These are complex questions for which we probably do not yet have universally definitive answers.

The slaughtering industry in the UK

In common with the situation in many developed countries there has been a gradual reduction in the number of red meat slaughter plants in the UK (Table 4.2). This trend is driven by the economies of scale, particularly in regard to the costs of more stringent hygiene requirements now imposed on slaughter plants. These requirements particularly apply in export plants. In 1995 in the UK, over 70% of animals of all red meat species were killed in plants approved by the European Union for the export of meat although these formed a minority of the total number of abattoirs killing each species (Table 4.3).

Some slaughter plants still process all three red meat species at the same site but this is becoming uncommon. About two-thirds of all pigs are killed at specialist pig abattoirs which process no other species and, traditionally, bacon producers killed all their own pigs for curing.

Table 4.2. The progressive reduction in the number of UK slaughter plants killing the different red meat species.

	Cattle	Sheep	Pigs
1981	965	989	808
1985	904	926	770
1990	698	717	578
1993	583	600	457
1995	436	452	334

Table 4.3. The numbers of slaughterplants killing cattle, sheep and pigs in the UK in 1995 (source: MLC, 1997).

	Cattle	Sheep	Pigs
Number of plants	436	452	334
Number of EU-approved plants	78	80	68
Number of animals slaughtered (millions)	3.3	19.3	14.4
% of total kill slaughtered in EU-approved plants	70.3	71.8	74.8

An average beef plant in the UK might kill 25,000 cattle, a pig plant 250,000 animals and a sheep plant 150,000–200,000 lambs a year. The largest specialist operations could have throughputs of 100,000 cattle or 500,000 pigs per year but these are still small in comparison with operations in, for example, North America.

Carcass Dressing, Post-mortem Inspection and Butchery

Carcass dressing

In a healthy animal the carcass tissues and the insides of the body cavities are effectively microbiologically sterile. In contrast, the skin of the animal, its body orifices and the inside of the gut are contaminated with soil, dirt and bacteria. The object of dressing the carcass is to remove the skin, together with the associated hair or feathers, and the gut, and the other non-edible parts of the body, in such a way as to prevent, or reduce to the minimum, contact of the carcass with this dirt. The ideal is to prevent microbiological contamination, so reducing the risks from pathogens and prolonging potential shelf life of the meat.

In modern slaughtering systems this has led to the dressing being carried out with the animal hanging by its hind legs from an overhead rail system from the time it has been exsanguinated. The change from traditional dressing on the floor, or on a cradle, to overhead rail systems with the carcasses suspended off the floor was an enormous advance in terms of both hygiene and throughput. Traditionally, one or several men would process a single animal at a time, carrying out all the procedures to produce the dressed carcass. Nowadays, the system operates as a production line with each man carrying out a single job. As well as being more efficient, this helps maintain carcass hygiene because, for example, the men removing the skin will not touch the insides of the carcass. All equipment and tools will also be restricted to use for one particular purpose and therefore will also not be a potential cause of cross contamination. Despite this, there is still apparently enormous potential for contamination of the carcass by organisms originally present on the hide or fleece of the animal. This has been elegantly demonstrated by the employment of 'marker' organisms, which are used deliberately to contaminate a site on the animal before the start of dressing. Subsequently the organism is looked for at other sites to define the degree of cross contamination. An example of the use of the technique was described by Hudson *et al.* (1998) who used a non-pathogenic strain of *Escherichia coli* K12 that was resistant to nalidixic acid. By incorporating nalidixic acid into the growth medium used to culture the swab samples, the naturally occurring strains of *E. coli* were eliminated allowing accurate detection of the marker strain.

The dressing of the carcass differs in detail for the different species and only the briefest general outline can be given here. Further information can be found in textbooks of meat inspection, for example Wilson (1998). In cattle and sheep the oesophagus is sometimes tied or closed with a clip to prevent backflow of the rumen contents (in cattle this is referred to as weasand tying). In these species, the head and feet are removed and the carcass is skinned. The head is normally removed at the occipito-atlantal joint and the feet below the carpals (knee bones) in the foreleg and tarsals in the hind leg. The feet thus include the cannon bones. Because of the dangers of contamination of the surface of the carcass with soil and dirt from the hide or pelt, skinning requires considerable care and skill. After the initial cuts with a knife, mechanical hide-pullers may be used to pull the hide or pelt from the carcass. As well as the benefits of ease and efficiency these are likely to improve hygiene by requiring less handling of the carcass.

Pigs are generally not skinned (except for making pigskin leather) but the hair is removed by scraping. This is facilitated by immersing the pig, after completion of bleeding, in a tank of water at 60°C for about 5 min (scalding). The hot water loosens the hairs and the outer layer of skin, which can then be scraped off, nowadays by passing the carcass between revolving metal-tipped paddles. The carcasses are washed and cleaned with revolving brushes and the toenails removed. Before washing the carcass may be singed. In this process the carcass passes through a gas flame which burns off any remaining hair and tightens up the skin. Both scalding and singeing to some degree kill bacteria on the surface of the body but this is not sterilized. The scalding tank tends to accumulate large quantities of dirt and bacteria. Vertical scalding, in which condensed steam is passed over the hanging carcasses, is sometimes used and may produce bacteriologically cleaner carcasses. The feet are left on pig carcasses and the head is only removed at a much later stage.

Before evisceration, the skinned or dehaired carcass is removed from the shackles that have up to now suspended it from the overhead rail if this has not been done previously. It is resuspended from the achilles tendons of the hind legs using a gambrel. To eviscerate the animal a cut is made around the anus allowing the rectum and the rest of the gut to be removed from the abdominal cavity through a ventral incision along the whole length of the carcass. This cut continues through the breastbone (sternum), allowing access to the thoracic cavity, to the throat. The sternum in mature cattle often needs sawing through (brisket sawing). The diaphragm is cut round and the trachea (windpipe), lungs, oesophagus (gullet), heart and liver are removed together as the 'pluck'.

The carcass is often then split into the two sides by sawing down the backbone. After trimming, and sometimes removal of kidneys and other parts, the carcass is inspected, further trimmed and placed in a chiller to cool. Immediately before chilling the carcass may be washed, weighed and graded. In North America, beef carcasses can be 'shrouded' prior to chilling. The sides are covered in a tightly applied cloth shroud wetted with salt solution. This improves the surface appearance of the carcass, especially that of the fat, and reduces evaporative weight loss. The shrouds are removed after the initial period in chill.

The trend in modern slaughtering practice is for more operations to be carried out by machine. This especially applies to hide and pelt removal but it seems likely that mechanical evisceration will be developed for red meat species as it has already for poultry. Particularly in countries such as Australia and New Zealand, there are increasing degrees of mechanization being developed in the dressing and automated boning of sheep and beef carcasses (Longdell, 1996). As well as reducing manpower requirements mechanization can improve carcass hygiene through reducing contamination, produce better hide and pelt quality, and give higher yields of retail joints when compared with manual methods.

Poultry processing

After stunning, poultry have the blood vessels in the neck severed to exsanguinate them. Usually this is carried out automatically with a knife with a rotating blade. A ventral neck cut should be used. In practice, many processors may use a dorsal cut to prevent severance of the oesophagus and trachea. This facilitates their removal from the neck flap when the carcass is eviscerated. Using a dorsal cut may only sever the blood vessels of one side and lead to slower bleedout. Because birds' brains are rather resistant to anoxia this will prolong the time to brain death unless, as often happens, the birds are killed by the stunning current passing through their heart.

To remove the feathers the birds are scalded, usually at a fairly low temperature (less than 55°C for broilers) for about 30 s. The hot water softens the skin so that the feathers are easily pulled out. Use of higher temperatures damages the skin and downgrades the appearance of the carcasses. Plucking is by rubber-fingered rotating cylinders. Geese and ducks are often dipped in molten wax, which is then cooled to harden it. The solid wax, together with the feathers, is then pulled off. The valuable soft down on the underside of the breast is removed before waxing to use as insulation for quilts.

Evisceration is physically separated from the defeathering process to reduce carcass contamination. The skin along the back of the neck is cut and the trachea and crop freed. The abdominal cavity is opened up by an incision around the vent (cloaca) to enable the viscera to be pulled out. These include the intestines, gizzard, liver and heart and reproductive system. The lungs lie tight under the vertebral column and need careful removal. The head, neck and feet are cut off and discarded, and the carcass is chilled either in cold air or in iced water. Water chilling tends to be used in North America and air chilling in Europe. The giblets, comprising the neck, liver, heart and gizzard, are sold with the carcass, usually packed inside it. The term 'New York-dressed' poultry refers to carcasses which are not eviscerated directly after plucking but are held refrigerated in an entire state until retailed. Although traditionally popular, this is unusual nowadays.

Poultry processing is now highly mechanized with most, if not all, operations carried out by machine. This includes evisceration. A potential problem is that any microbial contamination of the carcass, for example by accidental breakage of the gut, is likely to be spread to large numbers of other carcasses by the processing machinery.

Carcass washing

After the completion of dressing, carcasses are washed with a fine spray of water to remove surface blood, bone dust and any visible soiling. Unless prolonged, washing with cold water has little effect on bacterial numbers recovered from the carcass surface. Effectiveness may be increased by using hot (80°C) water or by including low concentrations of organic acids, chlorine or other agents in the water (see Chapter 9). The traditional practice of wiping carcasses with cloths is now considered unhygienic and is banned in some countries.

Post-mortem inspection

The carcass and viscera are inspected as soon as possible after slaughter. As in ante-mortem inspection, this is to identify abnormalities or disease that would make the meat and edible offal unfit for human consumption. To this end it is important that the carcass retains its identity with the parts and viscera removed from it. In modern systems this is often achieved by synchronized parallel line systems. Inspection is normally carried out by specially licensed veterinarians or meat inspectors. As well as inspection, they will often have other roles, including overseeing animal welfare and hygiene standards.

Tissues and organs are examined by visual inspection, palpation and incision. Considerable attention is paid to routine incision of lymph nodes to detect disease states. In infection, bacteria collect in the lymphatic system and are concentrated and destroyed in the lymph nodes. These occur at intervals throughout the system. In disease they become swollen and abnormal in colour, so alerting the inspector to look for the disease. Conditions such as pneumonia and tuberculosis have characteristic lesions. Parasitic diseases such as those caused by tapeworms (cestodes) are often manifested in cysts of the larval forms in the heart, liver and muscles. For example, *Cysticercus bovis* is the encysted intermediate stage of the beef tapeworm *Taenia saginata* that lives in the small intestine of man (see Chapter 9). 'Measly' beef and 'measly' pork were previously referred to in cases where there had been extensive infection with *C. bovis* and the pork tapeworm *Cysticercus cellulosae* respectively. Mature liver flukes (*Fasciola hepatica*), which are trematodes, can occur in the bile ducts of the liver of infected cattle, sheep, goats and pigs. The larval stage of the roundworm (Nematoda) *Trichinella spiralis* forms cysts in pork muscle, which, if eaten by man, can cause trichinosis (trichiniasis) if the meat has been undercooked. The larvae of the nematode parasite of pigs, *Ascaris suum*, may lodge in the liver and result in small foci of connective tissue giving rise to a condition known as milk spot liver. The adult worms live in the pig's small intestine.

Inflammation of the lining of the thoracic cavity (the pleura) or the lining of the abdominal cavity (the peritoneum) may indicate infection. Swine erysipelas, a bacterial disease caused by *Erysipelothrix rhusiopathiae*, produces characteristic, red, diamond-shaped marks on the skin of infected pigs. Abscesses, arthritic joint capsules and bruises may make meat unfit for human consumption. In the UK, The Fresh Meat (Hygiene and Inspection) Regulations 1995 list 46 specific conditions which, if found, render the whole carcass, offal and blood unfit for human consumption. Various findings may require condemnation as unfit of parts of the carcass and, if necessary, trimming of tissue. Details of meat inspection procedures can be found in standard textbooks (Gracey and Collins, 1992; Bremner and Johnston, 1996). In modern production systems the emphasis is on presenting only healthy animals for slaughter, controlling the levels of parasites and of infectious diseases largely by measures taken at the farm.

Carcass butchery

Carcasses are sold whole, or as sides, or may be cut into smaller 'primal' or 'retail' joints. The exact way a carcass is butchered into joints varies between countries, within countries and depending on the particular use that may be made of the meat. Three ways of dividing up a side of beef into primal joints are shown in Fig. 4.5. These illustrate the variation between countries. In particular, in the French system, the carcass is cut into many more joints. This reflects the way retail joints in France are often based on individual, or small groups of adjacent muscles, dissected from others along the natural lines of separation between muscles. This allows inherent differences in the quality characteristics of different muscles, particularly tenderness, to be best exploited. In the systems used in the UK and USA, the differences in inherent quality are still recognized. For example the high value cuts of the loin and hindquarter (sirloin, rump, topside and silverside) are distinguished from lower value cuts such as those of the shoulder, brisket and flank, but the differentiation is less detailed. In the UK and USA, retail joints tend to be cut with less regard for differences between individual muscles, the cutting lines being across muscles rather than between them.

The smaller carcasses from pigs and lambs are cut into fewer primal joints. In the pig, after removal of distal ends of the legs, the carcass is cut into four main primal joints, the loin, belly, hind leg or ham, and the foreleg/shoulder. In North America the foreleg/shoulder is cut into the 'butt' and the 'picnic'. An excellent account of the different cutting systems is given in Swatland (1994).

The Operation of Abattoirs

Abattoir design

Traditionally, abattoirs would often kill all red meat species. This is uncommon nowadays and specialized plants are more usual. Where cattle, sheep and pigs are killed at the same site, it is also usual to have separate lines and, especially for pigs, separate buildings. The majority of pigs are killed in specialized bacon factories or pork plants that also process the carcasses into cured and other processed products. The production of meat in a suitable form for retail sale, especially for supermarkets, and including packaging and value added products, is increasingly common in all slaughtering operations. Poultry processing plants are usually run as separate operations from red meat plants. A good description of the details of operation of slaughter plants is given in Gracey (1998).

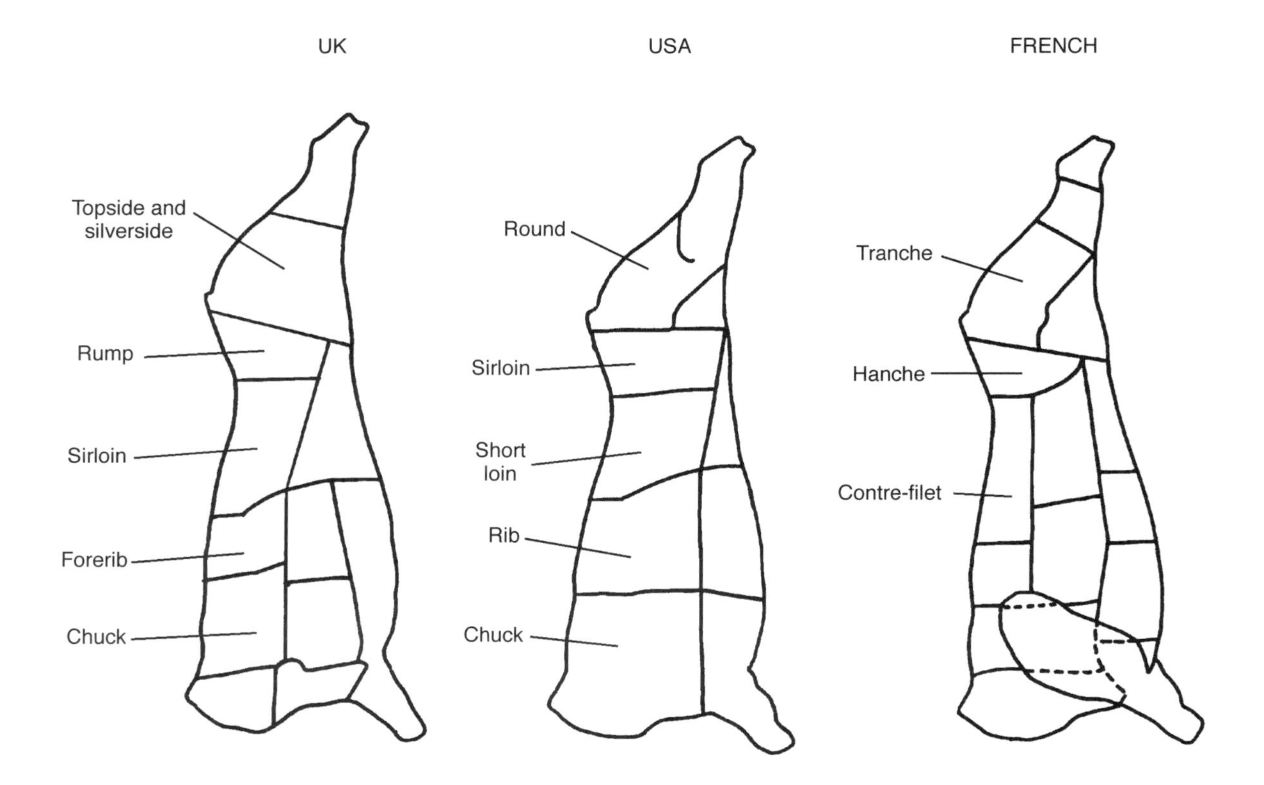

Fig. 4.5. Three methods of butchery of a side of beef into primal joints (based on information in Strother, 1975).

A major factor governing the design of modern slaughterplants is hygiene. The hygienic and other requirements are often laid down in legislation. In the UK, the requirements for the construction, layout and equipment of slaugherplants, meat cutting premises and cold stores are specified in The Fresh Meat (Hygiene and Inspection) Regulations 1995. These regulations also require the licensing of premises and give responsibility for ensuring compliance with hygiene, and animal and meat inspection requirements, to Official Veterinary Surgeons (OVSs) appointed by Central Government.

To maintain hygiene there must be clear separation of inherently dirty and clean areas, and the personnel who work in them. Therefore, the lairage and area up to the point of completion of bleeding is separated from subsequent areas to segregate live animals from carcasses and reduce to a minimum the chances of contamination of the clean areas. For the same reason, the entry of vermin, birds and insects, especially flies, must be prevented. Parts of the animal that are likely to be dirty, or potential sources of contamination, such as hides, skins, pelts, feet and guts need to be removed from the carcass dressing area as directly and quickly as possible. In poultry plants, stunning and bleeding, and scalding and plucking, should be carried out in separate rooms. Similarly, the evisceration of poultry must be in a separate room or at least in an area widely separated from other areas and partitioned off from them.

The lairage must be large enough to enable a sufficient reservoir of animals to be held while allowing a long enough resting period to recover from their journey from the farm or market. It must be provided with facilities for watering, and if necessary, feeding animals, and a pen with separate drainage to hold diseased or injured animals isolated from other stock. There need to be effective removal and disposal systems for the manure from the lairage.

The guts must be cleaned of their contents in rooms set aside for that purpose. There need to be rooms for the storage of hides and pelts, horns, hooves, fat and other waste material, and rooms for the preparation and cleaning of offal. Hygienic facilities for the disposal of solid and liquid waste, and an adequate drainage system, are required.

Construction of the building must be appropriate. Floors need to be impermeable and non-slip, yet easily cleaned, walls impermeable and washable. All surfaces need to be impervious and easily cleanable with no areas that can retain dirt. Joints between walls and floors should ideally be rounded to facilitate cleaning. Equipment and fittings should be of durable, impermeable and corrosion-resistant materials such as stainless or galvanized steel or plastic. Wood is not acceptable.

Ventilation is important to provide good working conditions, prevent condensation and reduce the risks of contamination by aerosols. Even lighting with a minimum brightness of 220 lux in working areas, and 540 lux where meat inspection is carried out, is required. It is important that the light does not distort normal colours.

There must be adequate lavatories and washing facilities for personal hygiene, adequate supplies of clean, wholesome (potable) hot and cold running water and cleaning facilities. There must be adequate facilities for disinfection of knives, tools and other equipment, and the cleaning and disinfection of vehicles delivering animals or transporting meat. People working in meat plants must not be suffering from any diseases that could be transmitted to others via the meat or equipment they handle, or have open (undressed) cuts or abrasions. They must wear protective clothing and footwear, cover hair and beards, and maintain personal cleanliness. Activities such as eating and smoking are unacceptable.

Sufficient and adequate refrigeration facilities must be available. Within the EU, a Directive (64/433 EEC) specifies that all fresh meat that will be traded within the Union must be chilled immediately and kept at a temperature of +7°C or less for carcasses and cuts, and +3°C for offal. Frozen fresh meat must be maintained at −12°C or less.

Cleaning and disinfection

Plant and equipment hygiene is essential to the production of meat that is safe to eat. Two processes are necessary to achieve this. *Cleaning* removes dirt that could harbour or support the growth of micro-organisms. *Disinfection* kills remaining microbes, or at least reduces their numbers to safe levels. It may not kill bacterial spores, however. Cleaning obviously has other benefits in improving the working environment and reducing the chances of contamination of carcasses and meat with other foreign matter. The cleaning process usually involves a combination of physical and chemical removal of dirt. It is therefore facilitated by scrubbing and hosing with water, often hot water and with the addition of detergents and other cleaning agents.

Although their main action is to remove fat and protein deposits (organic dirt) detergents also need to be effective against non-organic material, such as the scale formed from hard water, since in practice dirt is usually a combination of organic and non-organic components. Important characteristics of detergents are surfactancy, or wetting power, dispersion and suspension. These characteristics enable the detergent to cover and penetrate the dirt, to break it up into small particles and to float these particles away from the surface. Alkaline detergents are very effective against organic dirt. They include caustic soda (sodium hydroxide), which is rather corrosive, and washing soda (sodium carbonate), which is less so. Acid detergents usually contain phosphoric acid and are particularly effective against non-organic dirt.

The most commonly used surfactants, or wetting agents, are anionic – forming a negatively charged active ion in solution. They are sometimes mixed with non-ionic surfactants to improve the cleaning qualities in commercially available detergents. When used with hard water (containing high levels of dissolved calcium and magnesium salts), anionic surfactants can form a scum. To prevent this, chelating agents such as EDTA (ethylene diamine tetra-acetic acid), or amino carboxylic acids, are added. These sequester, or 'lock up', the calcium and magnesium ions so preventing scum formation.

The commonest disinfectants (sanitizers) are based on compounds that release chlorine such as hypochlorous acid (HOCl) or sodium hypochlorite (NaOCl). Chlorine has strong oxidizing properties that kill bacteria. Advantages are its effectiveness against most microbes, its cheapness and its being unaffected by hard water. A slight disadvantage of chlorine is that it is quite corrosive to metal. Quarternary ammonium compounds are much less corrosive but cannot be mixed with anionic detergents and are more expensive than chlorine-based disinfectants. Neither are they as effective as chlorine against Gram-negative bacteria (see Chapter 9). They are, however, odour and taint free. A number of other types of disinfectant are available, often for specialist purposes.

Some cleansing systems are now based on foams. The foam sticks to surfaces and so increases the contact time, and therefore the effectiveness, of the system. Obviously, cleaners and disinfectants used in abattoirs must be non-toxic, must not lead to taints and should be as non-corrosive as possible. Also, after cleaning and disinfection it is important that all traces of the chemicals used are thoroughly rinsed away so no residues remain. It is important to clean plant and equipment throughout the daily operation as well as thoroughly at the end of the day. This can be done during, for example, refreshment and meal breaks so that normal operations are not disrupted.

By-products

In the early days of the meat packing industry in North America the offal, heads, guts and other parts removed from the dressed carcass were considered as waste products and thrown away. In Chicago in the early 1800s they were thrown into the local river until the smell became so bad that the city council forbade the practice. The material was then buried to dispose of it, or later, fed back to pigs. By the 1850s the value of the material previously considered waste was realized and plants would slaughter pigs for no charge except the right to keep the fat associated with the entrails and the bristles. Even now, the profitability of the slaughtering industry largely depends on the value of the by-products – the so-called 'fifth quarter' of the carcass.

By-products fall into four main categories. The most valuable are the edible by-products. These consist of livers, hearts, tongues, kidneys, spleens (melts), brains, blood, edible raw fat, pigs' feet and cattle diaphragms (skirts) and various parts of the stomach and intestines. The rumens and reticula of cattle, and sheeps' rumens, produce edible tripe, the intestines of pigs, chitterlings, and the small intestines of cattle, sheep and pigs various types of sausage casings. In North America, offals such as liver, hearts, kidneys, tripe and tongues are referred to as 'variety meats'. Gelatin is extracted from pig snouts and skin.

Cattle hides and pig skins go for the manufacture of leather. Sheep skins, known as pelts, are made into rugs, chamois leather and clothing. Various organs and glands are used to produce pharmaceutical products. Heparin, used to prevent blood clotting, is extracted from lungs; insulin, for the treatment of diabetes, is extracted from the pancreases of pigs and cattle. Cattle pituitary, thymus and thyroid glands are also valuable in this regard. Rennet, used for curdling the milk in cheese making, is extracted from calves' stomachs.

Edible bone, stomachs, lungs and spleens that are unsuitable for human consumption, are used for the manufacture of pet food, and blood, inedible fat and condemned carcasses and offal are processed into feed for livestock.

One of the most important factors determining the value of by-products is how well they are handled. Most are prone to rapid deterioration if not handled carefully and this leads to downgrading. A critical part of the handling is storage at low enough temperatures. Fats in particular are prone to oxidation and the development of rancidity.

Rendering

Waste tissues, including bones, meat and offal unfit for human or direct animal consumption, are disposed of by rendering. The material is cooked for an hour or longer with the aid of steam, sometimes under pressure, either in batch or continuous processes so that the fat melts and can be run off, and the remaining material breaks down. This produces tallow and, after the water has been boiled off, a residue known as greaves. The dried greaves are ground to produce meat and bone meal, which can be incorporated into animal feed as a protein source. The high temperature during cooking sterilizes the material.

The greaves will contain 10% or more fat. In some rendering processes they are further extracted with organic solvents. This increases the yield of tallow and reduces the fat content of the meat and bone meal. Hyperbaric rendering involves pressure-cooking the materials. Using pressures of 2–3 atm enables temperatures of between

120 and 130°C to be attained. The breakdown of the material is more effective and it is likely that all but the most resistant infective agents, such as those causing transmissable spongiform encephalopathies like BSE (Taylor *et al.*, 1998), are destroyed.

Abattoir effluent

Very large quantities of water are used in the operation of slaughter plants. This is mainly used for cleaning and becomes very dirty with a high load of organic matter. This dirtiness is measured as its biological oxygen demand (BOD). The BOD is the amount of oxygen required to oxidize, and therefore break down, the organic matter completely in a certain time and at a certain temperature. Abattoir effluent may have a BOD five or six times that of normal domestic sewage and is therefore expensive to purify and has a high potential for polluting water-courses. Normally the effluent is given an initial cleaning treatment before it leaves the plant. Solids are screened out and fat particles removed by air flotation. Bacteria are then encouraged to break down remaining material, either anaerobically or aerobically, while it is held in tanks or ponds.

Chapter 5

Post-mortem Changes in Muscle and its Conversion into Meat

A period of time normally elapses between the slaughter of an animal and consumption of the meat. In practical terms, the carcass cools down and becomes stiffer or 'sets', the surface dries and the fat becomes firmer. With time, the texture and flavour of the lean improve. These effects are accompanied by significant biochemical changes in the muscles: acidification, the development of rigor mortis and, later, the gradual resolution of rigor and tenderization of the meat by a process referred to as conditioning.

Muscle Metabolism in the Living Animal

Energy metabolism in muscles

The major function of muscles is to contract and, as we have seen, the energy for contraction, and also for maintaining the functional integrity of the muscle, comes in the form of the purine nucleotide, adenosine triphosphate (ATP). A major role of the enzyme systems in the sarcoplasm and mitochondria is to ensure an adequate supply of ATP to the contractile elements. ATP is also needed to fuel the calcium pump of the sarcoplasmic reticulum. In living muscles the fuels for producing this ATP are either free fatty acids or glucose from the blood, or glycogen which is stored directly within the muscle fibres. In the fed animal the circulating levels of free fatty acids are low and glucose is mostly used. In the fasting state, free fatty acids derived from the breakdown of triglyceride stores in the fat depots of the body are metabolized. Glycogen is mobilized only when the rates of breakdown of fatty acids and glucose cannot provide energy at a sufficient rate to meet the demands of contracting muscle. Glycogen is then used to supplement the blood-borne metabolites.

Glycogen and glucose are broken down essentially by the same process. This involves the operation of three interrelated processes: glycolysis, oxidative decarboxylation and oxidative phosphorylation. These together lead to the complete oxidation of one molecule of glucose ($C_6H_{12}O_6$) by six molecules of oxygen to six molecules of carbon dioxide (CO_2) and six molecules of water (H_2O). Overall, the reaction can be described as:

$$C_6H_{12}O_6 + 6\ O_2 \rightarrow 6\ CO_2 + 6\ H_2O.$$

In practice the whole process is extremely complex but only an understanding of the outline of the system is necessary for our current purposes. In glycolysis, a glucose molecule (or a glucose moiety from glycogen) containing six carbon atoms is broken down into two pyruvate molecules each containing three carbon atoms. The process generates either two or three ATP molecules and four hydrogen atoms carried as reduced nicotine adenine dinucleotide (NADH). The net yield of ATP differs between glucose and glycogen because the start of the glycolytic pathway requires that the hexose be phosphorylated. An ATP molecule is required to do this for glucose (the reaction is *endergonic*) but the phosphorylation of glycogen is *exergonic* and consequently an extra ATP is produced. The full pathway of glycolysis is shown in Fig. 5.1. In decarboxylation, the carbon atoms in the pyruvate are removed as carbon dioxide, in the process generating 20 hydrogens carried as NADH and on other carrier molecules (flavin adenine dinucleotide, FAD). This process operates as a cycle, known as the Krebs or tricarboxylic acid (TCA) cycle, the pyruvate first being converted to acetyl coenzyme A. It is at this point that fatty acids would enter the system, being first converted by β-oxidation to acetyl coenzyme A. The last process is oxidative phosphorylation. In this, the 24 hydrogens generated by glycolysis and oxidative decarboxylation are oxidized by molecular oxygen in the cytochrome system. For each pair of hydrogens, three ATP molecules are produced. Therefore, in total, breakdown of one glucose molecule produces a further 36 ATP in addition to those produced by glycolysis. A summary of the three processes involved in the production of ATP is given in Table 5.1.

Glycolysis takes place in the sarcoplasm; the enzymes which catalyse the other processes are located in the mitochondria. Operation of the whole system requires aerobic conditions – six oxygen molecules are needed to oxidize each glucose molecule. Under anaerobic conditions only the glycolytic part of the system can operate. Normally this only occurs during very heavy exercise. Under these conditions, the pyruvate is reduced by the accumulated NADH to form lactic acid, the reaction being catalysed by the enzyme lactate dehydrogenase. This

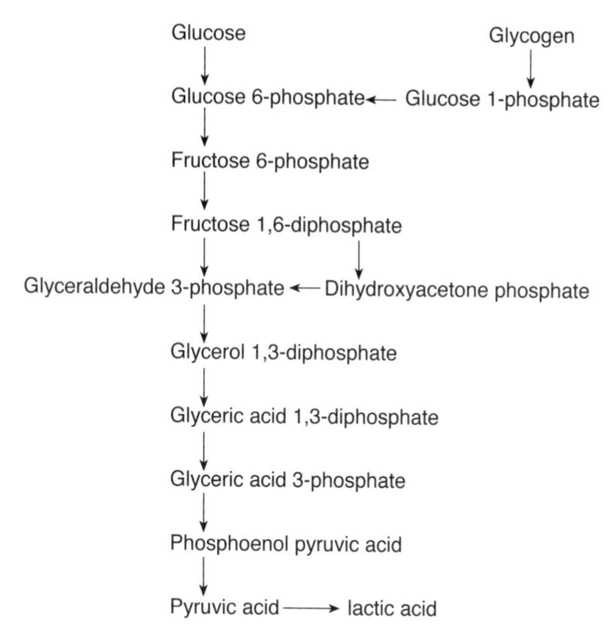

Fig. 5.1. The glycolytic pathway.

is what happens in a runner in a 100 m sprint race where the energy required by the leg muscles could not be produced oxidatively because of the inability of the blood to deliver sufficient oxygen to the muscles quickly enough. Instead, for every glycogen moiety, equivalent to a glucose molecule, two lactic acid molecules are produced:

$$\underset{\text{glycogen}}{(C_6H_{10}O_5)_n} + n\,H_2O \rightarrow \underset{\text{lactic acid}}{2n\,C_3H_6O_3}.$$

This level of muscular activity could not be sustained for very long because the build-up of lactic acid in the blood would lower its pH to an unacceptable level.

Mobilization of glycogen when it is needed

It is important that muscle glycogen can be broken down to release energy for contraction very quickly if, for example, the animal needs to

Table 5.1. The production of ATP from the oxidation of glucose.

1.	Glycolysis:	1 glucose	$\rightarrow$ 2 ATP + 4 H + 2 pyruvate
2.	Oxidative decarboxylation:	2 pyruvate	$\rightarrow$ 20 H + 6 CO_2
3.	Oxidative phosphorylation:	24 H + 6 O_2	$\rightarrow$ 36 ATP + 6 H_2O

run away from a threat like a predator. The hormone adrenaline (epinephrine), secreted in response to an external stressor (e.g. fear) promotes glycogen breakdown (glycogenolysis) through a series of steps which result in activation of the enzyme catalysing the first stage in glycogenolysis. This enzyme is phosphorylase. It catalyses the breakdown of glycogen to glucose-1-phosphate and is present in large amounts in muscle. It exists in two forms, an active form (phosphorylase a) and an inactive form (phosphorylase b). Conversion of phosphorylase b to phosphorylase a is by the enzyme protein kinase. Protein kinase is itself activated by cyclic adenosine monophosphate (cyclic AMP), produced when adenylate cyclase is converted into an active form by adrenaline. The overall chain of events leading to glycogen breakdown is therefore as summarized in Fig. 5.2.

Therefore, whenever glycogen is likely to be needed rapidly for energy production by glycolysis it is mobilized through the activation of phosphorylase and this can be through the secretion of adrenaline during a stressful episode. In non-stressful situations, phosphorylase b is activated by other mechanisms. These include increased concentrations of metabolites such as AMP and inorganic phosphate, and a decreased concentration of ATP. During normal muscle stimulation by the nervous system, calcium ions also promote the activation of phosphorylase.

Energy storage

ATP stores energy as an energy-rich phosphate bond. The energy is liberated by releasing the phosphate to give adenosine diphosphate

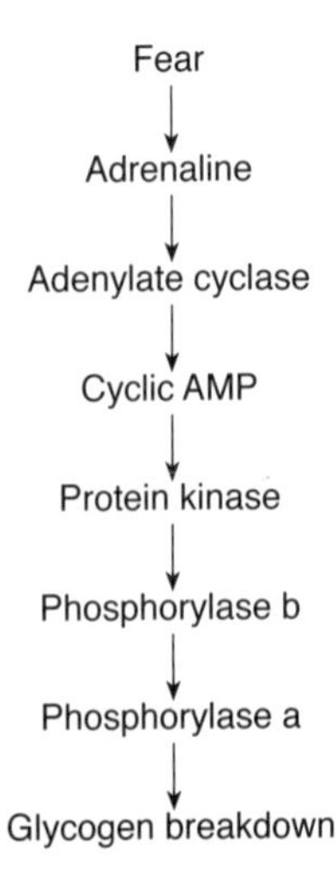

Fig. 5.2. The promotion of glycogen breakdown by adrenaline.

(ADP). As mentioned in Chapter 3, the reaction is in effect a hydrolysis and is reversible:

$$ATP + H_2O \rightleftharpoons ADP + H_3PO_4.$$

This is a simplified outline of the reaction. For example, ATP is actually complexed to magnesium ions. ADP can itself be hydrolysed to adenosine monophosphate (AMP). Perhaps surprisingly, bearing in mind its pivotal role in the operation of muscles, the concentration of ATP in the tissue is very low – only enough for a few brief 'twitches' or contractions. A typical concentration would be 5–7 mmol kg^{-1} of muscle and this would support contraction for only a few seconds at most. However, the concentration is maintained effectively constant by the reaction:

$$CP + ADP \rightleftharpoons C + ATP.$$

In this, creatine phosphate, or phosphocreatine (CP), reacts with ADP to form ATP and creatine (C). The reaction is reversible but the equilibrium is to the right at neutral pH so that, immediately ATP is removed, more is generated so long as CP is available. The reaction is catalysed by the enzyme creatine kinase (CK) which is abundant and active in muscle. Therefore, the ATP used in contraction is restored almost instantly. The levels of CP in muscle are much higher than those of ATP (Jeacocke, 1984), although they can drop during exhaustive exercise. They are replenished by a 'reversal' of the above reaction during a recovery period when ATP is generated from muscle glycogen, or from blood-borne metabolites, and the ATP:ADP ratio rises. The levels of glycogen in most muscles (10–20 mg g^{-1}) are sufficient for many thousands of 'twitches'. A full account of the biochemistry of energy production in muscles can be found in Newsholme and Start (1973).

Post-mortem Acidification and Rigor Development

Acidification of the muscles after the animal is killed

At the death of the animal the supply of oxygen (and glucose and free fatty acids) to the muscles ceases when the blood circulatory system fails. Any subsequent metabolism must be anaerobic and ATP can only be regenerated through breakdown of glycogen by glycolysis since oxidative decarboxylation and phosphorylation will no longer operate. As glycogen is broken down so lactic acid accumulates. Because this is not removed by the blood system the muscle gradually acidifies. In a muscle such as the m. longissimus dorsi of the ox, from a well-fed and unstressed animal, the pH value will typically fall from about 7.2 to around 5.5. The ultimate pH (pHu) finally reached varies between muscles. For example, in some 'red' muscles of the pig the ultimate pH may be closer to 6.0. The actual pattern of acidification also varies considerably. Typical patterns are illustrated in Fig. 5.3.

The process of acidification normally takes 4–8 h in pigs, 12–24 h in sheep and 15–36 h in cattle (Dransfield, 1994b). In poultry meat the initial pH fall may be relatively rapid. For example, in turkeys the pH in the breast muscle can have fallen to 6 by 10–15 min *post mortem*. However the pHu is often quite high (5.8) compared with that in many muscles in red meat species. The pHu is inversely proportional to the concentration of lactate and the initial glycogen concentration becomes limiting below about 10 mg g^{-1} muscle. This is illustrated for beef in Fig. 5.4. If glycogen is not limiting, the production of lactic acid ceases when the enzyme systems will no longer function at the low pH. Excellent, detailed accounts of the changes that occur in muscle after death are given in Bate-Smith and Bendall (1956) and Bendall (1973).

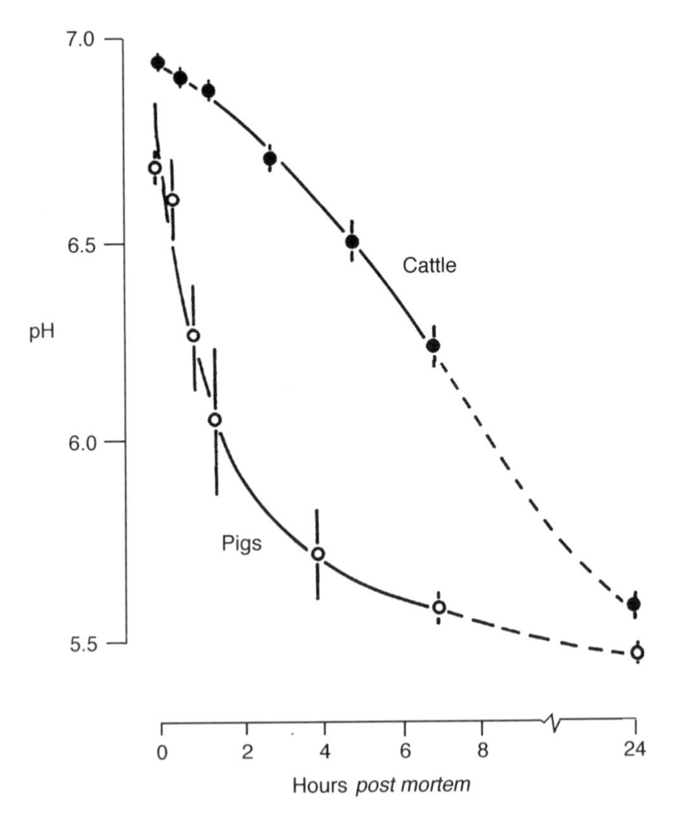

Fig. 5.3. The patterns of acidification of the m. longissimus dorsi in pigs and cattle. The curves are the average of 15 cattle and 30 pigs. The vertical bars are standard errors.

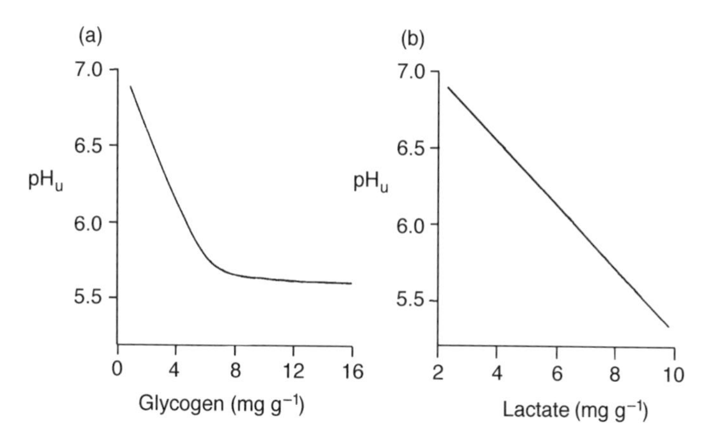

Fig. 5.4. The relationship between (a) initial glycogen and (b) final lactate concentration, and ultimate pH in the m. longissimus dorsi of the ox. Reprinted from Warriss *et al.* (1984), with permission from Elsevier Science.

Importance of acidification to the characteristics of meat

The muscle proteins tend to denature as the pH falls. This leads to a reduction in their power to bind water. Also, the myofibrillar proteins, myosin and actin, reach their isoelectric point. This is the pH at which the protein molecules have no net electrical charge and tend to lose the water that is normally bound to them. Both these phenomena lead to exudation of fluid from the muscle fibres. When the meat is cut the fluid also exudes onto the cut surface, which becomes moist. Eventually this exudate may produce drip, which can collect in the meat container or be lost, leading to weight loss. The change in the proteins increases the light scattering properties of the contractile elements of the muscle fibre. The meat changes from being relatively dark and translucent in the living animal to being opaque and paler (Fig. 5.5). These relationships between the physical characteristics of meat and pH are discussed in detail in Bendall and Swatland (1988). A detailed review of the effects of post-mortem changes occurring in muscles on their water-holding capacity and appearance is given in Offer *et al.* (1989).

The development of rigor mortis

In a resting muscle, ATP serves to keep the muscle in a relaxed state by preventing the formation of actomyosin. The muscle can also be stretched if put under tension. Only when ATP is hydrolysed to ADP does contraction occur. The ATP concentration is maintained by the breakdown of glycogen until lack of substrate or unsuitability of

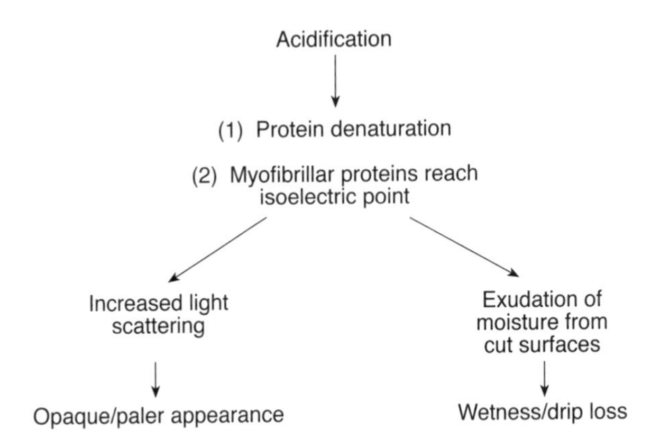

Fig. 5.5. The consequences of muscle acidification for the appearance and water-holding of meat.

conditions, particularly pH, for the enzymes, inhibits glycolysis. The level of CP then falls as it is used to regenerate ATP from ADP. Eventually however, the supply of regenerated ATP fails. Rigor mortis occurs when the ATP level falls below the very low level (~ 5 mmol kg^{-1}) required to maintain relaxation. When this happens, the actin and myosin molecules of the thin and thick filaments combine irreversibly to form actomyosin and extensibility of the muscle is lost. Cross-bridges form permanently and there is in effect a very weak contraction. Each muscle fibre goes into rigor very quickly once ATP is depleted, but the variation between individual fibres leads to a more gradual development of stiffness in the whole muscle as more and more fibres become inextensible (Fig. 5.6).

The time of onset of rigor will obviously relate to factors affecting the level of glycogen and creatine phosphate at death and the rate of post mortem muscle metabolism. For example, in animals that have undergone violent exercise at death, or in which glycogen has been depleted by longer-term stress preslaughter, rigor occurs faster. The rate of development will be reduced if the carcass is cooled quicker. Note that rigor onset is determined only by the availability of ATP, not the pH value of the muscle. It is possible to have rigor in muscle in which the pH is still high if the animal has been exhausted preslaughter. This has been referred to as alkaline rigor. However, the concentration of ATP below which rigor develops varies a little in different muscles and also it may be higher in alkaline rigor. On average, rigor takes different times to develop in the different species, ranging from about 4 h in the chicken to over 24 h in excised beef muscles (Etherington *et al.*, 1987).

There is some evidence that further breakdown of ADP occurs when ATP is exhausted. This may lead to the formation of AMP,

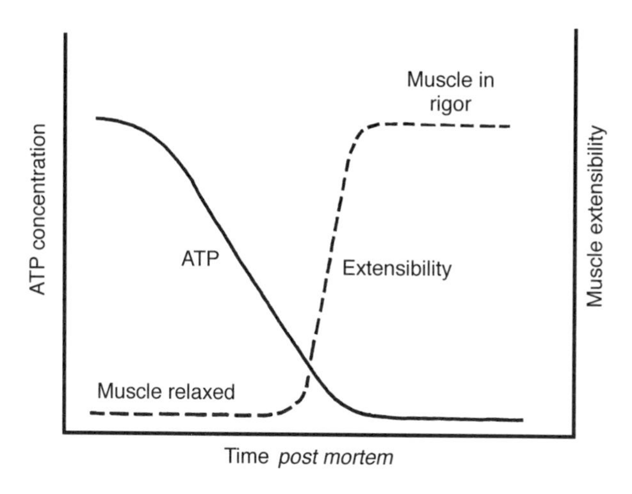

Fig. 5.6. The relation between ATP depletion and the onset of rigor mortis.

inosine monophosphate (IMP), inosine and eventually hypoxanthine. As more muscles enter rigor mortis the whole carcass becomes stiffer and 'sets'. This 'setting' is to a degree aided by the fat in the carcass becoming firmer as it cools.

The Resolution of Rigor Mortis and the Tenderization of Meat

The resolution of rigor

After a variable period of time there is a progressive 'resolution' of rigor when the muscles soften. The myofibrils become more easily fragmented by controlled homogenization of the muscle in aqueous solutions and this can be monitored by measurement of the 'myofibrillar fragmentation index' (see Chapter 12). In this, the degree of fragmentation is estimated from the opalescence of suspensions of myofibrils of equal protein content. Suspensions that are more opalescent indicate smaller particles, reflecting a greater fragmentation of the myofibrils. With longer times of ageing of the muscles after death of the animal the myofibrillar fragmentation index increases and the meat becomes more tender when it is cooked.

The rate of tenderization

The rate at which this tenderization occurs varies with temperature and in the different species. It is faster at higher temperatures. Every

10°C increase results in a more than doubling of the final tenderness achieved in a certain time. Chicken meat achieves 80% of its maximum tenderness about 8 h after death of the bird, whereas beef takes 10 days to reach the same level of tenderness (Table 5.2).

These differences in the rate of tenderization lead to different recommended ‘ageing’ times prior to cooking the meat. Keeping meat at refrigerated temperatures is expensive. There is the cost of the storage space, the cost of refrigeration and the inevitable weight loss from the surface of the carcass by evaporation of water, or the loss of exudate from butchered joints. A compromise has therefore to be reached commercially to produce meat with acceptable tenderness in a reasonable period of time (Table 5.3).

The ageing process continues irrespective of the size of the joints or at what stage of the marketing chain the meat has reached. Ageing time can therefore include time spent in distribution and retailing. However, it does not proceed in the frozen state but will continue on thawing if the normal ageing process was interrupted by the freezing. The optimization of the tenderization process was discussed by Dransfield (1994a).

The process of conditioning

Conditioning is the term applied to this natural process of tenderization when meat is stored or aged post-rigor. The tenderization could be attributable to two types of process: changes in the connective tissue components of the meat or weakening of the myofibrils. Nishimura *et al.* (1998) have suggested that conditioning takes place in two phases.

Table 5.2. The rate of tenderization of meat from different species [from Dransfield (1994a) based on figures in Dransfield and MacFie (1980) and Dransfield *et al.* (1981)].

Species	Days at 1°C to reach 80% of ‘maximum’ tenderness
Beef	10.0
Rabbit	9.5
Sheep	7.7
Pig	4.2
Chicken	0.3

Table 5.3. Recommended conditioning times (days) for pork, lamb and beef.

Pork	4–10
Lamb	7–14
Beef	10–21

There is a rapid first phase caused by changes in the myofibrillar component and a slower second phase caused by structural weakening of the intramuscular connective tissue. However, of these, the changes in the myofibrillar component are generally thought to be the more important and, in fact, only very small changes can be seen in the major connective tissue components such as collagen. Nevertheless, there is some cleavage of collagen cross-links and small structural changes can be seen under the electron microscope after extended ageing times.

In contrast, larger changes in the myofibrillar component can be seen. The attachments of the thin (actin) filaments to the Z discs show some breakdown (Boyer-Berri and Greaser, 1998) and there is an increase in the amount of water-soluble nitrogen compounds. However, the muscle does not become more extensible during conditioning and therefore the conditioning process is not associated with any dissociation of the actomyosin. The thick and thin filaments remain locked together by the myosin cross-bridges. Tenderization is *not* caused by the filaments regaining the ability to slide over one another.

The mechanism of tenderization

Calpains and cathepsins

Tenderization results from the activities of proteolytic enzymes present in the muscles. Their normal role is in the breakdown and recycling of proteins which occurs continuously in all living tissues. There are two main sorts of enzyme involved, cathepsins and calpains, of which, at least in red meat species and poultry, the calpains are thought to be more important. However, cathepsins may be more important in the post-mortem degradation of fish muscle and possibly in the tenderization that occurs in meat kept at high temperatures. Cathepsins occur in the lysosomes in the sarcoplasm. They are released *post mortem* and have maximum activity in mildly acid conditions. They are known to degrade troponin-T, some collagen cross-links and mucopolysaccharides of the connective tissue ground substance. They only appear to degrade actin and myosin below a pH of 5 so this is unlikely to occur under normal conditions in meat. The calpains are activated by calcium ions and have maximum activity in neutral to alkaline conditions. Originally they were referred to as calcium-activated sarcoplasmic factor (CASF). They occur in two forms, *m*-calpain activated by high (millimolar) concentrations of calcium ions (1–2 mM), and μ-calpain activated by low (micromolar) concentrations (50–100 μM). The relative importance of the two forms in promoting tenderization is a little unclear. It has generally been thought that the *m*-calpains were the more important. However, this view has recently been questioned in a paper which also gives an excellent review of our current knowledge of calpain biochemistry (Boehm *et al.*, 1998). The calpains are located in the region of the Z lines, which they degrade as well as promoting breakdown of other proteins such as tropomyosin and titin (connectin). The calpains are inhibited by calpastatin. High calpastatin activity reduces the extent of proteolysis in muscles.

Evidence for the importance of the calpains

There are various pieces of evidence supporting the importance of the calpains in the tenderization of meat by breaking down parts of the myofibrillar component of the muscle. Substances that inhibit proteolysis by calpains also inhibit tenderization. The rates of proteolysis in pork, lamb and beef correlate with overall differences in inherent tenderness. Thus, pork has the highest rate and in general is most tender. The extent of calpain-induced proteolysis in humped types of cattle (*Bos indicus*, e.g. Brahman) and European cattle (*Bos taurus*) correlates with texture. Proteolysis is greater in *B. taurus*, the meat from which is more tender. *Bos indicus* cattle have higher activities of the calpastatin inhibitor in their muscles (Shackelford *et al.*, 1991). The meat from animals treated with β-adrenergic agonists undergoes little or no proteolysis and is relatively tough (Wheeler and Koohmaraie, 1992). As we have seen previously (Chapter 2), β-adrenergic agonists are growth modifying compounds that enhance muscle development. It is likely that they do this by reducing the normal activity of the proteolytic enzymes involved in the continual processes of accretion and breakdown of the muscle proteins. This reduction in activity probably persists *post mortem*. The 'callipyge' gene in sheep causes muscle hypertrophy. However, meat from lambs carrying the gene is tougher than normal and undergoes conditioning at a slower rate. This has been attributed to the higher calpastatin activity in the muscles (Koohmaraie *et al.*, 1995). Stress just before slaughter may increase calpastatin levels and produce tougher meat through reduced conditioning (Sensky *et al.*, 1998).

Possible action of calpains post mortem

After exhaustion of ATP and the development of rigor mortis, the membrane systems of the sarcoplasmic reticulum and mitochondria no longer take up or sequester calcium ions. These are released into the sarcoplasm and bathe the myofibrils (Jeacocke, 1993). The increased calcium concentration activates the μ-calpains allowing proteolysis to proceed. Normally the calpains are inhibited by being bound to calpastatin. Calcium removes this inhibition. Calpastatin is itself eventually broken down by the calpains and the *m*-calpain may also be converted to μ-calpain by hydrolysis. Calpain activity is promoted by higher calcium levels, higher pH and temperature, and reduced calpastatin activity. From a practical point of view the enzyme activity in meat can be enhanced by infusing the carcasses *post mortem* with

0.3 M calcium chloride (see Chapter 8). Conversely, infusion of 10 mM EDTA (ethylene diamine tetra-acetic acid), which sequesters calcium, blocks enzyme activity. The effect of temperature is particularly important. From 0° to 40°C the rate of activity more than doubles for every 10°C rise. Keeping meat at high temperatures post-rigor can thus promote rapid tenderization. At 10°C, beef can be adequately aged in 4 days rather than the 10 days at about 1°C. However, these high temperatures are likely to have implications for spoilage. Koohmaraie (1996) gives a very good review of the biochemistry of tenderization.

Other possible mechanisms of tenderization

Many of the processes associated with tenderization, and especially the role and control of the calpains, are still poorly understood. Other mechanisms for tenderization that do not involve the calpains have been postulated. Calcium might, by stimulating muscle contraction pre-rigor, mechanically damage the meat structure and so make it more tender. Calcium might also cause disruption of the lysosomes and release cathepsins, which then could perhaps cause some protein breakdown.

Other Changes Occurring in the Conversion of Muscle to Meat

We have seen that the major changes occurring in muscles after the death of the animal are acidification and the development and resolution of rigor mortis. The acidification affects colour and water-holding capacity and the resolution of rigor results in tenderization. With time, the juiciness and flavour of the meat after cooking also often improve, although the reasons for this are poorly understood. The effect is illustrated by some Danish work. Bejerholm (1991) assessed the effects of ageing pork for up to 6 days. All characteristics improved significantly with longer times with the greatest effects between 2 and 3 days (Table 5.4).

Table 5.4. Effects of ageing pork on eating quality[a] (from Bejerholm, 1991).

	Ageing time (days)			
	1	2	3	6
Tenderness	−0.2	0	1.0	1.6
Juiciness	1.4	1.3	1.8	2.2
Flavour	1.9	1.8	2.2	2.3
Overall acceptability	0.4	0.6	1.5	1.8

[a] Slices of pork loin grilled to a final temperature of 65°C and scored using 11-point scales, where 5 was ideal, 0 was neither good nor bad and −5 was poor.

Chapter 6

Meat Quality

Agricultural systems go through three phases of development. Initially the aim is simply to produce enough to satisfy requirements. Secondly, when this aim has been achieved, production systems that are more reliable and efficient develop. Lastly, when we can produce enough and produce it efficiently, the quality of the product tends to be improved. First we learn how to rear enough pigs so everyone can eat pork, then we do it efficiently so the pork costs less, and last, we try and produce pork of better quality. The process is driven by the economics of competition since consumers always want to pay the least for the best. But, in regard to the production of meat, what does quality mean? In fact the term is rather difficult to define simply.

What Meat Quality Means

The concept of quality

Types of quality

Two overall types of quality can be distinguished. *Functional* quality refers to desirable attributes in a product. For example, we might want red meat to be tender and chicken to have good flavour. *Conformance* quality is producing a product that meets the consumer's specification exactly. An example of this type of quality might be that we want pork chops to be trimmed so there is exactly 5 mm of fat overlying the lean, or we want 'portion sized' chicken breasts to weigh exactly a certain amount. When most people talk about quality they tend to mean functional quality, but quality management often focuses on conformance quality. However, both types are important. No one really wants chicken breasts that are exactly the right weight but have poor flavour or texture.

Differences between people

Different people mean different things when they talk of functional quality depending on their cultural background, personal experience and where they stand in the production chain; whether farmer, processor, retailer or consumer. In other words, quality has a number of different components. While certain of these are of interest to everyone, others are only immediately important to some sectors. Meat yield mainly concerns the farmer and wholesaler, technological characteristics mainly the processor and palatability – what the meat is like to eat – the final consumer.

The cultural effect on quality perception is illustrated by the results of an interesting experiment in which the eating quality of meat from lambs produced in Spain and the UK was independently assessed by both Spanish and British taste panels (Sañudo *et al.*, 1998). The two panels were in agreement that odour and flavour were stronger in meat from the British lambs (which were older and heavier) and that juiciness was higher in the Spanish meat. However, when the members of the taste panels were asked which meat they *preferred*, the British panel best liked that from the British lambs and the Spanish that from the Spanish lambs. This shows how quality preferences can be determined by previous experience and possibly conditioning. In other words, people will often most like what they are used to.

Variation with time

Concepts of quality vary over time. The main purpose of rearing pigs was originally less for their lean meat and more for the lard they produced. Pigs were selected to grow large and fat because this produced most lard. In the early North American meat industry, instead of curing the pork, meat packers would often collect the fat, rather as used to be done with whale's blubber, by 'trying' it – heating the butchered carcasses in large vats or kettles to melt the fat which floated on the surface and could be ladled off. In contrast, modern North American and European pigs are relatively very lean, having been selected over the years to have less and less fat and proportionally larger muscles. At different times the highest quality has therefore been associated with both the fattest and the leanest pigs.

The major components of quality

Some components of meat quality – yield, technological properties and palatability – have already been mentioned. A full list of quality characteristics would include those in Table 6.1.

Table 6.1. The major components of meat quality (from Warriss, 1996c).

Yield and gross composition:	Quantity of saleable product
	Ratio of fat to lean
	Muscle size and shape
Appearance and technological characteristics:	Fat texture and colour
	Amount of marbling in lean (intramuscular fat)
	Colour and WHC of lean
	Chemical composition of lean
Palatability:	Texture and tenderness
	Juiciness
	Flavour
Wholesomeness:	Nutritional quality
	Chemical safety
	Microbiological safety
Ethical quality:	Acceptable husbandry of animals

Yield and composition

The yield of product is important because it determines how much you have to sell. Higher yields mean more product and potentially greater profit. In meat terms this could mean a higher proportion of carcass relative to the weight of the live animal (a higher killing-out percentage) or a higher yield of saleable lean and fat to non-saleable waste bone. As well as the absolute yield of lean and fat, the relative amount of lean is important. In general, a higher ratio of muscle to fat is preferred since the majority of consumers, at least in Europe and North America, want very little fat for reasons outlined in Chapter 1 and reviewed by Gibney (1993). However, fat is also associated with flavour development and so at least a minimal level is desirable. Above this level, fat will need to be trimmed leading to waste and reduced overall value. The shape of muscles is important, as well as the overall yield of lean, because this affects their attractiveness. Plump, rounded muscles are more attractive than thinner, flatter ones.

Appearance and technological characteristics

Appearance of the lean and its technological characteristics are often related. This is because factors that influence the microstructure of the muscle *post mortem* affect both aspects of colour and also water-holding capacity (WHC). Colour is a major determinant of appearance and WHC of technological value. Appearance is important because it is practically the only criterion the consumer can use to judge the acceptability of most meat at purchase. This presupposes that spoilage has not resulted in an unpleasant odour as it can in fish that is not fresh. Unlike, for example, many fruits, where the firmness or texture of the raw product is a good index of ripeness, the texture of raw meat usually tells little or nothing about that of the cooked material. The lean has a characteristic colour appropriate for each species and muscle but in general it should be bright in colour, and red or pink rather than brown, purple or grey. Moreover this colour should be stable to give the product a long shelf life.

There are three main reasons why waterholding capacity is important. First, the drip or exudate that results from poor WHC detracts from the appearance of the meat. This is especially so in modern retail packs where drip tends to collect, rather than draining away, and despite the frequent inclusion of absorbent pads in the bottom of trays to soak up the liquid. Second, loss of drip leads to weight loss in fresh meat, and in processed meats poor WHC may reduce water retention and therefore yield of product. Third, WHC is thought to influence the perceived juiciness of fresh meat after cooking. Meat with low WHC loses a lot of fluid in cooking and may taste dry and lack succulence. Problems with the colour and WHC of the lean are exemplified by the extreme conditions referred to as PSE (pale, soft, exudative) and DFD (dark, firm, dry) meat and which will be described later. The chemical composition of the lean, in particular its protein content may be important in determining the yield and quality of processed products.

The colour and chemical composition of the fat associated with the lean are important. Generally, the preference is for white or very pale pink fat over yellow pigmentation although the latter is accepted in certain cattle such as the Channel Island breeds, for example the Jersey. The yellow colour is caused by carotenes derived from green plants. It is therefore commoner in older animals and those that are grass-fed. The pigments are fat-soluble and the propensity to lay them down in the fat is genetically determined. Normally, firm fat is preferred over softer, oilier unsaturated fat. Soft fat may in fact be a problem in some modern very lean pigs but is beneficial in the Spanish breed of pig used to make Iberian hams. The pigs are fed on acorns from the locally grown cork oak trees and the pigs' fat is therefore unsaturated and soft. In the preparation of the hams this is taken advantage of, the subcutaneous fat covering being carefully smoothed over the ham surface. The fat characteristics may also contribute to the desirable distinctive flavour of the product. An important characteristic of fats is their resistance to oxidation. As we have seen in Chapter 3, this is also dependent on the degree of saturation of their component fatty acids.

Palatability

Palatability or eating quality encompasses three main characteristics. These are texture, juiciness and flavour/odour and, at least in red and poultry meats, their importance is usually in this order. In many developed countries, people prefer their meat to be tender and the value of different cuts or joints reflects this. Fillet steak is both the most tender and most expensive cut of beef. In some cultures this is not true. Many Africans prefer their meat 'chewy'. Good texture of fish flesh generally implies firm flesh, and a 'flaky' texture is sometimes perceived as desirable.

The extremes of juiciness are dryness and succulence. Modern meat is occasionally criticized for its lack of succulence and this is attributed to either poor WHC or low levels of intramuscular or marbling fat. Intramuscular fat has tended to be reduced with the selection of animals for overall greater carcass leanness, particularly in pigs. The human perceptions of tenderness and juiciness appear to be interrelated. Juicy meat may be perceived as more tender than a similar sample which has inherently the same texture (for example, as measured by an instrumental shear test) but is less juicy.

Flavour and odour are closely associated. Flavour is mainly determined by water-soluble constituents, odour by fat-soluble, volatile elements. Odour becomes very important if abnormal odours or taints are present. These override all other perceptions of quality. This is of obvious selective importance since meat that smells unpleasant often does so because it has spoiled and may therefore be unsafe to eat. Not all abnormal odours are produced by spoilage. An example is the odour associated with meat from some carcasses from entire male pigs (boars). This is referred to as boar taint and is often described as faecal in character or reminiscent of urine (see below). Women are more sensitive to certain components of boar taint and moreover find them more unpleasant than men appear to.

Wholesomeness

The wholesomeness of meat has two components. First, meat should be safe to eat, both in terms of freedom from parasites that may also infect humans, and microbiological pathogens and hazardous chemicals. People do not want to get food poisoning from eating meat. Neither do they want to be exposed to high levels of residues from previous veterinary medication of the animal, or from growth-promoting agents (Heitzman, 1996), or from adventitious contaminants such as pesticides.

Second, as well as this, people would prefer that meat was positively beneficial to their health in contributing minerals, vitamins and high value protein, and possibly essential fatty acids, such as eicosapentaenoic (EPA) and docosahexaenoic (DHA) acids (see Chapter 3), to their diet. The value of meat as a concentrated source of protein and energy is illustrated in Table 6.2. Only dried seeds like lentils have comparable protein contents, and only lentils or grains like rice are more concentrated sources of energy (because of their high carbohydrate contents). However, it should be remembered that the energy

Table 6.2. The protein, fat and energy content of some foods (based on data from McCance and Widdowson, 1997).

	Percentage protein	Percentage fat	Energy content (kJ 100 g^{-1})
Lean beef	20	5	517
Lean lamb	21	9	679
Lean pork	21	7	615
Skinless chicken	21	4	508
Herring	17	19	970
Potatoes	2	0.2	318
Peas	7	2	344
Carrots	1	0.3	146
Cabbage	2	0.4	109
Rice	7	3	1518
Lentils	24	2	1264

value of meat will vary somewhat with variation in its fat content. Much of the older information about the fat content of joints is based on analyses of meat that was much fatter than it is today. It came from fatter animals and was less closely trimmed of subcutaneous and intermuscular fat during butchery. For example, a boneless pork chop with 15 mm of subcutaneous fat might contain nearly 30% chemical fat. Trimming to 5 mm could reduce this to about 10% and some very lean pork may contain less than 3% fat. Carefully trimmed beef topside and rump steak may also now contain only 3–4% fat. As mentioned previously, meat is an important source of the B vitamins and various minerals (Table 6.3) including iron, zinc, phosphorus, potassium and magnesium.

Table 6.3. The concentrations of iron, zinc and five vitamins[a] in meat and vegetables (based on data from McCance and Widdowson, 1997).

	Iron	Zinc	Thiamine	Riboflavin	Niacin	B6	B12
Lean beef	2.1	4.3	0.07	0.24	5.2	0.32	2
Lean lamb	1.6	4.0	0.14	0.28	6.0	0.25	2
Lean pork	0.9	2.4	0.89	0.25	6.2	0.45	3
Potatoes	0.4	0.3	0.21	0.02	0.6	0.44	0
Peas	2.8	1.1	0.74	0.02	2.5	0.12	0
Carrots	0.3	0.1	0.10	0.01	0.2	0.14	0
Cabbage	0.7	0.3	0.15	0.02	0.5	0.17	0
Rice	1.4	1.8	0.59	0.07	5.3	–	0
Lentils	11.1	3.9	0.41	0.27	2.2	0.93	0

[a] Iron, zinc, thiamine, riboflavin, niacin and vitamin B6 concentrations in mg 100 g^{-1}; concentration of vitamin B12 in μg 100 g^{-1}.

In some regards, different types of meat may be better or worse in terms of their potential contribution to a healthy diet. This is exemplified by the characteristics of the fat in beef, lamb and pork, particularly the ratios of polyunsaturated to saturated fatty acids (the P:S ratio) they contain and the ratios of the $n-6$ to $n-3$ polyunsaturated acids (Wood and Enser, 1997). Values of 0.45 or above for the P:S ratio, and 4.0 or below for the $n-6$:$n-3$ ratio in dietary fats have been recommended in the UK. The ratios reported by Wood and Enser (1997) in UK meat are given in Table 6.4, together with their measurements of the proportion of dissectable fat in retail joints. Pork has the best P:S ratio (0.58), well above the recommended value, but the meats from the two ruminant species have the best $n-6$:$n-3$ ratios. However, the $n-6$:$n-3$ ratio for pork (7.22) is higher than desirable. Therefore, from one point of view pork is the healthiest of the three meats to consume, from another the least healthy.

Ethical quality

The last major component of meat quality, ethical quality, might be disputed by some. However, there is concern amongst many people that meat should come from animals which have been bred, reared, handled and slaughtered in ways that promote their welfare (see Chapter 10) and in systems which are sustainable and environmentally friendly.

Problems of conflicting requirements for different quality characteristics

Achieving some quality characteristics may be incompatible with achieving others. Juiciness is associated with higher levels of intramuscular (marbling) fat, but larger amounts of marbling are often found in meat that also has larger amounts of subcutaneous and intermuscular fat. As we have seen, consuming large quantities of fat is undesirable from the point of view of health. There is thus a potential dilemma that meat which is healthier for us to consume is likely to be

Table 6.4. The dissectable fat content, P:S and $n-6$:$n-3$ ratios of beef steaks, and pork and lamb chops in the UK (based on data in Wood and Enser, 1997).

	Percentage dissectable fat	P:S ratio[a]	$n-6$:$n-3$ ratio[b]
Beef	15.6	0.11	2.11
Lamb	30.2	0.15	1.32
Pork	21.1	0.58	7.22

[a] The ratio of polyunsaturated to saturated fatty acids.
[b] The ratio of $n-6$:$n-3$ polyunsaturated acids.

less juicy, and therefore have a poorer eating quality, than meat which is fatter and therefore less healthy. Health and palatability are to a degree incompatible, since the requirements for wholesomeness and eating quality are conflicting. It was mentioned that soft fat can be a problem in modern very lean pigs. This is because soft fat does not support the lean as effectively as firm fat and therefore may result in poorer muscle shape and less firm overall texture to the joint. However, softer fat contains a higher proportion of unsaturated fatty acids, which are healthier to eat. Again, one quality characteristic, appearance of the joint, is difficult to maintain while also achieving another, healthiness of the fat. A very effective way of improving carcass quality through reducing fatness is to use entire, rather than castrated, male animals, but the resulting lean meat may have less desirable eating qualities. The problem of boar taint has been mentioned and there is a suggestion that beef from young bulls may be less tender than that from steers (Morgan *et al.,* 1993).

Nitrite is used in the production of cured meats like ham and bacon (see Chapter 9). It reacts with the myoglobin to give the attractive characteristic pink colour of these products. It also inhibits the growth of pathogenic bacteria like *Clostridium*, but the consumption of nitrite has been implicated in the potential development of some cancers. Nitrite therefore has both beneficial and potentially undesirable characteristics as a meat additive.

Rapid carcass cooling inhibits the growth of microorganisms, so reducing potential spoilage, and also reduces weight losses by evaporation of water from the surface layers. However, cooling too rapidly may lead to less tender meat, either by reducing the activity of the naturally occurring proteolytic enzymes or by inducing cold shortening (see Chapter 8). There are thus both positive and negative consequences of rapid carcass chilling.

Ways to Improve Quality

Quality priorities

The dilemma of defining handling procedures where there are conflicting requirements for different quality characteristics may sometimes be solved by considering priorities. Some characteristics are more important than others. Kauffman *et al.* (1990) suggested there were three levels of quality. The first level, which had the highest priority, required that the meat be wholesome. It should be safe to eat and have nutritionally adequate levels of proteins, vitamins and minerals. If this could be achieved, the second level required the meat to show minimum shrinkage during processing, including cooking.

The third level also required the meat to have maximum attractiveness in terms of appearance, convenience and eating quality. It is likely that the first quality requirement, that of wholesomeness, would be agreed by all people. However, the choice of the second and third level requirements, while obviously desirable, would not necessarily be everyone's. Neither would the order of importance, and it is likely that different people in the meat production-consumption chain would have different views. For the final consumer, eating quality is likely to be the second priority after wholesomeness.

Strategies for improving quality

The first requirement is to identify what needs to be improved. In the USA, extensive surveys of beef tenderness (Morgan *et al.*, 1991) and pork quality (Cannon *et al.*, 1996) have been carried out to identify and prioritize problems. An essential output from such surveys is an estimate of the economic cost of the problems, allowing an assessment to be made of the cost of improvement in relation to the probable benefits. Of the many aspects of meat quality, some are easier to improve than others. Characteristics that are dependent on, and amenable to, human intervention can be controlled much more easily than those characteristics that are determined principally biologically. Examples of the first type are safety and wholesomeness. These can be achieved by careful control of hygiene during production and preparation. An example of the second type, which is much harder to control, is carcass fatness. We do not understand why there is variation in this largely because of the complexity of biological systems. We can reduce overall fatness in populations of animals by careful selection but we do not know how to reduce the variation. So, although the backfat thickness of pig carcasses has been very effectively reduced over the last 20 years (at an average rate of nearly 0.4 mm per year in the UK), there are still some carcasses that are too fat or too lean. This kind of variation extends to marbling fat, colour of the lean, WHC and eating quality.

The inherent, uncontrollable variation will always be likely to lead to a proportion of carcasses or joints that have unacceptable quality. Unfortunately, modern consumers have come to expect uniformity of product. At a level of about 5% of unacceptable product, consumers begin to be prejudiced against repeat purchases – they tend not to buy the product again. An approach to this problem of inherent variation is to try and reduce it as much as possible by strict control of all factors thought to influence it and then to monitor quality carefully to identify that product which is unacceptable. This product can then be marketed differently. For example, potentially tough meat would go for 'restructuring'. This could take the form of grinding, mincing or flaking it, and reforming the comminuted meat into burgers or restructured steaks (see Chapter 8).

In the UK in the 1990s, the Meat and Livestock Commission introduced 'Blueprints' to improve the eating quality of pork, beef and, later, lamb. These specified procedures for breed selection, rearing, husbandry, handling and slaughter of the live animal, and post-mortem handling of the carcasses and meat, which had been identified as optimal based on available knowledge. By optimizing each stage in the production chain, the resulting meat quality would on average be enhanced. Warkup (1993) described this approach and also provided evidence of its effectiveness. Pork produced using the blueprint was on average rated more tender, and less variable in texture, by a taste panel than that purchased from normal retail sources. The latter pork could have included samples produced according to some parts of the blueprint specification so it was not a true control sample. The improvements shown in texture were therefore possibly conservative.

It is important to note that there are inherent costs to quality improvement. There is the cost of controlling the factors that are thought to influence quality, the cost of measuring or monitoring quality, and the cost of the product that does not conform to the desired quality. The latter is both because of the cost of not being able to sell the product for its original purpose and the cost of reprocessing it.

Quality assurance schemes

The object of these is to certify that particular standards have been followed in the production of meat. Their purpose is to give consumers confidence in buying meat produced under the particular scheme, and to counter the confusion and concern that sometimes arises from general criticisms levelled at some production methods or aspects of quality. Because they are addressed to consumers, they focus on aspects perceived to be of major importance to them. There are three main areas: food safety and wholesomeness, ethical quality, and sensory or eating quality. Food safety concerns revolve, for example, around the possible presence of antibiotic residues, pathogenic bacteria and the contribution to a healthy diet. Ethical concerns include both animal welfare and environmental issues such as pollution from waste products and fertilizers. Sensory concerns include undesirable meat colour and texture. The aim of the quality assurance scheme is to guarantee to the consumer that these concerns are unfounded.

There is variation between different schemes in terms of what quality aspects are included or emphasized. Often, these are related to the potential concerns of the consumers in the target market, whether home or export. In the UK, considerable emphasis is placed on animal welfare. A quality assurance scheme originated by the Royal Society for the Prevention of Cruelty to Animals (RSPCA), and implemented through the company, Freedom Foods, specifies welfare standards for animals on the farm and through to slaughter. For example, in the standards for pigs, stalls and tethers are not allowed for dry sows (those without piglets). Piglets must not be weaned from their mothers before they are 3 weeks old, animals must be kept in stable social groups and have minimum areas to live in, and have access to straw. There must be no castration of male pigs if slaughtered at less than 90 kg live weight. Tail docking is prohibited except in certain circumstances and with the agreement of a veterinary surgeon. There must be a veterinary health plan. Pigs cannot be sold through live auction markets and must be slaughtered at the abattoir closest to the farm. Maximum transport times, and maximum times without food, are defined, and humane slaughter procedures specified.

Sometimes schemes relate to only one or two of the meat species and may focus on meat from stock in particular geographical regions. Farm Assured British Pigs (Gready, 1997; Webb, 1998), Farm Assured Scotch Livestock (Simpson, 1993) for lamb and beef, and Premium Quality Welsh Lamb (Zalick, 1993) are examples. In North America, the Pork Quality Assurance (PQA) programme was developed by The National Pork Producers Council (Lautner, 1997). In one sense the existence of different schemes might be considered undesirable in that a single, all-embracing scheme would be simpler for the consumer to understand. An element of standardization is, in any case, desirable. An essential aspect of all quality assurance schemes is monitoring compliance with the set standards and auditing them effectively. Obviously too, it is important that these functions should be performed by assessors who are independent of the scheme. A useful overview of quality assurance schemes is given in Wood *et al.* (1998).

Labelling and preconceptions

People may have preconceptions of the quality of certain products and this can influence the way they perceive the inherent or actual quality. An example of this is the interest, in some European countries particularly, in meat from animals reared non-intensively. Sometimes this is associated with the notion of 'organic' food. Organically grown food is produced with minimal or no use of 'chemical' fertilizers, pesticides, pharmaceutical products or medicines. Non-intensive rearing systems and organic methods of production are perceived by many people to be in the best interests of the animal and to lead to better quality of the product. The former is often probably true but the latter may not be. However, if meat is labelled as organically produced some consumers may be persuaded to believe that it will taste better, especially if, for ethical or other reasons, they normally buy meat from extensively or organically reared animals.

This effect is illustrated by the findings of a Dutch experiment. In the Netherlands some pigs are produced under a free-range, organic system (the animals are known as 'Scharrelvarkens'). It is prescribed that the animals must be kept in groups, sows must have access to the open air and that their diet must contain 10% roughage but no antibiotics or growth promoters, for example. This system is perceived to be beneficial to the welfare of the pigs and to produce better pork. Packs of this pork were compared with equivalent packs of pork but derived from pigs reared in the normal, commercial, intensive system. The pork was assessed by two groups of consumer. One comprised general members of the public, the other, people who normally preferred to buy meat from extensively reared animals. When the two sorts of pork were presented unlabelled to the consumers, practically no differences were detected by either consumer group. When the trial was repeated, but with the packs labelled as coming either from 'normal' or extensively reared pigs, the general public still did not detect material differences. However, the people who normally bought pork from extensively reared animals recorded very significant improved eating quality in this meat, but the results of the first trial with unlabelled packs had shown that there were really no inherent differences in quality between the two types of pork. The implication is that the consumers who normally bought meat from extensively reared animals had unwarranted preconceptions about its palatability and their assessments reflected these. Because they *expected* the meat to taste better they persuaded themselves that it *actually* did. This is an example of a general phenomenon. Deliza *et al.* (1996) have shown that consumers change their rating of the sweetness and bitterness of pure solutions of sucrose or quinine after being given (erroneous) information about them which led to expectations that the solutions were more or less sweet or bitter than they really were.

Some Specific Quality Concerns in Beef and Pork

The factors that are currently thought to influence meat quality fall into three time periods: on-farm, ante-mortem and post-mortem. Traditionally, inherent or on-farm factors have been considered to be the most important but, under modern production systems, the greater significance and importance of ante-mortem handling of the animal and post-mortem handling of the carcass have been recognized.

Beef quality

On-farm factors include breed, rearing system, feeding and nutrition, and age and maturity at slaughter. The effects of breed have perhaps been overrated in the past. There are genetic influences on meat quality factors but they usually relate to very specific characteristics. The best beef is often thought to come from the traditional beef breeds of cattle like the Hereford and Aberdeen Angus rather than the dairy breeds like the Friesian, Holstein and Jersey. Certainly, as we have already seen (Table 2.6), the beef breeds produce carcasses with better conformation and bigger muscles. The Hereford and Angus are early maturing breeds so they start laying down subcutaneous and intramuscular (marbling) fat earlier. At a fixed slaughter weight they therefore tend to have more such fat than the later-maturing dairy breeds. This effect is emphasized by the fact that at the same level of fatness dairy breeds also tend to store most of their fat internally as abdominal fat rather than associated with the muscles. Marbling fat contributes to juiciness and tenderness so on average, meat from the beef breeds should have better eating quality at the same carcass weight. However, if slaughtered at the same *overall* level of fatness, rather than at the same weight, the dairy breeds often have higher amounts of marbling in their meat. In practice, the eating quality of meat from beef and dairy breeds seems very similar and, in fact, the latter may even be better (Knapp *et al.*, 1989; Thonney *et al.*, 1991). The beef from humped cattle (*Bos indicus*) tends to be tougher than that from European breeds (*Bos taurus*). As we have seen (Chapter 5), part of the reason for this is that the post-mortem proteolytic breakdown of the myofibrillar system is less in meat from *B. indicus* because of differences in the activities of the calpains and calpastatin.

Pork quality

Major factors influencing pork quality are those that influence whether the muscle shows PSE or DFD characteristics, whether it has an abnormally low ultimate pH, and the level of intramuscular fat present. Major genes associated with the factors influencing muscle pH are the halothane gene and the RN^- gene. A review of the production factors known to affect meat quality in pigs is given in Wood *et al.* (1992). An excellent review of the genetic factors is that of Sellier and Monin (1994).

The halothane gene

The halothane (Hal^n) gene is so called because its presence in a pig as the double recessive genotype confers susceptibility to the common anaesthetic gas halothane. Susceptible pigs, referred to as halothane-positive, exhibit a characteristic response when they breath the gas through a face mask. Their limbs become extended and rigid and they develop a raised body temperature or hyperthermia. The hyperthermia gets progressively worse and is referred to as 'malignant'. If the response is not rapidly rectified the pigs die. The halothane test only identifies animals with the double recessive genotype (nn), not the heterozygote (Nn). These carrier animals, like the normal homozygote (NN), are not influenced adversely by halothane, and go into a relaxed state of stable anaesthesia. They are referred as halothane-negative. The inability of the halothane test to identify the heterozygote was a considerable disadvantage in attempts to control the presence of the gene in pig breeds by selective breeding. This situation was made worse by difficulty in interpretation of the test results. The length of exposure to halothane in the test was restricted to 3–5 min to reduce deaths in positive animals but this might not be sufficient time to detect some positive pigs. Also, the physiological state of the animal seems to affect the test. This is important since some stress is inevitably associated with carrying out the test itself. However, recently a DNA-based test has been developed which enables exact differentiation of all three genotypes (NN, Nn, nn). This test is based on detection of the ryanodine receptor gene (*Ryr*). The ryanodine receptor is the calcium release channel of the sarcoplasmic reticulum and a single mutation of the gene controlling it has been identified by Fujii *et al.* (1991) as likely to be the cause of halothane sensitivity in pigs.

The halothane gene was early on discovered to be closely associated with the occurrence of stress-susceptibility in some pig breeds or strains. Susceptible breeds showed difficulty in coping with stressful episodes, relatively high mortality during transport and produced carcasses that exhibited a high prevalence of PSE meat. These characteristics are sometimes referred to as the porcine stress syndrome (PSS). However, halothane sensitivity was also associated with the positive attributes of muscularity and good carcass conformation, undoubtedly the reason for its inadvertent selection for in some breeds, notably the Pietrain and Belgian Landrace in Europe and the Poland China in North America. Because of the recessive nature of its inheritance it was thought at one time that the benefit of the halothane gene – better carcass quality – could be exploited while eliminating the problems of poorer meat quality – a high level of PSE meat – by producing a carefully controlled heterozygous slaughter generation. This would be done by retaining a halothane-negative, homozygous population of the female parent (gilts and sows) and a halothane-negative, but heterozygous, population of boars. When crossed together these would produce a halothane-negative slaughter generation of half normal homozygotes and half heterozygotes:

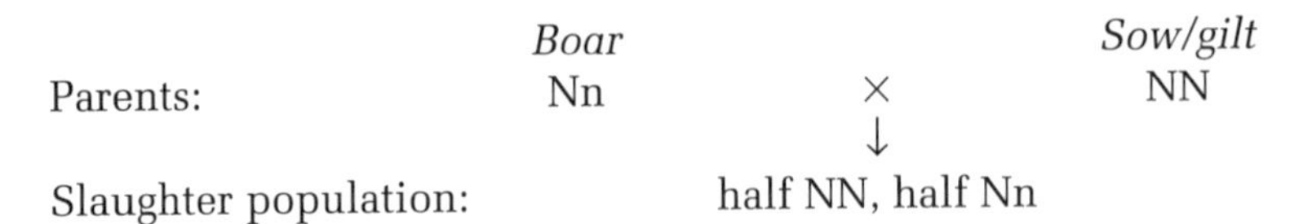

Unfortunately, the meat quality in the heterozygote is in fact generally not as good as in the normal, halothane-negative pigs. In other words, the gene is not fully recessive in its effects on these traits. Therefore, the strategy adopted by most pig-breeders appears to be to eliminate completely the recessive mutation from their herds, aided by the DNA-based test. An example of the differences that have been found between pigs exhibiting the three halothane genotypes is given in Table 6.5.

The RN^- *gene*

The RN^- gene has been identified in certain strains of Hampshire pigs, particularly in France and Sweden (Monin and Sellier, 1985; Lundström and Enfält, 1997). The name of the gene reflects a major effect in its dominant form, that is, to reduce the yield of cooked, cured ham, and the names of the originators of the technique used to measure this yield. Hence, RN^- refers to 'Rendement Napole', rendement from the French word for 'yield', and Napole from the initial letters from the surnames of N. Naveau, P. Pommeret and P. Lechaux. The yield is measured by curing and cooking a sample of 100 g of the m. semimembranosus under defined conditions. The three genotypes are RN^-RN^-, RN^-rn^+ and rn^+rn^+ (normal). The yield of muscles from pigs carrying the RN^- gene (either homozygotes or heterozygotes) is reduced by up to 8%.

Table 6.5. Growth and carcass and meat quality characteristics of British Landrace pigs selected as halothane-positive, halothane-negative, or their crosses, and fed *ad lib.* (data from Simpson and Webb, 1989).

	Halothane-positive (nn)	Crosses (Nn)	Halothane-negative (NN)
Daily live weight gain (kg)	0.91	0.94	0.89
FCR (food eaten/weight gain)	2.40	2.51	2.58
Average backfat (mm) thickness	22.4	23.8	23.2
LD cross sectional area (cm^2)	34.0	33.4	32.6
Killing-out percentage	76.6	76.7	75.9
Conformation score[a]	7.4	7.1	7.1
Reflectance of LD (EEL units)	51	43	42
Percentage of carcasses visually scored as pale, wet, or PSE	51	16	6

[a] Ten-point visual scale, higher is better.
FCR, food conversion ratio; LD, m. longissimus dorsi; EEL, Evans Electroselenium Reflectance meter; PSE, pale, soft, exudative.

The RN^- gene is thought to increase the glycogen content of the muscles, particularly those with a high complement of white, glycolytic fibres, redder muscles being little affected. The gene also produces lower ultimate pH values, resulting in higher drip losses and paler meat, and lower muscle protein concentrations. There may also be effects on eating quality and carcass composition, although this is not clear. The lower ultimate pH values have led to the use of the term 'acid meat', and its association with the Hampshire breed, the 'Hampshire effect'.

Intramuscular fat

The potential role of intramuscular (marbling) fat in promoting juiciness and tenderness has already been mentioned. Several studies suggest that low levels of intramuscular fat reduce eating quality. In contrast higher levels are beneficial. Wood (1995) has suggested several reasons for this. Improved tenderness may be because the soft fat 'dilutes' the effects of tougher myofibrillar elements so reducing shear force, or the fat may reduce the 'rigidity' of the muscle structure or it may allow fibre bundles to separate from one another more easily. Improved juiciness may be because fat promotes the flow of saliva in the mouth and better flavour may derive from reactions of the fat during cooking. A good illustration of this relation between fat level and eating quality is a study carried out in Denmark by Bejerholm and Barton-Gade (1986). They aged pork loins for 7 days then cooked slices to an internal temperature of 65°C before evaluating them using an experienced taste panel. They also made objective measurements of shear force using an instrumental method after cooking to 72°C (Table 6.6).

Table 6.6. The effect of fat content on the eating quality[a] of pork (from Bejerholm and Barton-Gade, 1986).

Average percentage intramuscular fat	Tenderness score	Flavour score	Overall acceptability score	Shear force	Percentage of samples with acceptable or better quality
0.86	0.6	0.8	0	100	71
1.24	1.7	1.6	1.2	86	87
1.73	1.9	1.7	1.4	78	89
2.37	2.2	1.9	1.9	79	97
2.76	2.7	2.5	2.3	76	100
3.94	2.7	2.3	2.3	69	100

[a] Measured using 11-point hedonic scales where +5 was ideal, 0 was neither good nor bad and −5 was poor.

With increasing fat levels, tenderness, flavour and overall acceptability increased. Samples judged more tender by the panel also had lower shear values. As the fat level increased the percentage of samples judged as having acceptable or better eating quality increased. However, overall, there was relatively little improvement in quality above an intramuscular fat concentration of about 2%. Higher intramuscular fat was also found to improve the eating quality of PSE pork, although overall panel scores were lower than for normal pork. Similarly, studies in North America by DeVol *et al.* (1988) found significant correlations between eating quality, and instrumentally determined shear force, and fat concentration in the muscle. When they grouped samples according to their instrumentally determined texture they found that higher fat levels were associated with more tender pork (Table 6.7).

The levels of intramuscular fat measured in both the Danish and American studies were high compared with concentrations measured in UK pigs. These seem to average about 1% or less, perhaps reflecting the reductions in the overall fatness of the carcasses. At these very low intramuscular fat levels, eating quality may well be less than optimal. An important consideration is the method used to extract the fat. Fat solvents like diethyl ether do not extract phospholipids present in the cell membranes and therefore underestimate the true total fat content of the muscle (Chapter 11). At low fat concentrations this underestimation may be a significant fraction of the whole.

The beneficial effects of fat on the eating quality of fresh pork are reflected in similar effects in minced (ground) meat products. In fact, since the range of fatness can be greater, because fat is added to levels of up to 20%, the effects are more pronounced.

Different breeds of pig have different inherent amounts of intramuscular fat. The Duroc is generally credited with having the highest levels and has been used in breeding schemes in Denmark and the UK to improve pork eating quality because of this. The benefits of incorporating Duroc genes on increasing intramuscular fat content and eating quality are illustrated in Table 6.8. In fact, Duroc pigs may have

Table 6.7. The association between instrumentally determined texture and intramuscular fat (from DeVol *et al.*, 1988).

Average shear force (kg)	Average percentage of fat in muscle
5.1	2.4
4.0	3.3
3.6	3.2
3.2	3.4
2.6	3.6

Table 6.8. The effect of incorporation of different proportions of Duroc genes on the intramuscular fat content and eating quality of fresh pork from gilts and boars fed *ad lib.* (from MLC Stotfold Pig Development Unit, Second Trial Results, 1992).

	Percentage Duroc genes			
	0	25	50	75
Intramuscular fat (%)	0.70	0.86	1.08	1.27
Tenderness[a]	5.0	5.0	5.3	5.4
Juiciness[a]	4.1	4.1	4.2	4.4
Pork flavour[a]	3.9	4.0	4.0	4.0

[a] Taste panel scores based on 1–8 scales, 1 being extremely tough, dry or weak in flavour, 8 being extremely tender, juicy or strong in flavour.

intramuscular fat levels which are too high (>3–4%) for both consumer acceptability of fresh pork (because of the preference for lean-looking pork) and for processing into cooked hams. The benefits of the breed are therefore normally used in a cross containing up to 50% of Duroc blood.

The relationship between intramuscular fat levels and eating quality is undoubtedly complicated by other factors, notably the influence of breed *per se*. This is illustrated by the results from a comparison of the eating quality of pork from a number of breeds carried out by Warriss *et al.* (1990c, 1996). The overall acceptability of meat from the different breeds compared with the concentration of intramuscular fat in the muscles is shown in Table 6.9. Although the

Table 6.9. The levels of intramuscular fat and eating quality (overall acceptability) of pork from 10 breeds of pigs killed at an average live weight of 62 kg (from Warriss *et al.*, 1990c, 1996).

Breed	Eating quality[a]	Percentage of fat in the muscle[b]
Pietrain	1.60	1.2
Gloucester Old Spots	1.67	1.3
Landrace	1.71	1.4
Berkshire	1.90	2.1
Large White	1.91	0.9
Large Black	2.01	1.6
Saddleback	2.10	1.4
Hampshire	2.51	1.3
Duroc	2.56	2.2
Tamworth	2.81	1.5

[a] Overall acceptability taste panel scores based on a scale of −7 to +7 with higher scores indicating better quality.
[b] Diethyl ether-extractable.

Duroc breed had nearly the highest rated eating quality and the greatest amount of intramuscular fat, the best quality pork came from the Tamworth, a traditional, relatively unselected breed with only moderate amounts of marbling fat. The Berkshire, another traditional breed, had high levels of fat but only moderate eating quality. The Pietrain had low amounts of intramuscular fat, although not as low as the Large White, but very poor eating quality possibly to some degree because of the generally poor WHC of the meat of this breed. This tends to produce dry-tasting meat lacking in juiciness.

Breed effects

This work comparing quality characteristics of different breeds also serves to illustrate other changes in meat quality that have occurred with selection in the modern commercially-important breeds such as the Pietrain, Large White, Landrace, Hampshire and Duroc in comparison with the 'traditional breeds'. Table 6.10 shows the characteristics of the meat from the breeds grouped under three headings. Group I comprises the six traditional breeds from Table 6.8, Group II the Large White, Landrace, Hampshire and Duroc, and Group III the Pietrain which perhaps represents the extreme case of selection for carcass muscularity. Improvements in carcass quality are associated with some less desirable characteristics of the meat. That from the improved breeds tended to be paler in colour (higher reflectance values) and to lose more exudate during storage than that from 'traditional' breeds. These differences were attributable to a reduced initial muscle pH (pH_{45}). There were also progressive increases in the coarseness of the grain of the muscles.

Fat firmness

In the early days of the European settlement of North America the colonists allowed their pigs to run wild in the woodlands to feed off

Table 6.10. Meat quality characteristics in different types of pig breeds (from Warriss *et al.*, 1996).

	Group I	Group II	Group III
pH_{45} in LD muscle	6.48	6.34	5.83
Muscle colour[a]	46.3	47.8	60.1
Water-holding capacity[b]	7.3	10.4	12.9
Graininess of muscle[c]	2.1	2.3	2.9

Group I = Large Black, Berkshire, Tamworth, Saddleback, Gloucester Old Spots; Group II = Hampshire, Duroc, Large White, Landrace; Group III = Pietrain

[a] Measured as reflectance (EEL units); higher values indicate paler muscle.

[b] Measured as the percentage loss of exudate from stored meat.

[c] Subjective score based on a scale of 1 = fine, 4 = coarse.

the natural foods. However, pigs fattened entirely in this way, although they grew well, did not produce good pork. It was soft, oily and hard to preserve even though its flavour was originally good if eaten directly. To overcome this, the pigs were rounded up and housed, being fed corn for several weeks before going to market. This resulted in their meat becoming solid and their fat white and firm. Corn-fed pigs therefore fetched a higher price than those fattened only on naturally available food. The softness of the fat from the naturally fattened pigs was caused by the unsaturated nature of the fats in the nuts and acorns they consumed. The unsaturated fat would have been prone to oxidation and rancidity so the meat would not store well.

Another disadvantage of soft fat is that it does not contribute to the firmness of joints of meat so detracting from their appearance when displayed for sale. This is a problem that has been associated with modern, very lean pork. The reduced fat firmness leads to meat that butchers refer to as not 'setting' well. The problem is caused both because there is less fat to support the lean tissues and because the fat is softer. As well as this softness, the fat layers tend to separate from the underlying muscle. The fat is softer because it is less saturated and because the adipose tissue contains more water and therefore proportionally less lipid.

Use of entire males (boars) for pork production

As we have seen, raising entire male animals, rather than castrating them soon after birth, is one of the most effective ways of reducing carcass fatness. Because lean is cheaper to deposit than fat in energy terms, entire males eat less food for the same weight gain. They also tend to grow faster. Compared with castrates, boars have shown improved daily live weight gain and food conversion efficiency of the order of 10% in some studies, although figures rather less than these are perhaps more usual in modern lean breeds of pigs. To exploit these advantages fully boars must be fed at high levels – probably *ad lib*. The carcass yield from boars is very slightly reduced: on average killing-out percentages are about one percentage point lower. This is generally attributed to the weight of the testicles (Table 6.11).

As well as these production benefits of rearing boars the castration procedure is avoided. Very young pigs are usually castrated without anaesthetic or analgesia and many people who are concerned with animal welfare therefore find the procedure unacceptable.

All these benefits led to the percentage of male pigs left entire (uncastrated) in the UK rising from less than 5% in 1976 to more than 30% in 1986 and 49% in 1991. In other words, by 1991, almost all male pigs were left uncastrated. Ireland and Spain also rear boars for slaughter but worldwide this is unusual. The reason for this is that there are also potential disadvantages associated with the production of boars. These fall under several headings. The first is that boars are more aggressive than castrates or gilts. Because of this they tend to fight more, especially when mixed with unfamiliar animals as can often happen when batches of pigs are made up from separate rearing pens prior to being sent to slaughter. On average, carcasses from boars always show higher levels of skin blemish caused by fighting during this preslaughter period. This is illustrated in Table 6.12.

The prevalence of downgraded carcasses from boars ranged from 1.3 to 2.5 times that in carcasses from gilts and castrates and the plant with the highest frequency of downgrading overall (C) had the lowest ratio. The implication was that, at very low levels of downgrading, reflecting careful control over the amount of mixing of animals pre-slaughter, the effect of sex was more important than where handling was less careful and the frequency of downgrading was high. With poorer handling the differences between boars and non-boars were considerably reduced.

The average prevalence of downgrading in the study was 4.7%. Many more carcasses may show some skin blemish but at a level not severe enough to warrant downgrading. In the UK, up to about 40% of pig carcasses show some damage, albeit slight. As well as skin blemish,

Table 6.11. Growth and carcass characteristics of gilts, castrates and boars fed *ad lib.* (from the report of the MLC first Stotfold trial, MLC, 1989).

	Gilt	Castrate	Boar
Daily live weight gain (g)	796	823	862
Daily carcass gain (g)	642	656	676
FCR (food eaten/weight gain)	2.68	2.79	2.43
Killing-out percentage	76.9	76.3	75.4
Backfat thickness (P_2, mm)	12.1	14.6	11.6
% Lean in carcass	56.4	53.0	57.2
Cost (£) of producing 1 kg of lean	1.38	1.52	1.33

Table 6.12. The prevalence of carcasses downgraded because of skin blemish in three slaughter plants (from Warriss, 1984c).

	Frequency of downgrading		
Plants	Percentage non-boar carcasses	Percentage boar carcasses	Ratio of percentage downgrading in boars to that in non-boars
A	0.9	2.2	2.5
B	3.7	5.0	1.4
C	8.2	10.5	1.3

The differences between boars and non-boars are all very highly significant. Non-boars included gilts and castrates.

the carcasses from boars also tend to exhibit a higher prevalence of DFD meat. Undoubtedly this is caused by the combination of stress and physical activity associated with fighting which depletes muscle glycogen stores.

Partly because they are leaner, boars tend to have softer fat that is less saturated and contains more water than fat from gilts or castrates. The number of carcasses in which the fat is unacceptably soft is therefore slightly higher in boars. A potentially more serious problem with the fat in boar carcasses is the occasional occurrence of an abnormal and unpleasant odour or flavour when it is heated, such as obviously occurs during cooking. This is referred to as 'boar taint'. Boar taint is not restricted to the carcasses from boars but is very rare in those from castrates or gilts. Because the lean portion of the meat also contains some fat, even trimmed chops or steaks can have the unpleasant flavour (Table 6.13).

The cooked lean from boars had a weaker pork flavour but a more abnormal flavour. Similarly, the cooked fat had a weaker pork odour but a stronger abnormal odour. The apparent reduced 'normal' pork odour and flavour in boar meat may simply reflect a masking effect by the abnormal taint. Of the samples of lean from boars, 8.5% were given slightly to extremely strong abnormal flavour ratings compared with only 0.3% from gilts. Of the samples of fat, 11.7% from boars were given slightly to extremely strong odour ratings compared with 0.4% from gilts. Even though texture and juiciness of the meat did not differ

Table 6.13. Odour and flavour assessments in pork from gilts and boars (from Warriss *et al.*, 1993a).

	Gilts	Boars
Number of samples	300	300
Odour of fat		
Pork odour score	3.8	3.6[a]
Abnormal odour score	2.3	3.0[a]
Percentage with slight to extremely strong abnormal odour	0.4	11.7
Flavour of lean		
Pork flavour score	3.9	3.7[a]
Abnormal flavour score	2.8	3.2[a]
Percentage with slight to extremely strong abnormal odour	0.3	8.5

The figures are mean taste panel scores based on eight-point category scales in which higher ratings indicate stronger odour/flavour. They come from deboned, griddled chops cooked to an internal temperature of 80°C.

[a] Indicates that the difference between scores for gilts and boars was statistically highly significant.

between the sexes the overall acceptability of the pork from the boars was highly significantly lower, illustrating the importance of abnormal flavour and odour to palatability. These results suggest that about 10% of boars may produce meat exhibiting some level of taint. This figure agrees with estimates from other studies (Table 6.14) and implies that, in a mixed population of gilts and boars, about 5% of carcasses may be a potential problem.

Two compounds have been implicated in the production of boar taint (Fig. 6.1). Androstenone (5α-androst-16-en-3-one), originally identified by Patterson (1968), smells of urine or perspiration and is produced in the testicles of the male pig and concentrated in the salivary glands and fat, acting as a pheromone in the adult boar to stimulate the sow to mate. Not all people can smell the odour. Women are more sensitive to the compound than men and, when they can detect it, appear to find it more distasteful. Skatole (3-methyl-indole) in the pure state has a smell often described as like camphor (mothballs) but in combination with other compounds present in meat has an unpleasant faecal odour. It is produced by the bacterial breakdown of the amino acid tryptophan in the large intestine. Men and women seem equally sensitive to it.

For obvious reasons, androstenone concentrations are higher in the carcasses of boars. Perhaps surprisingly, so are skatole concentrations and it is not clear why this should be. However, it is probable that the subsequent metabolism of skatole absorbed from the large intestine is different in the two sexes. Thresholds for detection of the two compounds by humans vary with how they are presented, as well as between individuals. This makes it difficult to set maximum limits for the concentrations of the compounds in fat for carcasses to be deemed completely acceptable to consumers. A further complication may be that there is an interaction between the effects of skatole and androstenone so that levels of one compound may determine the importance of levels of the other. Nevertheless, concentrations of skatole in fat of between 0.20 and 0.25 $\mu g\ g^{-1}$ and of androstenone of 0.5–1.0 $\mu g\ g^{-1}$ have been suggested as maximum limits for acceptability. In different countries, skatole or androstenone may be perceived by consumers to be more or less important contributors to overall taint. In Denmark and Sweden skatole seems more important, in France,

Table 6.14. Prevalence of taint in carcasses from boars as estimated in various studies.

Country	Frequency (%)	Reference
Denmark	5–10	Sandersen, 1993
Norway	14	Froystein *et al.*, 1993
Canada	5–15	Xue *et al.*, 1996

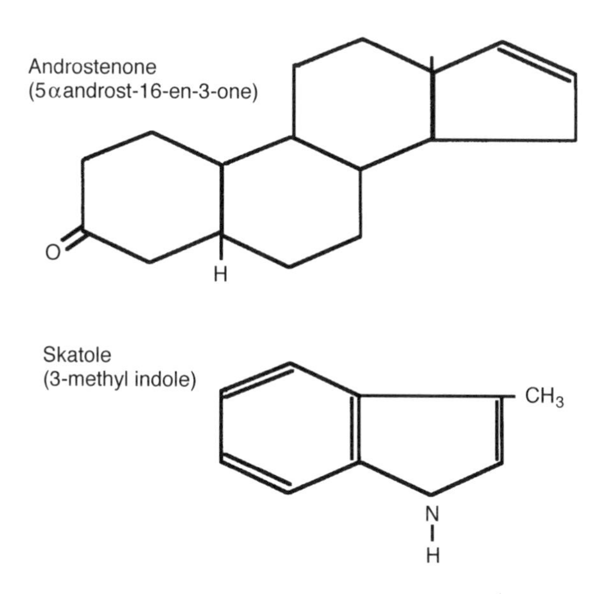

Fig. 6.1. The chemical structures of androstenone and skatole.

Germany and Canada androstenone. This may reflect variation in the levels of androstenone and skatole in different pig populations, differences in animal husbandry or cooking methods, or simply cultural differences in the way meat flavours and odours are perceived.

There is some evidence that taint is more prevalent in carcasses from some breeds such as the Duroc. Skatole levels in fat are generally proportional to skatole production in the gut. This depends on the amount of tryptophan in the diet and the conditions in the large intestine. Skatole levels are reduced in pigs fed some types of high-fibre diets, for example those containing sugarbeet pulp, in wet feeding systems, where food consumption is restricted, and in husbandry systems where the pigs are cleaner, for example on slatted floors where access to dung (which contains skatole) is reduced. Cooking methods may affect taint levels, with higher temperatures reducing perceived taint. The size of pig is important. As carcass weights increase, the proportion of boars starting to mature sexually increases. These animals are likely to have higher androstenone levels in their carcasses. Traditionally in the UK, pigs have been slaughtered at lower weights than in many other countries and this could be important in reducing the impact of boar taint in consumers.

The very significant production advantages of raising boars instead of castrates, together with benefits to animal welfare, must therefore be set against the disadvantages of higher skin blemish and poorer meat quality in a proportion of carcasses. At present most countries feel that the disadvantages outweigh the advantages, but new developments in nutrition to control skatole levels, or new techniques to control androstenone concentrations, for example by immunization, or better methods to detect tainted carcasses at slaughter, may change this. A good review of much of the early research on the use of uncastrated male animals in general is that of Seideman *et al.* (1982). The problems of boar taint are well documented in Bonneau (1993) and Lundström and Bonneau (1996).

Chapter 7

The Effects of Live Animal Handling on Carcass and Meat Quality

The efforts of farmers to produce animals with good carcass and meat quality may be wasted if they are handled in less than optimal ways before slaughter. The importance of pre-slaughter handling in affecting quality is therefore increasingly recognized. Getting animals to slaughter (marketing) involves several stages. On the farm they may be individually selected, drafted and sometimes weighed and, in the case of pigs, tattooed to identify them. Groups of marketable animals may be made up from different rearing pens. Most transport is nowadays by road vehicles although in the past railways were important. Vehicles are usually specially designed. Ventilation requirements are very important, particularly when carrying stock at high ambient temperatures. Very low ambient temperatures may also be a problem. In parts of northern Europe, such as Finland, winter temperatures may drop below −20°C and the advantages of vehicles with completely controlled ventilation have been demonstrated (Honkavaara, 1993).

The Marketing Process

Live animal handling

Loading and unloading animals can be difficult and stressful. Some vehicles require the use of steep loading ramps which animals find difficult to negotiate. Pigs, especially, are more easily loaded and unloaded using vehicle tailboard hoists or tail-lifts. Animals may be reluctant to move out of pens or through races. Advantage can be taken of their natural behavioural characteristics both in the design and the operation of handling facilities. Much of our knowledge in this area, and particularly its practical application, comes from the work of Temple Grandin in North America (Grandin, 1991). An excellent series of papers covering various aspects of the handling of livestock both during transport and in slaughter plants is given in Grandin (1993).

The harvesting of poultry consists of catching the birds and placing them in transport crates (cooping). Broiler chickens are mostly reared on litter such as wood shavings in sheds housing many thousands of birds. Hens are often housed in battery cages and removal from these at the end of their laying life is more difficult than catching broilers. Older designs of battery cage do not allow easy access. Catching hens from 'alternative' systems, such as percheries, which give the birds more choice of movement, is also difficult because of the large amount of furniture, perches and nest boxes which restrict access.

Birds are picked up manually by teams of catchers or by mechanical 'harvesters' in which rotating rubber fingers collect and encourage the birds onto moving conveyors (Berry *et al.*, 1990). There is considerable economic pressure to harvest birds quickly so that it is difficult to accord to each individual the care that is desirable to prevent physical damage. Mechanical harvesters may help to reduce damage although little information is available on the extent of the improvement.

The crates may be loose or form the drawers of 'modules'. A module is a metal framework that can be handled and loaded onto a flat bed lorry by a forklift truck. The crates are of different heights for the different species, for example they are taller for turkeys. A module might carry 12 drawers each holding 20–25 broilers. A single vehicle might transport 6000 birds. The closely stacked crates restrict airflow and ventilation may be poor. Birds on the inside of a load may suffer hyperthermia while those on the outside may become very cold. In cold weather, side curtains may be used to protect these birds. However, there is a high probability of thermal stress being suffered by at least some birds in transit (Webster *et al.*, 1993; Kettlewell *et al.*, 1993).

Animals may be sent directly from the farm or production unit to the slaughter plant, or may be sold via collecting stations or live auction markets. The latter options increase the time between leaving the farm and slaughter, and the chances of different groups of animals being mixed together. The introduction of computer auctions, where animals are sold based on a description, and without the need to take them to central collection points, may be beneficial if the duration of handling is thereby reduced.

Times spent between leaving the farm and slaughter

Animals can spend considerable times in transit. Total marketing times of over 12 h have been recorded for poultry, and times over 30 h for pigs and sheep in the UK (Warriss, 1992). Marketing times for cattle reared extensively under 'range' conditions can be very long. In Australia, such animals may travel for up to 2 weeks. Pigs have been exported from The Netherlands in northern Europe to southern Europe, journeys of 1500 km that can take up to 40 h. As the slaughtering industry in many countries becomes centralized into fewer, larger plants, marketing times and the distances animals must travel to slaughter are likely on average to increase and will tend to continue to do so.

On arrival at the plant, animals are held for various lengths of time before slaughter in a lairage or stockyard. They need to be supplied with water and, if appropriate, bedding and food. Generally, the conditions in the lairage need to be conducive to the animals resting so that ideally they recover from the rigours of transport. Most animals spend between 1 and 24 h in lairage. In some countries a minimum period – often 24 h – is prescribed, in others a maximum. In the UK the maximum time is 72 h.

The stresses associated with marketing

Even when carried out with care and consideration the marketing process is inherently stressful to animals in that it involves removal from their home environment, loading and unloading onto vehicles, often long journeys and holding in unfamiliar surroundings. This results in their being potentially exposed to physical stresses such as extremes of temperature, vibration and changes in acceleration, noise, confinement and crowding. There are also psychological stresses such as the breakdown of social groups and mixing with unfamiliar animals, unfamiliar or noxious smells and novel environments. Because animals are not usually fed before and during transport, and because water may not be available all the time, they may suffer from hunger, thirst and fatigue.

The effects on carcass and meat quality

The way the animal responds to these stresses, and the effects associated with them, can influence carcass and meat quality. In many cases, carcass quality equates to carcass yield and is therefore relatively easy to relate to economic loss. For example, total loss results if an animal dies during transport. Losses of variable size may occur if the carcass is damaged through bruising, haemorrhage, fighting or other trauma necessitating removal of the damaged tissue. Smaller, but economically significant losses occur if animals are subjected to a period of food or water deprivation and the stresses associated with transport. The most commonly recognized consequences of poor pre-slaughter handling on lean meat quality are pale, soft, exudative (PSE) meat in pigs and dark, firm, dry (DFD) meat in pigs and cattle. The full economic consequences of lean meat quality defects are difficult to quantify accurately.

Carcass Quality Effects

Mortality of animals during transport

Death of an animal results in total loss of value. The problem affects mainly pigs and broiler chickens; ruminants seem to be generally more resilient (Table 7.1). The high figure for sheep in Australia relates to animals exported by sea to the Middle East. The sheep are sometimes in a poor state before shipping, the journey is long and the conditions are arduous. Sometimes they will not eat.

In European countries the number of pigs dying during or shortly after transport ranges from about 0.1% to above 1%. Two major factors influence the incidence: environmental temperature and genotype. In northern Europe, below an average daily temperature of 10°C the incidence is very low, between 10° and 18°C it rises, and above 18°C there is a very rapid increase in mortality (Fig. 7.1). This leads to a well-defined seasonal effect with most deaths during the hottest months. However, pigs reared in hotter countries appear to be tolerant of higher temperatures to some degree. Stress-susceptible breeds of pig, which often have better carcass conformation and greater muscular development, are much more prone to dying in transport. This largely explains the variation between countries, many more pigs dying in places where genes from stress-susceptible breeds are widely disseminated.

In studies carried out in the UK, the mortality of transported broilers has ranged up to nearly 0.6%. The average is around 0.2%. Although this appears relatively low, because of the large numbers of broilers transported every year (750 million), the loss equates to over a

Table 7.1. Some recorded mortality rates during transport.

Species	Country	Mortality (%)	Reference
Pig	UK	0.07	Warriss and Brown, 1994
Broiler	UK	0.19	Warriss *et al.*, 1992
Hen	UK	0.2–0.5	Swarbrick, 1986
Sheep	UK	0.02	Knowles *et al.*, 1994a
Sheep	Australia	1–2.5	Higgs *et al.*, 1991

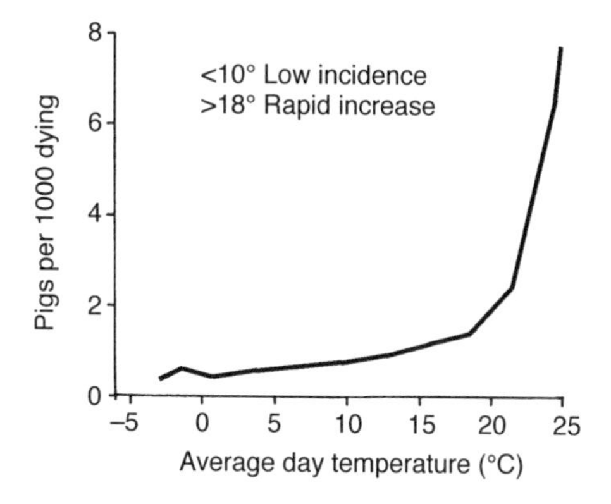

Fig. 7.1. The influence of temperature on transport deaths in pigs (based on data in Allen and Smith, 1974).

million birds. The mortality is higher in longer journeys (Fig. 7.2). As in pigs, higher ambient temperatures are associated with higher mortality. In both species adequate ventilation of the transport vehicles is therefore of paramount importance. In confined conditions birds lose heat (thermoregulate) at high temperatures largely by panting. At high humidities the effectiveness of panting is reduced or nullified. Hot, humid conditions therefore limit the bird's ability to lose body heat.

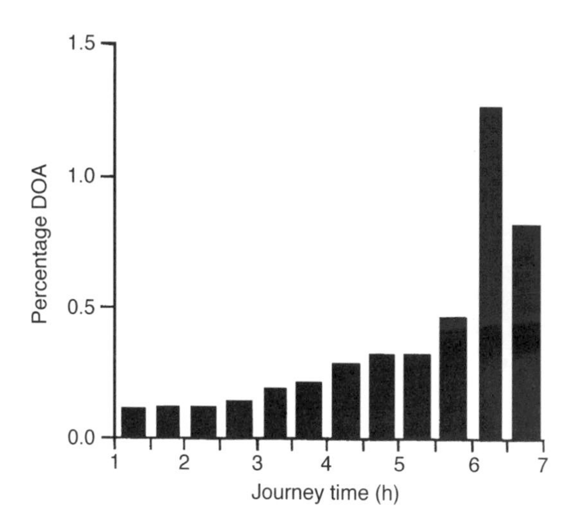

Fig. 7.2. Influence of journey time on the percentage of birds recorded as dead on arrival (DOA) at a poultry processing plant. The data relate to 3.2 million birds transported in 1113 journeys (based on information in Warriss *et al.*, 1992).

Carcass damage

Carcass damage can take the form of bruising and haemorrhages, skin blemishes or, particularly in poultry, broken bones. Bruising can occur at any point in the marketing chain from handling on the farm, through transport, to the time immediately after stunning but before the animal is bled out. In a bruise, blood from damaged blood vessels accumulates. Bruised tissue therefore looks unsightly and is usually trimmed, reducing yield as well as frequently leading to downgrading. The cost of this downgrading may be greater than the value of the trimmed meat. Surveys have shown that about 2% of pork hams are bruised in the USA and that over 30% of bulls and 80% of cows show some bruises.

In terms of quality, in red meat species bruising is an aesthetic rather than a hygiene problem. Bruised tissue probably has no greater initial microbiological load than normal tissue. However, because it tends to be handled more, for example at inspection and trimming, it may pick up a higher microbial load. For poultry the situation may be different, but for reasons that are unclear, and bruising can be associated with a higher susceptibility to spoilage. Although in the fresh state bruised tissue may be aesthetically undesirable, its use in processed products may be acceptable. The microbiological and organoleptic properties of bruised meat have been described (Gill and Harrison, 1982; Gill, 1994).

Bruising can occur in pigs by misuse of slap markers (used to tattoo an identification mark on the animal's back), by rough handling, and internally. This occurs when injuries are caused by the pig's back legs slipping apart on poor or wet surfaces. In cattle it can be caused by animals slipping and falling, or through the inappropriate use of sticks. An important cause of bruising in cattle is the agonistic behaviour, such as butting and mounting, which occurs on mixing animals from different rearing pen groups. This is a particular problem with young bulls.

Bruising is often caused by trying to move animals too quickly, particularly over uneven or slippery floors. Too high or too low a stocking density during transport can cause bruising. Understocking allows animals to be thrown about when the vehicle is moving. This is especially important for adult cattle which, except on the longest journeys, may not lie down. In the close confinement of holding pens or vehicles, horned cattle can be a problem in causing damage to other stock. Cutting off the tips of the horns before transport, known as 'tipping' has not been found to reduce bruising. Other factors that have been shown to increase the level of the problem in cattle are long periods without food, and chronic stress. Marketing animals through live auctions increases the levels of bruising in both sheep and cattle (Table 7.2). This may be because it increases the number of journeys the animals make or because of the handling that occurs in the market.

Table 7.2. The effect of marketing through live auctions on the prevalence of bruising in sheep and cattle.

		Method of marketing	
Species	Country	Directly from farm	Through live auction
Sheep	UK	12	20[a]
Sheep	UK	1.1	1.4[b]
Cattle	UK	4.8	7.0[c]
Cattle	Australia	2.8	3.5[d]

[a] Cockram and Lee, 1991; [b] Knowles *et al.*, 1994b; [c] McNally and Warriss, 1996; [d] Eldridge *et al.*, 1984. The figures represent the percentage of carcasses showing bruising in studies a, b and c, and the numbers of bruises per animal in study d.

The differences in overall levels of bruising in the two studies on sheep are because of the different recording methods used. Cockram and Lee (1991) recorded all bruises, Knowles *et al.* (1994b) recorded only bruises severe enough to be commercially important in that they led to economic loss. The studies on cattle also recorded only commercially significant bruising.

McNally and Warriss (1997) found that the prevalence of bruising varied with the particular market. It ranged from 2 to 18%. Distance travelled from market to slaughterplant could not explain the variation. However, there was a correlation between bruising and the amount of stick-marking on the carcasses. This suggested that the greater bruising was caused through less careful handling by the drovers and stockmen, rather than poorer facilities, since greater stick-marking is caused by people hitting animals more.

Bruises can vary both in number and severity or size. Various methods of assessing bruising have been developed. An example is the Australian Bruise Scoring System (Anderson and Horder, 1979). Attempts to estimate the age of bruises, in order better to identify the factors causing them, have not been very successful. The characteristic colour changes seen are caused by the breakdown of the red haemoglobin in the blood to bilirubin (yellowish) then to biliverdin (green) but they are relatively insensitive indices of bruise age. More sensitive methods to estimate bruise age have been based on measurement of the concentration of bilirubin (Hamdy *et al.*, 1957) or histological changes (McCausland and Dougherty, 1978).

Skin blemish in pigs

A related problem is the superficial skin damage caused by fighting in pigs, particularly between unfamiliar animals. This takes the form of unsightly lacerations (Fig. 7.3) and detracts from the appearance of rind-on products (those sold with the skin on). Pigs reared together develop stable social hierarchies. When animals are selected for slaughter, pigs from different rearing pens are frequently mixed together to make up batches of individuals with similar live weights. They may also get mixed in lairage. This disrupts the established hierarchies and individuals, particularly the more dominant ones, will often fight to establish new dominance orders. The fighting can be severe and leads to the lacerations on the skin, particularly on the shoulders and, usually to a lesser extent, along the loins and hams. In extreme cases it may lead to the carcass being downgraded. Surveys in the UK have shown about 5–7% downgraded carcasses (Warriss, 1984c; MLC, 1985). The problem is more common in boars than gilts or castrates, this reflecting the more aggressive nature of the uncastrated male pig (see Table 6.12).

Petherick and Blackshaw (1987) reviewed the factors that affect agonistic behaviour in pigs. Competition for food and, by implication,

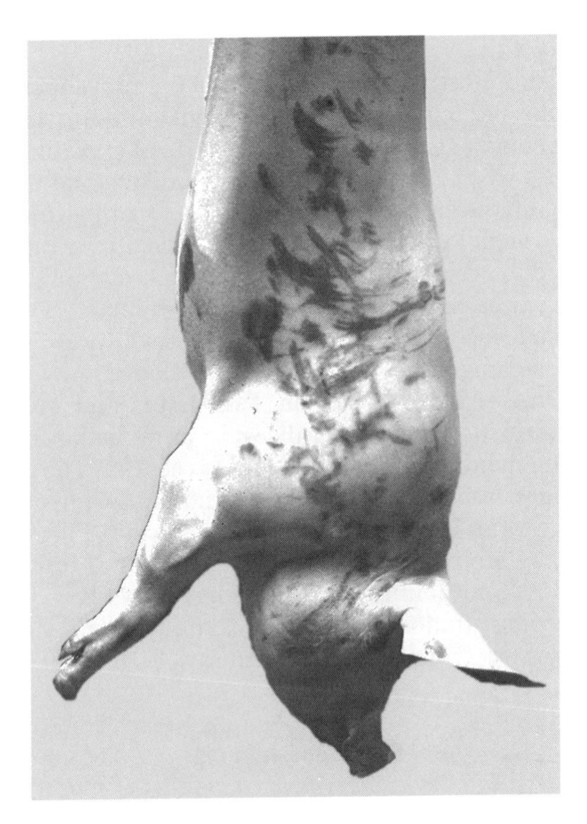

Fig. 7.3. Lacerations on a pig carcass caused by fighting pre-slaughter.

factors that promote hunger, increase aggression. So also does competition for space. Having sufficient space to be able to easily retreat from aggressive congeners is important. It is known that pigs use pheromones to communicate, particularly in relation to potential aggression. Androstenone may be an important pheromone and there is evidence that spraying it on pigs can reduce agonistic behaviour. Interestingly, Grandin and Bruning (1992) have found that the presence of a sexually mature boar in a group of slaughter-weight pigs reduced the incidence and intensity of fighting. It has been suggested that odour-masking substances, particularly those with a very strong smell, could help reduce aggression, but there is little or no evidence that they are effective. Tranquillizers such as azaperone will reduce fighting but their use in slaughter pigs is precluded by the need to ensure that carcasses and meat are free from residues.

Broken bones and bruising in poultry

Broken bones are a particular problem in poultry, and especially in culled hens. Gregory and Wilkins (1989b) found that 29% of battery hens in the UK had broken bones at slaughter. A corresponding survey of broilers indicated a level of 3%. The high level in hens is attributable to the weakness of the skeleton caused by demineralization of the bones and a restricted opportunity to exercise (Knowles and Broom, 1990). The situation is exacerbated by lack of sufficient care as the birds are removed from the battery cages when they are culled at the end of lay. Broken bones may cause bone splinters in the meat. These can be dangerous to the consumer if not detected after deboning.

Bruises in poultry may be caused by both ante-mortem handling or by stunning at slaughter. For example, red wingtips can be associated with severe flapping *ante mortem* as well as certain stunning procedures. The reported levels of bruising vary widely from about 2 to 20%. Most bruises occur on the breast, followed by the legs and wings, then the backs and thighs. Strain of bird, season, degree of muscling, care during handling, particularly being picked up by one leg, and struggling on the shackles used to suspend the birds before slaughter, have all been suggested as factors influencing the level of the problem. Modern strains of turkeys, which are bigger but younger at slaughter, are very prone to carcass damage (Barbut *et al.*, 1990).

Reduction of live weight and carcass yield by inanition and transport

It is inevitable that animals be deprived of food for some time before slaughter. Losses in live weight are due to loss of gut fill and excretory losses. Losses in carcass weight are caused both by mobilization of tissues to provide energy for maintaining the vital functions of the body, and dehydration which often accompanies fasting and transport. These losses in live or carcass weight are sometimes referred to as 'shrinkage'. Shrinkage is loss of potential yield.

Loss of live weight in pigs begins almost directly after feed withdrawal; the rate of loss is about 0.2% h^{-1} (Warriss, 1985). The time when carcass loss begins is less clearly defined but is probably between about 9 and 18 h after the last meal. This reflects the rapid passage of food through the gut in pigs, food reaching the small intestine 4–8 h after ingestion, and most nutrient absorption occurring within 9 h. The rate of carcass loss is about 0.1% h^{-1}. What this can mean in practice is that keeping pigs in lairage overnight without food may result in a reduction of 1.4% of potential carcass weight. This is nearly 1 kg in a 90 kg pig. On long journeys dehydration is probably an important factor. Although the influence of transport on yields is less well defined than that of fasting, a loss of 2% of carcass weight after a 6 h journey in hot weather has been recorded in pork pigs.

Because of their proportionally larger guts, ruminants are less susceptible than pigs to short periods of inanition. However, in sheep, economically significant losses in carcass yield can be detected after periods of food deprivation that occur during normal marketing. There is also a progressive loss of liver weight and, initially, a large part of this is attributable to loss of stored glycogen, which the animal uses as an energy source. With longer fasting, muscle glycogen stores are also mobilized.

In adult cattle the gut contents can account for 20% of the body weight and a large proportion of the loss in live weight over the first 24 h of food deprivation is attributable to loss of faeces. Gut fill is larger in animals on high roughage pasture than in those fed grain diets, and in animals that have recently drunk. Previous diet and access to water are therefore important influences on the patterns of live weight loss in cattle. Based on data collected from 26 publications, Shorthose and Wythes (1988) produced a relationship showing mean losses of live weight ranging from about 7% after 12 h to 11% after 72 h (Fig. 7.4). The effects of inanition on carcass yield are poorly defined. Various reports have recorded loss starting between 17 and 48 h after the beginning of a fast. Reported losses in carcass yield after 48 h range from 1 to 8%. Much of the research on the effects of transport on shrinkage in cattle has been carried out in North America and Australia. Animals have lost between 6 and 12% of their live weight in journeys of 500–2000 km. Losses in carcass weight range from 0 to 4% in journeys up to 2000 km.

Food and water deprivation in broiler chickens lead to live weight losses averaging about 0.2–0.3% h^{-1}. Veerkamp (1986) pointed out that from estimates of a bird's heat production (5 W $kg^{-0.75}$) and the

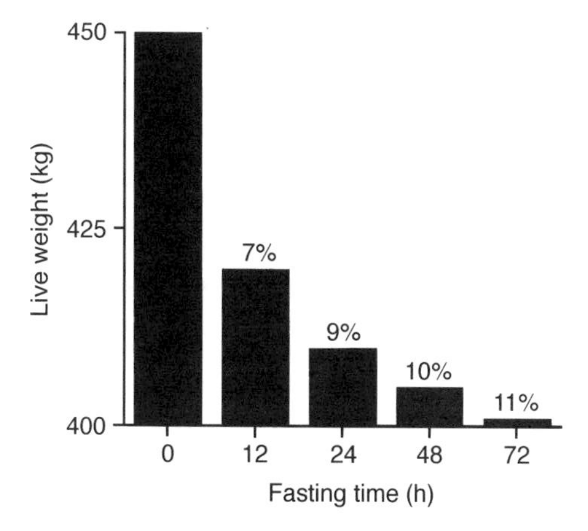

Fig. 7.4. Liveweight loss in fasted cattle based on information derived from 26 studies by Shorthose and Wythes (1988) as summarized by Warriss (1995).

energy value of animal tissue (7500 J g^{-1}), one would expect a loss of 0.22% h^{-1} body weight. At high ambient temperatures the loss is greater because the bird's heat production will increase and more moisture will be lost by evaporation from the respiratory tract. The size of carcass yield losses is poorly defined.

Other important quality implications of food and water deprivation

As well as affecting carcass yield, the times for which animals are deprived of food and water before slaughter may have other implications for quality. Pigs fed too soon before transport show a slightly increased mortality rate. Because of this, pigs should not have access to food within 4 h of loading on to the vehicle. Also, food that will not have had time to be digested will be wasted. To minimize carcass yield losses, however, the total time from last feed to actual slaughter should ideally be not more than about 12 h in pigs, and certainly not more than 18 h (Warriss, 1996a).

With longer food deprivation periods the stomach contents of ruminants become more watery, increasing the chances of head, tongue and carcass contamination, either through regurgitation or through accidental cutting of the gut wall during carcass dressing. Very full guts, however, make their handling and hygienic removal more difficult so a compromise must be reached. The disposal of large quantities of gut contents at the abattoir is also costly because they increase the dirtiness of the effluent water, incurring greater processing costs before discharge into the sewerage system.

In sheep and cattle subjected to long periods without water, the removal of skin or hide is more difficult. This may result in greater tearing of the underlying tissues and a poorer appearance to the carcass surface. If the flaying is done by hand the greater effort required may increase chances of contamination of the carcass with dirt from the skin.

In red meat species there is some evidence that long food deprivation can lead to a build-up of pathogenic bacteria such as *Salmonella* in the gut. However, increased times between leaving the farm and slaughter also tend to increase the prevalence of *Salmonella*-infected cattle (Grau *et al.*, 1968) and keeping pigs in lairage for 2–3 days prior to slaughter increased the incidence of *Salmonella* even when the pigs were fed (Hansen *et al.*, 1964).

With poultry, the risk of contamination of the carcass with *Salmonella* and *Campylobacter* is perhaps greater. The transport of birds in stacked crates, often with perforated floors, gives great potential for faecal contamination of the outsides of the live birds. Fasting periods of up to 10 h have been recommended for poultry but even prolonged food withdrawal will not completely prevent defaecation. Paradoxically, longer feed withdrawal may increase the prevalence of *Salmonella* in the crop of laying hens (Humphrey *et al.*, 1993) and has also been associated with a higher prevalence of birds testing positive for *Campylobacter jejuni* in cloacal swabs before slaughter and caecal swabs after (Willis *et al.*, 1996).

Lean Meat Quality

Poor ante-mortem handling can produce PSE or DFD meat and may influence eating quality in more direct but as yet little understood ways. There is also some evidence that stress pre-slaughter may predispose animals to showing bloodsplash in their muscles and other tissues.

PSE and DFD meat

PSE and DFD meat are two of the major quality problems facing the meat industry. PSE affects pigs and DFD occurs in all species. However, PSE-like characteristics, particularly pale colour, have been reported in some turkey (Sosnicki, 1993) and chicken (Boulianne and King, 1995) meat recently. Also, some of the deep muscles of the leg of the beef carcass may cool sufficiently slowly under some conditions to lead to characteristics reminiscent of PSE pork and PSE has been found in beef m. longissimus dorsi, although the prevalence is very low

(Aalhus *et al.*, 1998). The names describe the characteristics of the muscle in comparison with normal meat. Having said this, there is no universally accepted definition of either condition in terms of objective instrumental measurements.

Often, they are defined by the pH value of the meat at specific times (Table 7.3). PSE meat is commonly defined as having a pH at 45 min *post mortem* of <6. However, in some countries, particularly where the prevalence is high, a stricter criterion, for example a pH of <5.8, may be used. DFD meat is often defined as having an ultimate pH – measured after 12–48 hours *post mortem* (depending on the species), of $\geqslant 6$. Again, a value of 6.2, rather than 6, may be used. However, particularly where the meat is to be stored in vacuum packs, a lower figure of 5.8 may be preferred. These limit values do not take account of variation between different muscles of the carcass. For 'redder' muscles in pig carcasses, especially those found in the neck and shoulder region, much higher values are appropriate. For example, values of <6.3 are considered normal for the pig m. semispinalis capitis.

Using objective indices of PSE and DFD tends to produce higher estimates of the prevalence of the conditions in a population than using subjective assessment. Perhaps this is a reflection of the lower sensitivity of the subjective approach where only more extreme examples of the conditions are recognized. Beef that is DFD is sometimes referred to as dark cutting (DC) or dark cutting beef (DCB).

Prevalence and cost to the meat industry

Surveys have suggested an increasing prevalence of the problems. In the UK there is some evidence that up to one-quarter of all pork may show PSE characteristics. In other words it may be too pale, or too wet, or both. About a tenth may show DFD characteristics – it may be too dark, too dry or both. A recent large survey in the USA showed 10% of pork to be PSE, 4% to be DFD and 13% to suffer from two-toning. The total cost of PSE to the American pork industry was estimated at 30 million dollars in 1992, that of DFD pork 0.2 million dollars and that of two-toning 23 million dollars. Two-toning is a poorly defined condition in which either parts of a muscle are too dark and other parts too pale, or in which adjacent muscles in the carcass show these

Table 7.3. Typical 'limit' pH values for PSE, normal and DFD pig m. longissimus dorsi.

	PSE	Normal	DFD
pH_{45}	<6.0	6.4	6.4
pH_u	5.3	5.5	$\geqslant 6.0$

contrasting characteristics in an abnormal way. It is described in more detail later. Some reported prevalences of PSE and DFD pork are shown in Table 7.4.

Surveys of DCB have shown widely different incidences in different countries and between different classes of stock (Warriss, 1990). Young bulls are particularly prone to the condition, with prevalences of over 25% having been recorded in some countries. The problem also occurs in veal calves.

Problems associated with PSE and DFD meat

The colour of meat is one of the most important criteria consumers use to select meat. Meat which is too pale or too dark is discriminated against in preference to normal coloured meat (Topel *et al.*, 1976; Wachholz *et al.*, 1978). The large amount of exudate (drip loss or purge) from PSE meat, especially if it collects in the packaging, also contributes to the undesirable appearance. This exudate leads to weight loss and therefore reduced yield both of fresh meat and of processed products like hams and bacon (Kauffman *et al.*, 1978; Smith and Lesser, 1982). DFD meat has poor processing characteristics with slow or uneven formation of cured meat pigments. Flavour development is poor in processed products and flavour is poor in cooked fresh DFD meat. PSE pork tends to taste dry and have poor texture after cooking (Bennett *et al.*, 1973; Jeremiah, 1984).

DFD meat has a high spoilage potential, so does not keep well and has a short shelf life (Newton and Gill, 1981). This is for two reasons. DFD meat is caused by glycogen depletion *ante mortem* and is therefore characterized by very low levels of carbohydrates in the muscle. The low levels of carbohydrates present in the meat restrict the growth of lactic acid-producing bacteria and this encourages the growth of bacteria that metabolize amino acids and proteins. These produce unpleasant smelling waste products. The high pH value of the meat promotes this bacterial growth. The spoilage risk is a serious problem in processed raw (uncooked) products. Meat with a high pH can be a

Table 7.4. Estimates of the prevalence of PSE and DFD pork.

Country	Percentage PSE	Percentage DFD	Reference
USA	16	10	Cassens *et al.*, 1992
Australia	10	15	Warner and Eldridge, 1988
Australia	32	15	Trout, 1992
Canada	20–90[a]	–	Fortin, 1989
Portugal	30	10	Santos *et al.*, 1994
Various[b]	≤20	≤35	Warriss, 1987

[a] Pale meat.

[b] Reported in various studies.

problem if vacuum-packed. A green coloration may develop due to the formation of sulphmyoglobin. This is caused by the haem pigment myoglobin reacting with hydrogen sulphide produced by bacteria under the anaerobic conditions (Taylor and Shaw, 1977).

Causes of PSE and DFD meat

Both PSE and DFD meat are caused by stress experienced by the live animal at and before slaughter. Acute (short-term) stress around the time of slaughter leads to PSE meat by stimulating the rate of acidification of the muscles immediately *post mortem* so that low pH values are reached in the muscle when the temperature of the carcass is still high (Fig. 7.5). In Fig. 7.5 the patterns of acidification are idealized. In practice, the pattern varies enormously even in normal meat. Measured series of pH values from a particular muscle often do not fall on smooth curves. The ultimate pH reached in DFD meat can vary considerably, the important point being that it is higher than normal.

As we have seen, stress-susceptible genotypes of pigs are much more prone to producing extreme PSE meat than normal animals. Poultry white muscles such as the breast muscle (m. pectoralis) also tend to acidify rapidly *post mortem*. In broiler chickens the carcass cools quickly and therefore the combination of low pH and high temperature needed to produce the PSE condition rarely occurs. However, because of their greater bulk, turkey muscles cool more slowly and the temperature can still be 40°C or more when pH values

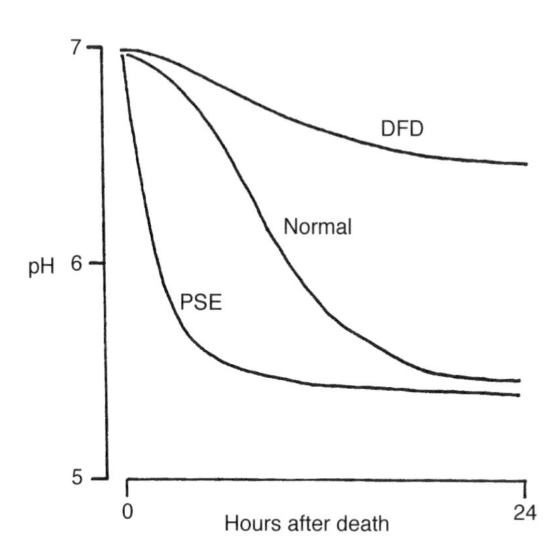

Fig. 7.5. The pattern of acidification in PSE, normal and DFD meat illustrated schematically.

of around 6 are reached. This may well predispose them to PSE-like characteristics.

In PSE meat the combination of low pH and high temperature causes denaturation of some of the muscle proteins leading to a reduction in the amount of water they bind. Shrinkage of the myofibrillar components (the myofilament lattice) expels the resultant fluid into the extracellular space (between the muscle fibres) which increases in volume. When the muscle is cut the extra fluid exudes to produce the exudate (drip or purge) seen in all meat to some extent, but especially associated with PSE pork. The large amount of exudate reflects a poorer water-holding capacity. Light scattering from the meat surface is probably caused by differences in the refractive indices of the sarcoplasm and myofibrils. The larger the difference, the higher the scattering and the paler the meat appears. The shrinkage of the myofilament lattice increases the amount of light reflected from the meat. At high light scattering the amount of absorbed light is low and the importance of the haem pigments (myoglobin) in selectively absorbing green light, and therefore looking red, is reduced. This makes PSE meat look less red and more yellow. The low pH also tends to promote oxidation of the haem pigments from the purple or red myoglobin (Mb) and oxymyoglobin (MbO_2) to the brown metmyoglobin (met Mb).

The acidification that occurs in muscle *post mortem* is caused by the breakdown of glycogen to lactic acid (Chapter 5). If glycogen is depleted by chronic (long-term) stress before slaughter then less lactic acid can be formed and the meat does not acidify normally, the ultimate pH remaining high. The relationship between glycogen concentration in beef and ultimate pH reached is shown in Fig. 7.6. Muscle that will produce meat with a normal pH contains about 10–20 mg g^{-1} (1–2%) glycogen. Reducing the glycogen to below around 8 mg g^{-1} results in elevation of the ultimate pH, and the greater the reduction, the higher the pH.

The high pH results in relatively little denaturation of the proteins, water is tightly bound and little or no exudate is formed. There is little or no shrinkage of the myofilament lattice and the differences in refractive index of the myofibrils and sarcoplasm are reduced. The muscle presents a closed, translucent structure that absorbs rather than reflects light. This makes the meat appear dark. The closed structure reduces the diffusion of oxygen into the muscle from the surface and any oxygen that does reach the interior is used up by the high cytochrome activity encouraged by the high pH. This results in only a very thin surface layer of bright red oxygenated myoglobin (MbO_2) allowing the purple colour of the underlying reduced myoglobin (Mb) to show through (see Chapter 8). A summary of events leading to PSE and DFD meat is shown in Table 7.5.

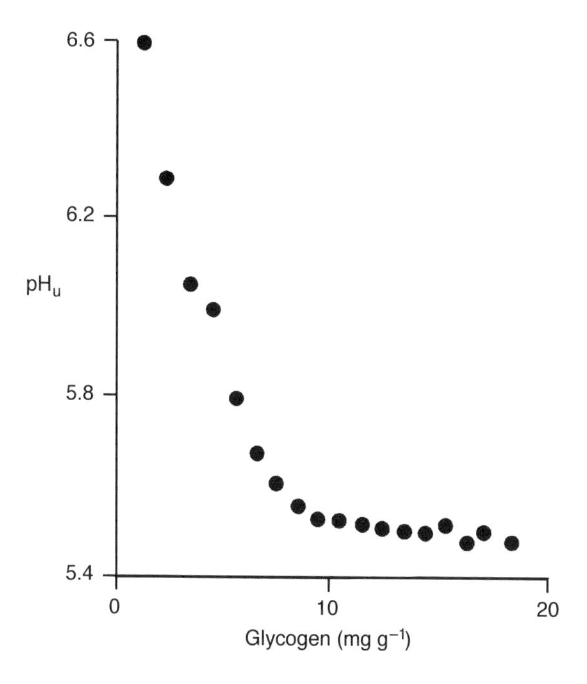

Fig. 7.6. The relationship of ultimate pH (pH_u) to the concentration of glycogen present in the muscle (m. longissimus dorsi) of cattle at death. Each point is the mean of a large number of values. Overall there were 2345 observations. Reprinted from Warriss (1990) with permission from Elsevier Science.

Table 7.5. Summary of events leading to PSE and DFD meat.

PSE	DFD
• Acute stress	• Chronic stress
• Rapid initial acidification	• Reduced glycogen
• Low initial pH at high carcass temperature	• High ultimate pH
• Proteins denature	• Proteins do not denature
• Low water-holding capacity	• High water-holding capacity
• 'Bound' water lost	• Water held by proteins
• Muscle fibres separate	• Fibres tightly packed
• Large extracellular space	• Small extracellular space
• Light scattering high	• Light scattering low
• Surface appears pale	• Surface dark
• Low pH promotes Mb oxidation	• O_2 diffusion inhibited by closed structure
• Reduction in absorption of green light by Mb	• O_2 used up by high cytochrome activity
• Meat looks less red	• MbO_2 layer thin and underlying Mb (purple) shows through

The propensity of muscles to become PSE or DFD can be influenced by metabolic type as reflected in their fibre type composition. Red, oxidative fibres have a relatively low concentration of glycogen, which is easily depleted. Muscles containing a high proportion of them, like the m. adductor of the pig, therefore tend to be more prone to producing DFD meat. In contrast, muscles with a large complement of white, glycolytic fibres, like the pig m. longissimus dorsi, which have a high glycogen content and high glycolytic capacity, are prone to the PSE condition. It is important to realize that the concentrations of the haem pigments are not different in PSE and DFD meat; it is the changed structure of the muscle that causes the difference in appearance. A summary of actual measured differences in the colour and drip loss of normal, PSE and DFD pork is shown in Table 7.6.

In this table, colour is defined in terms of lightness, hue and saturation, and reflectance. These measurements are described fully in Chapter 11. Essentially, however, lightness and reflectance measure how pale or dark the colour is, hue whether it is yellow, orange, red, green etc., and saturation or chroma, the purity of the colour. It can be seen that, not only is PSE meat darker, but the other characteristics of the colour also differ. So, DFD meat looks dull and more purple than normal meat while PSE meat has a more yellowish colour. However, in extreme cases the colour may appear grey. Although there is an obvious general correlation between colour and drip loss, this is not absolute. It is possible to get pork that is pale but not exudative, or normal coloured but exudative. This has led to some researchers constructing more complicated systems of subjective categories (Kauffman *et al.*, 1993; Warner *et al.*, 1993).

Two-toning

In general it may be said that chronic pre-slaughter stress leads to DFD meat and acute pre-slaughter stress leads to PSE meat. This is an oversimplification because to some degree different pre-slaughter handling

Table 7.6. Colour and loss of exudate in pork (m. longissimus dorsi) of different quality (from Warriss and Brown, 1993).

	Pork quality assessed subjectively				
	Extremely DFD	Slightly DFD	Normal	Slightly PSE	Extremely PSE
Lightness (L*)	42	48	54	60	66
Hue (°)	1	22	38	48	53
Saturation (chroma)	3	5	7	9	12
Reflectance (EEL)	20	32	44	56	67
Drip loss (%)	0	5	10	13	15

factors interact, and also different types of muscle tend to be more or less susceptible to PSE or DFD. For example, if muscle glycogen is depleted by chronic pre-slaughter stress, then the ultimate pH in that muscle will be high. The muscle cannot exhibit the PSE condition even if the pig is of a breed predisposed to producing PSE meat and is subjected to acute stress as well. Also, as pointed out previously, 'white' muscles such as the m. longissimus dorsi in the back tend to be less susceptible to glycogen depletion than 'red' muscles such as are found in the ham. So, occasionally, a single carcass may show both PSE and DFD conditions in different muscles. This leads to so-called 'two-toning' if adjacent muscles are affected. Two-toning is particularly apparent in the ham. Confusingly, the term has also been used to describe the occurrence of both dark and pale coloured areas in the same muscle. This is a rare condition and its physiological and biochemical basis is rather unclear.

The development of both PSE and DFD meat can be associated with earlier development of rigor mortis. This is because ATP levels and the sources of ATP regeneration – creatine phosphate and glycogen – will be depleted in both conditions. In DFD meat the depletion of glycogen will have occurred before death and, in PSE meat, immediately after death by enhanced rates of glycolysis. Some pigs whose carcasses will subsequently show extreme PSE characteristics in the muscles may go into rigor even before the completion of dressing. A simple way of detecting this is to lift the forelimb of the hanging carcass. Stiffness of the shoulder joint indicates that rigor has set in.

Practical causes of PSE and DFD meat

PSE. The type of acute stress that can lead to PSE pork is that often occurring in the period immediately before stunning. The problem is greater in stress-susceptible genotypes. The increased size of modern slaughter plants has led to animals being killed and processed at higher line speeds since line speed is related to plant size. This is illustrated for pig slaughter points in Fig. 7.7. A plant killing 900 pigs h^{-1} has to deliver on average one pig to the slaughter point every 4 s. Even with carefully designed handling systems this may require considerable use of coercion and lead to high levels of stress in the animals. Pigs slaughtered in larger plants can also be stressed by the types of enclosed race systems and restraining conveyors, which immobilize and carry the pig forward, to deliver animals to the slaughter point. Pigs find the close confinement and restraint inherent in these systems stressful. This is particularly true if electric goads are used to move them in the races.

Troeger (1989) measured plasma adrenaline levels in pigs after different pre-slaughter handling procedures. Adrenaline is an index of stress. Compared with resting levels, careful driving of a group of

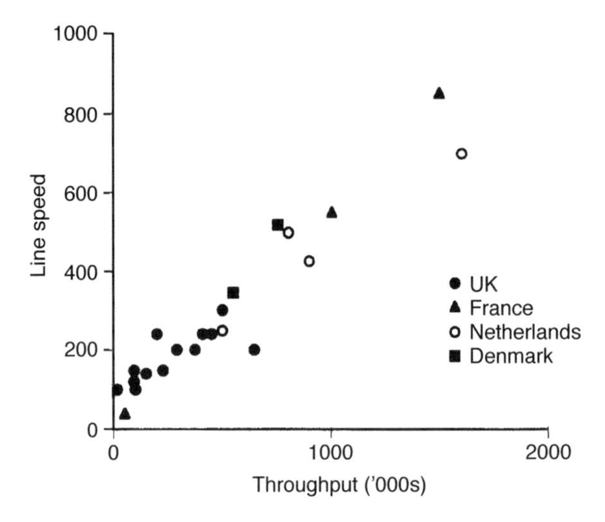

Fig. 7.7. The relationship between line speed (animals per hour) and size of plant based on 22 pig abattoirs in four European countries.

animals more than doubled adrenaline levels. Using coercion increased them fivefold while moving the pigs through a single file race increased them sevenfold. Passage through a V-shaped restraining conveyor elevated adrenaline concentration 12-fold. There is direct evidence that increased levels of stress at this time result in poorer meat quality. Pigs killed in plants operating handling systems subjectively assessed as producing high levels of stress in the animals had higher levels of lactic acid and the enzyme creatine kinase (CK) in their blood and produced paler, wetter meat (Table 7.7). Lactic acid and CK are also objective indices of stress.

Table 7.7. Indices of stress and meat quality in pigs killed in plants assessed as having low-stress or high-stress handling systems (based on Warriss *et al.*, 1994).

	Pigs killed in low-stress systems	Pigs killed in high-stress systems
Blood lactic acid (mg 100 ml^{-1})	64	140
Blood CK (U l^{-1})	965	1436
Percentage of pigs with lactic acid concentrations >100 mg 100 ml^{-1}	5.8	69.4
PQM probe value[a]	3.8	4.7
Percentage of carcasses with PQM probe values ≥6	7.5	16.8

[a] The PQM probe value is a measure of the electrical characteristics of the meat. Higher values are associated with paler, wetter meat.

DFD. Examples of chronic stress that can produce DFD meat are long periods without food (fasting), fatigue caused by very long transport under poor conditions, or the fighting that occurs when unfamiliar pigs are mixed together (Table 7.8). In this study, carcasses were categorized according to the amount of skin blemish. Pigs producing carcasses with greater damage had higher levels of the stress hormone cortisol and CK in their blood at slaughter, and had muscles that had higher ultimate pH and darker colour (lower FOP value), indicative of more DFD meat.

The major cause of dark cutting in cattle is allowing unfamiliar animals to mix pre-slaughter. The resulting agonistic behaviour directed at re-establishing dominance hierarchies takes the form of butting, pushing, mounting and 'chin resting'. The physical exertion associated with this, together with the effects of the psychological stress, depletes muscle glycogen. Handling procedures which prolong the time during which mixed cattle can interact, such as long lairage times, increase the prevalence of the problem. This is illustrated by data collected by Whittaker (1997) who compared the frequency of dark cutting in cattle killed on the day of arrival at the plant with that in animals held for 1 day or longer (Table 7.9). The greater effect in bulls is noticeable. Kreikemeier *et al.* (1998) found the incidence of dark cutting doubled from 0.8 to 1.6% in cattle held over a weekend or holiday rather than being killed within 12 h of arrival at the plant. Animals sold through live auction markets also show higher levels of dark cutting, presumably because of the greater chances of their being mixed with unfamiliar animals and the prolongation of the time for which they are mixed (Table 7.10).

In young bulls a correlation has been found between the severity of dark cutting and the level of physical activity shown when mixed with unfamiliar animals (Warriss, 1984b; Kenny and Tarrant, 1987). Muscle

Table 7.8. Effect of fighting on stress, as measured by circulating levels of cortisol and creatine kinase (CK) in the blood, and indices of meat quality (from Warriss, 1996d).

	Skin damage score[a]			
	1	2	3	4
Cortisol ($\mu g\ 100\ ml^{-1}$)	15	16	19	22
CK ($U\ l^{-1}$)	517	716	1119	1372
pH_u in m. longissimus	5.55	5.60	5.66	5.68
pH_u in m. adductor	5.77	5.88	6.03	6.15
FOP in m. adductor[b]	35	31	27	25

[a] Higher scores indicate worse damage/more fighting.
[b] Fibre optic probe measurement; lower values indicate darker meat.

Table 7.9. Effect of lairage time on the percentage of dark cutting in cattle (Whittaker, 1997).

	Animals killed on day of arrival	Animals held 1 day	Animals held 1.5 days or more
Bulls	4.7	10.0	12.5
Steers	2.4	3.3	3.7
Heifers	2.2	3.5	3.3

Table 7.10. Effect of source of animal on prevalence (%) of dark cutting in cattle (Whittaker, 1997).

	Animals sold direct from farm	Animals marketed through live auctions
Bulls	5.9	10.8
Steers	2.1	4.2
Heifers	1.9	4.0
Overall	2.4	4.4

glycogen stores are depleted when blood-borne metabolites, such as glucose and free fatty acids, are inadequate to fuel the intense or prolonged activity. Different muscles in the carcass exhibit dark cutting to different degrees. The m. longissimus dorsi tends to be worst affected, together with the larger muscles of the hindquarter. The forequarter muscles are largely unaffected. The are probably two reasons. First, the loin and hindquarter musculature is made greater use of during the physical interactions that occur between animals, particularly in pushing and mounting behaviours. Second, glycogen depletion patterns are different in white and red fibres. Depletion is more likely in fast red fibres as found in the m. longissimus and m. semimembranosus than in white fibres. Redder muscles therefore tend to be more prone to dark cutting.

As well as mixing unfamiliar animals, longer transport also sometimes increases dark cutting (Jones and Tong, 1989) but the effect is small. There is high variation between the prevalence of the problem at different plants for reasons that are unclear (Kreikemeier *et al.*, 1998). After glycogen depletion, the time taken for full recovery of muscle glycogen reserves in cattle is peculiarly long (McVeigh and Tarrant, 1980). Between 3 and 11 days are needed, although sufficient glycogen repletion occurs in 2 days' rest with access to feed and water to produce near-normal ultimate pH values in mixed groups of young bulls (Warriss *et al.*, 1984).

DFD in lambs is a problem in some countries. Sheep in New Zealand are washed pre-slaughter by swimming them through water. This may be repeated with very dirty animals so they are washed up to three times. The process leads to higher ultimate pH in the muscles of some animals and, when washing is combined with other stresses, the level of DFD meat may be very high. Carcasses from underfed sheep that had been sheared and washed showed a level of about 80% DFD compared with 12% in control animals (Bray *et al.*, 1989).

Measures to reduce the prevalence of PSE and DFD meat

Prevention of PSE and DFD meat relies on avoidance of stresses pre-slaughter. This is easier said than done since all animals are likely to be subjected to some stressors even with the most careful handling. Particularly regarding pigs, avoidance of the use of genotypes that are stress-susceptible would obviously be beneficial. Many specific handling procedures have been put forward to reduce stress. These include container transport to reduce loading and unloading stress and the use of controlled temperature vehicles.

Keeping animals in their rearing groups to prevent the problems associated with mixing unfamiliar animals is obvious but often difficult to achieve in practice. For mixed pigs the use of odour-masking substances is often suggested but there is little evidence of their effectiveness. Water sprays may reduce fighting and reduce the prevalence of DFD; by cooling pigs they may also reduce the occurrence of PSE. To prevent the mounting associated with aggressive interactions between young bulls the use of electrified wire grids above the lairage pens has been proposed.

Many administered substances have been suggested to alleviate or reduce quality problems. Sugar feeding in lairage to replenish muscle glycogen levels will prevent DFD pork and there is some evidence that molassed water will similarly reduce DFD in cattle – but presumably by a different mechanism since the molasses would simply be fermented by the rumen microorganisms. Pork quality has been reported to be improved by the use of tranquillizers such as azaperone, the β-adrenergic blocking drug carazolol and magnesium salts such as magnesium aspartate hydrochloride and magnesium fumarate. The use of pharmacological agents is limited by problems of administration and potential residues remaining in the meat. Pre-slaughter administration of electrolytes has shown some benefits in cattle and the use of sodium bicarbonate loading has been demonstrated to partially alleviate metabolic acidosis in pigs and reduce the rate of post-mortem glycolysis in the muscles (Schaefer *et al.*, 1990, 1992).

Poultry meat quality

Pre-slaughter handling can potentially influence several important quality characteristics of poultry meat, either through influencing the pattern of acidification or the time of rigor development. However, the exact effects of different ante-mortem handling treatments on birds are poorly understood (Uijtenboogaart, 1996). Glycogen in the redder muscles of the leg, such as the m. biceps femoris, can be depleted by prolonged food withdrawal and transport with corresponding increases in ultimate pH. As mentioned above, poultry breast meat (white muscle) can exhibit properties similar to PSE pork (Barbut, 1996; Boulianne and King, 1995) and Sosnicki (1993) suggested that in turkeys heat or cold stresses, or stress associated with transport, could cause rapid post-mortem glycolysis. Heat stress, struggling at slaughter and pre-slaughter injection of adrenaline have been associated with tougher turkey meat.

Because poultry carcasses are relatively small they can be chilled very rapidly *post mortem*. Small differences in chilling regimen, and the consequences for the fall in muscle temperature, can therefore have important effects on muscle characteristics. It is also likely that the interaction between events before slaughter and post-mortem processing contributes to the variation seen in final meat quality and the difficulty in defining exactly the influences of ante-mortem stressors in poultry compared with red meat species. A series of papers summarizing current knowledge on many aspects of poultry meat quality can be found in Richardson and Mead (1999).

Other Effects on Quality

Direct effects of handling on lean meat quality

As well as the role of pre-slaughter stress in causing PSE and DFD meat there is some evidence that poor handling can be detrimental to beef palatability directly. The effects vary in size and the causes are unclear. A series of papers by Wythes and her colleagues from Australia (see Wythes *et al.*, 1989) has demonstrated the benefits of quietly resting cattle with feed, either in transit or in lairage, on meat tenderness. Similarly, Canadian work (Jeremiah *et al.*, 1988; Jones *et al.*, 1990) has demonstrated potentially very important influences of stress, and food and water deprivation, on eating quality in beef. The overall palatability of pork also seems to be higher in pigs subjected to less stress (Warriss, 1994).

Bloodsplash

Bloodsplash (blood spotting, ecchymosis) is not of concern from the point of view of hygiene but, because it detracts from the appearance of meat, is an important problem economically. It takes the form of discrete spots of haemorrhage ranging from pin-head size to about 1 cm in diameter. It is frequently seen on the inside of the thoracic cavity but may occur in any muscle and is also found in the walls of the intestines. It occurs most commonly in lambs and less commonly in older sheep, but is also found in pigs and young cattle although rarely in calves. Despite considerable interest having been shown in the problem, its cause is not understood although various factors have been found to influence the incidence. Animals slaughtered without prior stunning appear to show little or no bloodsplash. All stunning methods increase the incidence but to varying degrees. There is good evidence that one of the main reasons for this is the several-fold increase in blood pressure immediately after the stunning procedure (Kirton *et al.*, 1978). The rise in blood pressure increases the chance of capillaries rupturing, and reducing or preventing the rise by exsanguinating the animal within about 6–10 s from the end of stunning reduces the incidence of bloodsplash. However, since the problem cannot be completely prevented even by sticking animals before stunning, some other factor must predispose the capillaries to weakness so they rupture. Selenium and vitamin E deficiencies have been postulated. It has also been suggested that the capillaries may be ruptured mechanically. Preslaughter stress has been implicated in causing bloodsplash. For example, use of electric goads has been shown to be responsible in pigs (Calkins *et al.*, 1980). Variations in the stunning current have also been suggested as causing the problem in pigs. In this case, constant current stunners, in which the voltage is varied automatically to ensure only a set current is delivered, may be helpful. To prevent changes in current flow, careful application of the stunning electrodes, especially in handheld tongs, is also important in this respect.

Chapter 8

Post-mortem Handling of Carcasses and Meat Quality

As well as inherent characteristics of the animal, and how it is handled before and at slaughter, the way the carcass is processed subsequently can influence quality. A particularly important factor is the rate at which the carcass is cooled.

Temperature Effects

Carcass chilling

At death, animals have a body temperature of between about 37 and 39°C. After carcass dressing the temperature drops as heat is lost to the surrounding air. The rate of loss will depend on factors such as the size of the carcass, the covering of subcutaneous fat and the circulation of air over the surface. Larger carcasses cool more slowly and thicker fat acts as an insulation layer because its thermal conductivity is low compared to muscle or bone. Modern practice has been to speed up the process of chilling using refrigerated air in order to reduce microbial growth on the carcass surface and to reduce evaporative weight losses. At 35°C the bacterium *Escherichia coli* divides every 25 min or so whereas at 7°C the generation time is more than 25 h. Rapid chilling can reduce weight loss from the 2–3% of carcass weight in normal chilling to less than 1% over the first 24 h of storage. Rapid chilling may also reduce the manifestation of PSE (pale, soft, exudative) pork, improving water-holding capacity (WHC) and lean colour. Conversely, keeping the temperature high (>30°C) during rigor development can promote PSE pork in carcasses that would not otherwise be susceptible.

In conventional chilling systems the carcasses are placed in chill rooms held at about 1°C as soon as possible after they have been dressed, washed and inspected. Because of the large amount of hot carcass meat, and therefore the large amount of heat that needs to be dissipated, the air temperature in the chiller may rise above 1°C for periods while hot carcasses are being loaded. Modern refrigeration systems can, however, allow much lower chiller temperatures to be achieved – well below freezing point – so that much faster chilling is possible. 'Blast chilling' for 1 h using air at −25°C can reduce pork carcass temperatures to 24°C at 2 h *post mortem* compared with 32°C in carcasses subjected to a standard 1°C chill (McFarlane and Unruh, 1996). In some systems the surface of the carcass is frozen by very cold air when combined with high air speeds. After such extreme blast chilling the carcasses may be tempered at higher temperature (1°C). This allows equilibration to a higher uniform meat temperature equivalent to that achieved over a longer time in normal chilling. Normal practice is to achieve a meat temperature of 7°C or below before further handling such as butchery, or transport from the plant. Rarely, carcasses are not chilled immediately after washing and inspection but are held at relatively high temperatures while they are hot processed (see p. 166).

The influence of temperature on muscle metabolism

The rate of cooling of meat has other implications besides its effects on microbiology, weight loss and WHC. Because the activity of enzymes is temperature dependent, different cooling rates can affect the rates of pH fall through lactic acid production, the disappearance of creatine phosphate and adenosine triphosphate (ATP), and the speed of onset of rigor mortis.

Between the *in vivo* pH of about 7 and a value around 6.1, the rate of pH fall in beef muscles is approximately linear with time. The rate of fall depends on the muscle temperature. The minimum rate occurs at about 10°C. As the temperature gets closer to 0°C the rate increases. Also, as the temperature increases to 37°C the rate increases, producing overall a curvilinear relationship between rate of pH fall and temperature (Fig. 8.1). There is evidence that the increased rates above and below about 10°C are both caused by activation of the actomyosin ATP-ase that results in muscle contraction. However, the increase above 10°C is caused by increasing activation of calcium-independent ATP-ase but the increase below 10°C is caused by a calcium dependent ATP-ase. The calcium ions that stimulate this come from the sarcoplasmic reticulum, which loses its ability to sequester calcium at low temperatures.

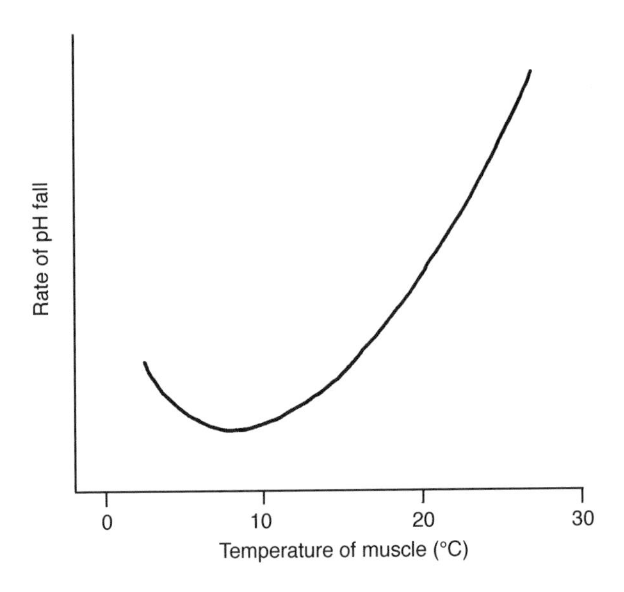

Fig. 8.1. Relation of rate of pH fall to muscle temperature in beef muscle (based on Jeacocke, 1977a).

Temperature also influences the rate of ATP depletion *post mortem* and therefore the time of onset of rigor mortis. Characteristically, ATP depletion follows a biphasic pattern (Fig. 8.2). There is an initial 'delay' phase where ATP that is used up by the normal energy-consuming processes in muscle is wholly or partly replenished by resynthesis from creatine phosphate and through glycolysis. This is followed by a phase in which the processes of resynthesis cannot maintain the ATP concentration, which consequently falls in a more or less linear fashion. The length of the delay phase is temperature dependent with a maximum at about 10–15°C. At lower and higher temperatures the delay phase is shorter. The rate of the second phase, where ATP levels fall significantly, is apparently relatively independent of temperature.

A shortening of the delay phase reduces the time to the onset of rigor. If the muscle is maintained at temperatures around 0° or 30°C there is effectively no delay phase and rigor occurs relatively rapidly. In practice, interpretation or prediction of the course of events is complicated by other factors. Normally, the temperature of muscles is falling progressively with time after death and the fall will not be exactly the same throughout either the muscle, or the carcass, since temperature gradients will be set up during chilling. Muscles differ in their fibre composition and tendency towards oxidative or glycolytic metabolism. This can affect the rate of acidification and rigor development. Events immediately

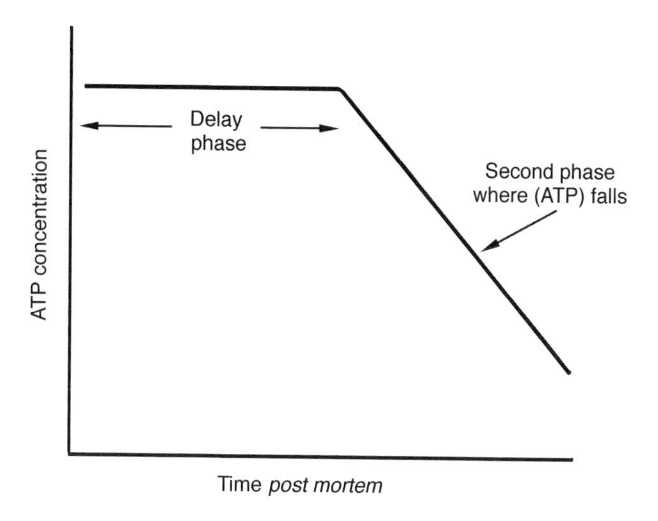

Fig. 8.2. The biphasic pattern of ATP depletion *post mortem.*

pre-slaughter, such as prolonged fasting, or struggling at slaughter, can deplete glycogen reserves and reduce the length of the delay-phase of ATP depletion.

Three practical implications of different rates of carcass cooling, and therefore muscle temperatures *post mortem*, are cold shortening, thaw rigor and, to a lesser degree, heat shortening. Cold shortening and thaw rigor are consequences of wanting to cool muscle too quickly.

Cold shortening

If muscle is cooled below about 10°C before the onset of rigor the subsequent meat is tough after cooking. The phenomenon is referred to as cold shortening (Locker and Hagyard, 1963). Above freezing, the effect is greater the lower is the temperature. The problem is therefore likely to be most acute in situations where rigor development is delayed and where small volumes of tissue are being chilled. Species such as chickens and pigs, because they have relatively rapid rates of rigor onset, are less prone to cold shortening even though their carcasses are small (Møller and Jensen, 1993). Beef carcasses tend to cool slowly because of their bulk and are again less prone. Lamb carcasses are small enough to cool rapidly and generally do not enter rigor quickly. They are therefore most prone to shortening. This is an oversimplification since modern, very fast chilling regimes can cool some muscles, particularly those near the surface of the carcass, rapidly enough to shorten in all species. Different muscles in the carcass will also be differently predisposed to cold shortening because of inherent metabolic differences. So, while the m. longissimus dorsi is very prone to cold shortening, the m. psoas is hardly affected. Variation in ante-mortem handling may also deplete glycogen stores or speed up post-mortem glycolysis.

The mechanism of cold shortening is thought to be stimulation, by the low temperature, of massive release of calcium ions from the sarcoplasmic reticulum without subsequent sequestration. This is because the calcium pump of the sarcoplasmic reticulum does not appear to function very well at low temperatures. The calcium ions activate the actomyosin ATP-ase and lead to muscle contraction. 'Red' (oxidative) muscles tend to have a less well developed sarcoplasmic reticulum than 'white' (glycolytic) muscles and, in the pig at least, appear to be more prone to cold shortening, perhaps because of the consequent potential reduced ability to sequester the calcium. This calcium ion sequestering ability also seems to be less reduced at low temperatures, particularly below about 10°C, in 'white' fibres. An exception is the pig m. longissimus dorsi, which does seem to be prone to cold shortening despite being composed largely of these glycolytic fibres. Mitochondria also sequester calcium ions. However, under anaerobic conditions at low temperature this ability is reduced. 'Red' muscle fibres have more mitochondria. In redder muscles, the mitochondria release calcium ions that are not sequestered, so also promoting contraction. The relative involvement of the sarcoplasmic reticulum and mitochondria in cold shortening is not completely clear. The question has been addressed by Cornforth *et al.* (1980).

Contraction of muscle that is not followed by relaxation produces shorter sarcomeres and tougher meat (Marsh and Leet, 1966). The shorter sarcomeres reflect greater overlap of thin (actin) and thick (myosin) filaments. Under normal conditions, muscles cooked pre-rigor are tender, become tough as rigor develops in the first 24 h *post mortem* and then progressively tenderize with longer storage times *post mortem* (Wheeler and Koohmaraie, 1994). If muscles are physically prevented from shortening after slaughter until they have entered rigor, both sarcomere length and texture after cooking (shear force) remain constant (Koohmaraie *et al.*, 1996). This illustrates the fundamental importance of sarcomere length to meat texture. The relationship between the temperature at which muscles are held pre-rigor, the degree of their shortening, and the relation of this shortening to meat texture after cooking, was studied by Locker and Hagyard (1963). The effects are illustrated in Fig. 8.3. The apparent decrease in toughness at very high degrees of muscle shortening is thought to be because the overlap of thick and thin filaments in each sarcomere is so great under these conditions that some cross-bridges are no longer able to function. In practice, muscles that cold shorten show uneven contraction with localized areas of shortening interspersed with adjacent areas of non-shortened or stretched muscle. This results in cold-shortened meat having more variable texture as well as being tougher overall. The extent of tenderization through conditioning decreases as muscles shorten more in relation to their resting length. Therefore, meat with shorter sarcomeres tends to tenderize least.

Normally therefore, cold-shortened meat appears to undergo little or no tenderization during ageing (Davey *et al.*, 1967; Locker and Wild, 1984) but for reasons that are not completely clear. The effects of cold shortening cannot then be overcome or ameliorated by long conditioning times. However, Locker and Daines (1975) recorded an interesting phenomenon. They cold-shortened excised beef sternomandibularis muscles by holding them at 2°C. This resulted in a 33% shortening of the muscle length. However, if they subsequently held the muscles at 37°C until rigor was completed they did not become tough, the texture being equivalent to that of control muscles held at 15°C and not cold shortened. The effect could not be attributed to ageing effects at the high temperature since Z discs remained intact. Instead, they suggested that the temperature of the muscle at the time rigor mortis developed was the important factor and in some way affected the molecular bonding between myosin and actin, reducing its strength.

In normal beef, cold shortening can be prevented by ensuring that muscle temperature does not fall below 10°C until the muscle pH has reached 6.1, which would normally take about 10 h. By this time, the progress of rigor will be sufficiently advanced to prevent cold contracture. In pork it is now relatively common commercial practice in some

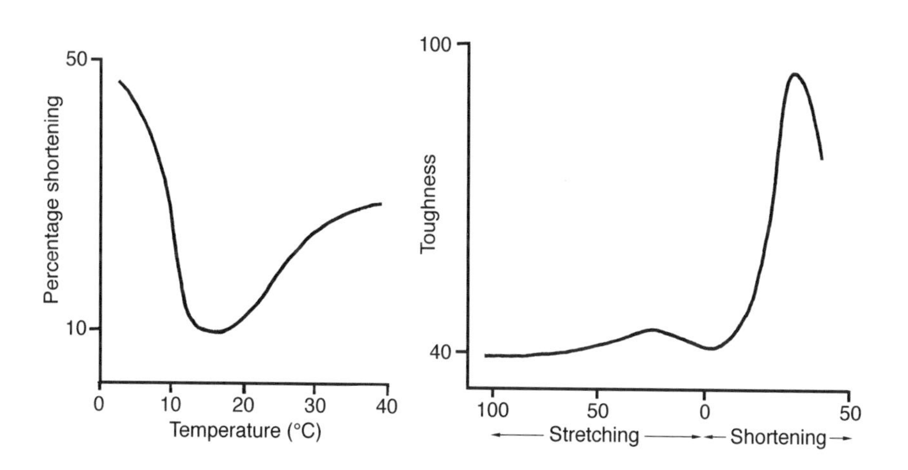

Fig. 8.3. The relationship between temperature at which muscles are held pre-rigor, degree of shortening and toughness (based on Locker and Hagyard, 1963).

countries to chill carcasses very rapidly using blast chilling with air at temperatures of −20°C or lower. There is evidence that this may induce some cold shortening in muscles such as the m. longissimus dorsi but the effect on the texture of the cooked meat is seemingly small and possibly of little practical consequence. The subject of cold-induced toughening of meat was reviewed by Locker (1985).

Heat ring

The phenomenon of so-called 'heat ring' sometimes occurs in beef subjected to relatively fast chilling. In particular, the part of the m. longissimus dorsi that is nearer the outside of the carcass cools more quickly than the inside so the rate of pH fall is reduced. This leads to a darker band of muscle forming. This has an unattractive appearance.

Very fast chilling

Recently, based on earlier observations that, under some conditions, expected cold shortening did not occur (Sheridan, 1990) so-called very fast chilling (VFC) of meat has been investigated more fully (Joseph, 1996). In this procedure the rate of chilling is extreme, with the carcasses held in intensely cold air (−70 to −20°C) moving at high speeds. Despite initial concerns, this can lead to tender meat in some circumstances, rather than the toughening associated with cold shortening. The reasons for this are unclear but several possibilities have been put forward. A hard crust formed by the frozen surface of the meat could prevent shortening of the underlying muscle by virtue of the physical restraint. The differential freezing might cause fractures or breaks in the meat structure, so tenderizing the meat, or the massive release of calcium ions caused by the low temperature might promote proteolysis by stimulating the calpain system.

Thaw rigor

If the rate of cooling of the carcass is sufficiently high and the meat freezes before the onset of rigor then, on thawing, the muscle shortens severely (to up to 50% of its length if unrestrained) and becomes very tough after cooking. Additionally, very large amounts of drip or exudate (30% of muscle weight) are lost during thawing. This is known as thaw rigor. It is thought that, on thawing, glycolysis is completed very rapidly and ATP breakdown is extremely rapid. This rapid metabolism is accompanied by a very strong contraction – unlike the relatively weak contraction, if at all, associated with normal rigor. The contraction is probably stimulated by the rapid and massive release of calcium ions from the sarcoplasmic reticulum on thawing. The effect is greater with muscles that have been frozen very quickly (slow freezing may of course produce cold shortening before freezing). The breakdown of ATP is probably through the activation, by freezing and thawing, of the contractile (actomyosin) ATP-ase, rather than the non-contractile ATP-ase that causes ATP breakdown in normal rigor development. This leads to the strong contraction seen in thaw rigor and accounts for the very high ATP-ase activities (×10) seen.

As in cold shortening, physical prevention of contraction and shortening of muscles can reduce the toughening effects. Physical prevention may be through restraint on the carcass or by thawing being so slow that ice prevents contraction. At temperatures below freezing the activity of actomyosin ATP-ase and the levels of ATP are gradually reduced in storage so that on thawing the effects seen in 'normal' thaw rigor may also be reduced.

Heat shortening

If muscles are stimulated, and allowed to contract and shorten, at high temperatures, without subsequent relaxation, then they may subsequently become tough if they enter rigor in this state (Locker and Daines, 1975). This so-called heat shortening may be a problem if hot processing is practised.

Carcass Handling Procedures to Improve Quality

Electrical stimulation

Because cold shortening can only occur in pre-rigor muscles, accelerating rigor development can enable faster chilling without the meat toughening. One way to do this is by electrical stimulation (Carse, 1973). Electrical stimulation of carcasses at various times after slaughter speeds up the normal post-mortem processes by causing intense muscle contractions. These use up glycogen and creatine phosphate, promoting a rapid pH fall and earlier development of rigor mortis (Bendall, 1976). Because the carcass temperature is still high, after stimulation ceases, the sarcoplasmic reticulum can take up the calcium previously released and the muscle goes into rigor in a relaxed state. After rigor the muscle can no longer respond by contraction to the cold stimulus caused by rapid chilling and there is no danger of toughening. In beef carcasses, the fall in pH to about 6.0 could take 10–12 h under normal conditions. Electrical stimulation may reduce this time to only 1–2 h. The effectiveness of electrical stimulation for lamb carcasses was demonstrated by Chrystall and Hagyard (1976), and for beef carcasses by Davey *et al.* (1976). Table 8.1 shows the improved tenderness of lamb muscles caused by stimulation.

As well as preventing cold shortening, electrical stimulation also appears to tenderize the meat *per se* and improves appearance and possibly flavour. This is even true in pork, which is rarely cold shortened by normal chilling rates (Taylor *et al.*, 1995). The reasons for these effects are not completely understood. It has been suggested that tenderization could be caused by several mechanisms. The intense contractions might physically disrupt and so weaken the muscle structure (Savell *et al.*, 1978). Calcium released during contraction might stimulate the calpains, at a time when muscle temperature and pH were high, and cause greater proteolytic breakdown. Rather less likely, the lysosomes might be disrupted, allowing the release of their enzymes, which could also cause proteolytic breakdown. The colour of beef from electrically stimulated carcasses is brighter, perhaps because the rapid muscle acidification leads to some protein denaturation, causing greater reflectance of light from the meat surface. The occurrence of 'heat ring' is also reduced. These effects improve beef carcass grades in North American systems (Smith, 1985).

The influence of electrical stimulation on potentially dark cutting meat is a little unclear. Inadequate muscle glycogen concentrations at slaughter should reduce or remove any benefits of faster glycolysis and consequent pH fall. However, there is evidence that electrical stimulation does influence the biochemistry and ultrastructure of dark cutting beef (Fabiansson *et al.*, 1985) and could potentially have beneficial effects on colour, although work by Dutson *et al.* (1982) indicated none in practice.

Electrical stimulation may improve flavour by affecting the concentrations of flavour precursors and enhancers, such as nucleotides, in the muscles. Mikami *et al.* (1993) have shown that

Table 8.1. The effect of electrical stimulation on the texture of lamb muscle (from Chrystall and Hagyard, 1976).

Muscle	Unstimulated carcasses	Stimulated carcasses
m. longissimus dorsi	77	37
m. biceps femoris	49	21
m. semimembranosus	76	36
m. gluteus medius	57	22

Texture was assessed by shear force measurements made with a tendermeter. Shear force values of 30–40 were considered marginally tender with 40 the maximum acceptable level for palatability. Values above 50 were very tough.

electrical stimulation of beef leads to the accumulation of peptides and glutamic acid which are thought to contribute to better flavour. The flavour enhancement has been seen in beef (Smith, 1985) and pork (Warriss *et al.*, 1995a).

Numerous different forms of electrical stimulation have been developed. The voltages used normally range from 20 to 1000 V. However, low- and high-voltage stimulation systems are generally differentiated (Table 8.2). Low-voltage stimulation is usually considered to be up to 100 V, high-voltage greater than about 500 V. The time of application can be almost immediately after death to up to 60 min *post mortem*. The current can be applied through various combinations of electrodes but usually flows between the muzzle or nose of the animal, or the chest, and the hind legs. The electrodes are often clips or rubbing bars. Low voltage systems are usually applied immediately after exsanguination and work by stimulating the musculature via the still-living nervous system. High-voltage systems can be applied much later and do not rely on the animal's nervous system but stimulate the muscles directly. Usually the current is applied as a series of pulses of 1–2 s duration and for a period of up to 90 s.

The advantage of high-voltage stimulation is that it is less reliant on accurate timing of the application. However, stringent safety precautions are required and the investment to fulfil these may be too expensive to justify in small, low-throughput plants. Low-voltage systems obviously also require attention to safety but the necessary compliance costs are generally lower. However, good electrode contact is more critical than in high-voltage stimulation and the final results may not be as consistent.

Electrical stimulation is generally only applied to carcasses from sheep and cattle. Cold shortening is less of a potential problem with pork carcasses because of the much more rapid rigor development. However, with very fast chilling procedures, stimulation may be beneficial. It appears that timing of the stimulation is important (Taylor, 1996c). Stimulating pigs within 5 min of slaughter results in very rapid pH fall in the musculature leading to loss of large amounts

Table 8.2. Low- and high-voltage electrical stimulation.

Low voltage	High voltage
20–100 V	500–1000 V
≤ 1 amp	> 5 amps
For up to 20 s	For up to 90 s
Applied immediately after exsanguination (within 5 min of stunning)	Applied up to 60 min *post mortem* (but more usually earlier than this)
Stimulates muscles via nervous system	Stimulates muscles directly

of drip from the meat, reminiscent of the PSE condition. By contrast, stimulating at 20 min after slaughter seems to prevent the excessive exudation. Stimulation even at 20 min *post mortem* without very rapid chilling results in paler, more watery meat from pigs, as might be expected in view of their predisposition to PSE (Table 8.3).

Hot processing

Conventional systems chill the whole carcass to a temperature of 7°C or less before subsequent cutting into smaller parts and further processing. This can be wasteful of chiller capacity, and energy consumption, if, on butchery, much bone and fat is removed and discarded since it will have been cooled unnecessarily. Additionally, because of their size and irregular shape, whole carcasses cool unevenly. A solution is to process the carcass when it is still hot, before chilling. Because the processing largely involves removal of muscles from the skeleton it is often referred to as hot boning, hot deboning or hot cutting. As well as saving refrigeration space and energy, the system may require less labour and reduce the time needed to produce

Table 8.3. Effect of electrical stimulation on conventionally chilled pig carcasses (from Warriss *et al.*, 1995a).

	Unstimulated	Stimulated[a]
Temperature in the m. longissimus dorsi at 45 min *post mortem*	35.5	36.0
pH at 45 min *post mortem*	6.31	5.92
Ultimate pH	5.55	5.51
Lightness (L*)	53.3	55.2
Percentage drip loss	7.1	9.3

[a] Carcasses were stimulated 20 min after exsanguination using 700 V applied for 2 min at 12.5 cycles s^{-1}. After slaughter the carcasses were held at ambient temperature for 2 h before chilling at 2°C. All differences between stimulated and unstimulated carcasses were statistically significant.

Table 8.4. Advantages and disadvantages of hot processing.

Advantages	Disadvantages
Reduced refrigeration costs	Abnormal shape of joints
Energy saving	Difficulty of handling and butchering pre-rigor carcasses
Increased meat yield	Decreased tenderness
More uniform colour	Carcasses cannot be graded using normal post-chill systems
Better water-holding capacity, less drip	

marketable meat. In regard to yield and meat quality there are advantages and disadvantages (Table 8.4).

Meat yield can be improved by up to about 2% (Taylor *et al.*, 1981) because of the reduction in evaporative and drying losses. The meat also tends to have better WHC, so loses less drip during storage and colour is more uniform. Both these effects can be attributed to faster, more uniform cooling of the smaller meat pieces, compared with whole carcasses. Because the muscles are removed before they have gone into rigor, their shape is not fixed by the skeleton and the presence of other muscles of the carcass. The corresponding joints of meat do not therefore have the characteristic shapes associated with normal post-rigor butchery. This can be a disadvantage as the appearance is novel to the consumer but, on the other hand, allows the processor to control the shape of the final joint by appropriate packaging. Handling soft pre-rigor carcasses and meat is more difficult for butchers used to traditional techniques developed for dealing with firm bodies of meat.

A more serious disadvantage of hot processing is that the meat may be slightly tougher. This is true for both beef (Babiker and Lawrie, 1983) and pork (Van Laack and Smulders, 1989). There are several likely reasons for this. The meat may heat shorten because of the stimulation associated with boning and manipulation pre-rigor. It may cold shorten because of the speed with which it can be cooled when compared with whole carcasses. Lastly, this relatively rapid cooling may reduce the tenderizing effects of the proteolytic enzymes involved in the normal conditioning processes. This is because they are working at a high temperature for only a short time.

A compromise solution to enable the processor to take advantage of hot processing while minimizing the disadvantages may be to hot-process some parts of the carcass and to retain normal processing for others. Hot processing is especially suitable for beef forequarter meat, which has inherently lower value. In contrast the high-value hind quarter cuts may benefit from conventional processing where the traditional appearance of joints is more important and palatability is at a premium. Hot processing could influence the microbiological characteristics of the meat. Exposure of a large surface area allows the potential for the contamination by bacteria from the operative's hands and tools, and contamination at a time when the meat temperature is high and the meat surface is wet or sticky. This might predispose hot-processed meat to faster spoilage or the growth of pathogenic bacteria associated with food poisoning. However, provided that the hot processing is carried out with due regard for hygiene, and that chilling is rapid, these concerns may be unfounded (Gilbert *et al.*, 1977; Taylor *et al.*, 1981).

Novel carcass suspension methods

The conventional way to suspend carcasses during chilling is by the hind legs using a hook passed behind the Achilles tendon. The weight of the carcass puts many muscles into tension so stretching them as they pass into rigor. This stretching may increase sarcomere lengths and produce more tender meat. While some muscles are in tension others are free to contract because of the antagonistic way in which many groups of muscles operate. If, instead of hanging the carcass from the Achilles tendon, it is hung from a hook placed into the obturator foramen, then the valuable m. longissimus dorsi, and the muscles on the outside of the hip, such as the m. semimembranosus and m. semitendinosus, are stretched when they enter rigor. The obturator foramen is the hole in the skeleton of the pelvic girdle between the ilium, ischium and pubis bones. This is referred to by butchers as the aitch bone because of its shape. The process is called pelvic suspension or hip free suspension. The stretching of the muscles results in more tender meat after cooking. It was originally described for beef carcasses in North America (Hostetler *et al.*, 1970, 1975) and became known as the 'Tenderstretch' method. A disadvantage is that although some muscles become more tender, others toughen. However, these are usually either the less valuable ones, or muscles like the m. psoas, which is inherently very tender anyway so the slight toughening is of little importance. Another problem is that the carcasses are unconventional in shape after pelvic hanging and take up more space in the chillers. The different shape makes butchery more difficult and alters the appearance of the joints. It is possible to rehang small carcasses, such as those of pigs, from the Achilles tendon after rigor has developed while in pelvic suspension. This returns the carcasses to near-normal shape and gives the benefits of pelvic suspension without the disadvantage of altered carcass shape. It is, however, not a popular technique in practice because of the considerable extra labour required to rehang carcasses while in the chiller. Taylor (1996c) has given an interesting comparison of the benefits of pelvic suspension and electrical stimulation in pig carcasses.

Meat Packaging

Packaging in controlled gas mixtures

In traditional butchers' shops meat is often displayed unpackaged. However, the trend to distribution of meat as primal cuts, central preparation of retail cuts, and the selling of meat by supermarkets has highlighted the importance of appropriate packaging. This has three main functions. It protects the meat from contamination and inhibits microbial growth, it reduces or eliminates evaporative weight loss and surface drying and it may enhance the appearance of the product. Bacteria such as *Pseudomonas* can grow below 5°C under aerobic conditions. Including high concentrations of carbon dioxide in the pack restricts this growth and encourages the proliferation of lactic acid-producing bacteria, which are far less likely to cause spoilage. This sort of packaging may therefore delay spoilage and prolong shelf life. Consumers like meat such as beef and lamb to appear bright red because they associate the colour with freshness. The red is produced by reaction of the muscle haem pigments with oxygen. Covering meat with plastic films of different gas permeabilities can affect this reaction and so alter the colour of the meat surface.

Reaction of the haem pigments with oxygen

To understand how this occurs it is necessary to discuss the way oxygen reacts with myoglobin and haemoglobin. Myoglobin (Mb), oxymyoglobin (MbO_2) and metmyoglobin (met Mb), and their three haemoglobin equivalents, are the common forms of the pigments that occur in meat. The formation of oxymyoglobin from myoglobin involves the attachment of an oxygen molecule (O_2) to the myoglobin molecule. Oxygen is referred to as a ligand. Various other molecules can act as ligands. Examples are carbon monoxide (CO), which reacts to form carbonyl compounds, and nitric acid (NO) which reacts to form the compounds associated with the characteristic pink colour of cured meat. The formation of metmyoglobin from myoglobin or oxymyoglobin does not involve reaction with a ligand. Instead, there is a change in the oxidation state of the iron atom at the centre of the haem molecule. In myoglobin and oxymyoglobin the iron is in the ferrous state (Fe^{2+}) whereas this is oxidized to ferric iron (Fe^{3+}) in metmyoglobin (Fig. 8.4).

The reduction of metmyoglobin only occurs to a limited extent, particularly in meat that has been aged for a long time *post mortem* and in which the reducing activity of the muscle enzymes is consequently low. The importance of these changes to the colour of meat is that the three compounds have different colours. Myoglobin is purple, oxymyoglobin is bright red and metmyoglobin is grey–brown. The colours of myoglobin and oxymyoglobin are analagous to those of the corresponding haemoglobin compounds that occur in deoxygenated venous blood (purple) and oxygenated arterial blood (bright red) in the living animal. To consumers the bright red of oxymyoglobin is desirable as the colour of fresh meat whereas the purple and particularly the grey–brown of the other two forms of the pigment are less desirable.

A freshly cut surface of meat is purple because the pigment is in the deoxygenated form. On exposure to air, the myoglobin in the surface to a depth of 2–6 mm (or more) reacts with oxygen to form the desirable,

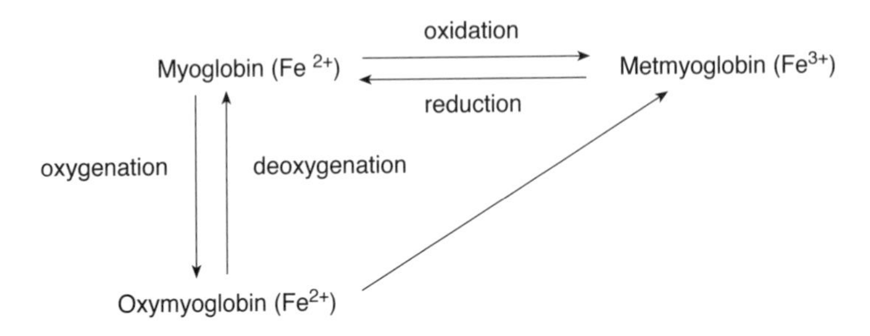

Fig. 8.4. The relationships between myoglobin, oxymyoglobin and metmyoglobin.

bright red oxymyoglobin, the process taking between about 15 min to 1 h. This is known as 'blooming'. The depth of the oxymyoglobin layer depends on the extent of penetration of oxygen from the atmosphere. The oxygen oxidizes various reduced substances, particularly coenzymes, present in the muscle. Below the layer of oxymyoglobin a very thin layer of oxidized metmyoglobin forms (Fig. 8.5). This is because *oxidation* is favoured over *oxygenation* at low partial pressures of oxygen. Metmyoglobin formation is maximal at partial pressures of oxygen between 6 and 7 mm in beef semitendinosus muscle stored between 0° and 7°C (Ledward, 1970). Oxymyoglobin is more resistant to oxidation than is deoxygenated myoglobin.

The depth of the oxymyoglobin layer varies slightly between muscles because of their different metabolic characteristics, particularly the activity of the various enzyme systems, which continue to be active for a time after death of the animal. The layer is thinner in muscles with high activities of reducing system enzymes, particularly the cytochromes. The reducing activity is high in fresh meat and low in aged meat. It also decreases with temperature more than does the ease with which oxygen diffuses through the tissue. The thickness of the oxymyoglobin layer is therefore greater, and meat colour is brighter, at lower temperatures of storage.

After about 2 or 3 days in air the oxymyoglobin at the meat surface gradually starts to oxidize to brown metmyoglobin. When around 20% of the surface pigment has oxidized, the change in colour of the meat can be enough to cause consumer discrimination. Colour stability is very sensitive to temperature. The difference between storage of meat at 0°C compared with 5°C is significant, browning of the surface being postponed from perhaps 48 h to 1 week. The factors that affect discolouration of meat have been reviewed by Renerre (1990) and Kropf (1993).

Controlling gas atmospheres

The major role of plastic films in influencing the appearance of meat is to control the gas atmospheres in contact with its surface and so

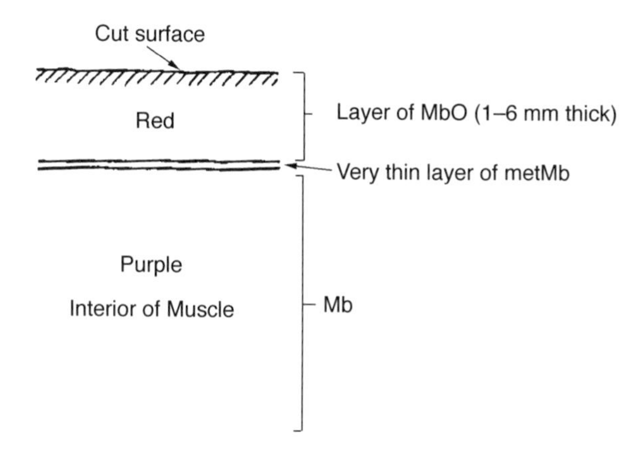

Fig. 8.5. Schematic cross section of muscle showing layers of myoglobin, oxymyoglobin and metmyoglobin in relation to the surface in contact with atmosphere.

influence the reaction of the haem pigments. The gases of importance are oxygen, carbon dioxide and nitrogen. Oxygen oxygenates or oxidizes the pigments and influences the differential growth of aerobic and anaerobic bacteria. Carbon dioxide inhibits undesirable bacterial growth (Gill and Penney, 1988) mainly by extending the lag phase (see Chapter 9). Nitrogen is inert and is sometimes used as a 'ballast' gas to overcome the problem of the high solubility of carbon dioxide in water, and therefore in meat. If large amounts of carbon dioxide dissolve in the meat, the pack may collapse. Carbon dioxide and oxygen are often used for fresh red meats. For cooked, cured and processed meats, the gases are carbon dioxide and nitrogen, oxygen being excluded to prevent the development of rancidity and colour fading. Different types of plastic film have different properties of gas, and, to a lesser degree, water permeability. Taylor (1996a) lists the oxygen and water transmission properties of a variety of plastics used in meat packaging. Different plastics can be laminated together to benefit from their combined properties – polyethylene for its sealing ability, ethyl vinyl alcohol or polyvinylidene chloride for gas impermeability, and nylon for strength.

Using very gas-permeable plastic film to overwrap meat in trays allows oxygen from the air to penetrate the pack easily and react with myoglobin to give bright red oxymyoglobin. The colour is, however, stable for only a short time – often only 1 or 2 days – before oxidation to metmyoglobin becomes a problem. To extend shelf life, modified atmosphere packaging (MAP) is used. In MAP the atmosphere over the meat is modified by inclusion of more oxygen, or more carbon dioxide, than in air. Although the gas atmosphere is fixed when introduced into the pack it may change over the life of the product because of interaction with the meat. A relatively impermeable plastic film is employed and the pack is filled with a gas mixture containing, for example, 60–80% oxygen in carbon dioxide. The enhanced oxygen concentration (compared with the 20% in normal air) encourages penetration of oxygen into the meat for a much greater distance from the surface. The depth of oxygen penetration is proportional to the square root of its concentration. A fourfold increase in the oxygen level from 20 to 80% therefore doubles the depth of the oxymyoglobin layer. This thicker layer of bright red oxymyoglobin might reach 10 mm after a day's storage and delays the progress of metmyoglobin formation so that shelf lives of a week at 1°C are possible. The high carbon dioxide concentrations in the pack inhibit undesirable microbial growth and so also prolong microbiological shelf life.

A potential concern is that the increased shelf life could enable the growth of pathogenic bacteria to levels that would make the meat unsafe. This is especially true for cooked, ready-to-eat products, and for bacteria that can grow at refrigerated temperatures such as *Listeria monocytogenes*, or those that grow at low oxygen concentrations, or anaerobically such as *Clostridium botulinum* and *Clostridium perfringens*. Inhibition of non-pathogens can also encourage the proliferation of pathogens.

To prevent the unsightly accumulation of exudate from the muscle when displayed for the longer times possible with modified atmosphere packaging, the trays in which the meat sits are often furnished with an absorbent pad which soaks up any drip that is formed. In these packs it is important that there is a space between the top meat surface and the overwrapped plastic film to allow the gas mixture access to the meat. These more stringent packaging requirements can make modified atmosphere systems expensive compared with simple overwrapping.

In vacuum packing, joints are sealed in bags in which the plastic is effectively impermeable to gases. Before sealing, residual air is removed from between the meat and the plastic by carrying out the process under a partial vacuum. The plastic pack or pouch is therefore very closely applied to the meat surface. Enzyme systems in the muscle continue to use any available oxygen. Oxygen penetrating the surface is consumed and carbon dioxide is given off. This process 'mops up' or scavenges any residual oxygen in the packs, which quickly become in effect anaerobic. The layer of oxymyoglobin at the surface of the meat is therefore non-existent or extremely thin. Instead, the normal oxidized layer of metmyoglobin layer increases in thickness and, together with the underlying deoxygenated myoglobin, produces a dark purple appearance. This makes the method less suitable for retail display but ideal for storing and transporting boneless primal joints of meat where the appearance is unimportant. As oxygen is consumed so carbon dioxide is generated. This inhibits spoilage by undesirable Pseudomonad growth and encourages lactic acid-forming bacteria. With good hygiene, vacuum-packed meat can be stable for 5–6 weeks, or even more, when kept at 1°C. On removal from the packs and cutting into retail joints or steaks the meat surface 'blooms' normally.

The size of the meat cut or joint can influence the effectiveness of vacuum packing. In retail-sized packs the ratio of meat volume to residual air volume may be undesirably small. Vacuum packing is therefore of most use for larger joints at the wholesale level. The same is true of controlled atmosphere packaging (CAP). This is like MAP but the atmosphere is periodically monitored and controlled at its initial specified level, if necessary by the addition of fresh gas. It is therefore suitable for bulk storage purposes.

A key advantage of MAP is in allowing the development of centralized cutting operations, removing the need for butchery facilities at the retail level. It also allows 'portion control' and the pack can be made attractive to the consumer to aid marketing. An obvious requirement of all packaging systems is that the packs are sealed. Stringent quality control systems must therefore be in place to identify leaking packs. Excellent reviews of both modified atmosphere and vacuum packaging are given by Taylor (1996a, b).

Use of Antioxidants

During the storage of meat, oxidation can be detrimental to both colour and flavour. Colour is affected through the formation of unattractive brown metmyoglobin and flavour is compromised by lipid oxidation leading to rancidity. Various mechanisms and substances in the body protect against oxidation, including vitamin C (ascorbic acid) and vitamin E (α-tocopherol). Recently there has been considerable interest in using these antioxidants to extend the shelf life of meat by protecting its appearance and inhibiting lipid oxidation. Various other antioxidants have been employed in food products. Three synthetic antioxidants are commonly used. These are propyl gallate, butylated hydroxyanisole (BHA) and butylated hydroxytoluene (BHT). For example, Green *et al.* (1971) found that butylated hydroxyanisole or propyl gallate, in combination with ascorbic acid, retarded pigment and lipid oxidation in ground beef. However, use of these substances is sometimes prohibited by legislation and may also meet with consumer resistance because they are synthetic rather than naturally occurring. Obviously, both vitamin C and vitamin E occur naturally. Vitamin C is soluble in water. Vitamin E is fat soluble and occurs in cell membranes, which are largely composed of lipids, protecting them from oxidative damage. Because of this, vitamin E levels in meat take a relatively long time to both increase and become depleted in response to changes in dietary vitamin E.

The difference in solubility between vitamins C and E has led to slightly different ways of using them. Vitamin C is usually either incorporated directly into processed products or has been investigated as a 'dip' – steaks are dipped into an aqueous solution. It should be noted, however, that legislation in some countries actually prohibits its use in fresh meat. Nevertheless, in one of the original studies on the efficacy of vitamin C in beef, animals were injected 5–10 min pre-slaughter with a very large dose of sodium ascorbate to produce final levels of 100–200 mg kg^{-1} in the meat (Hood, 1975). This was an attempt to overcome the disadvantage of surface application, which is that the vitamin must diffuse into the meat to have an effect. Obviously this is not a problem in minced or comminuted products.

In contrast, vitamin E has generally been used as a dietary supplement in the live animal because of the need to incorporate it within the cell membranes. It has been successfully employed in poultry (Webb *et al.*, 1972; Bartov and Bornstein, 1977), pigs (Buckley and Connolly, 1980) and cattle (Faustmann *et al.*, 1989). In pigs, vitamin E supplementation may reduce drip loss from pork, and even prevent the development of PSE characteristics in some stress-susceptible animals according to Cheah *et al.* (1995). These authors provided evidence that the effect was produced by the vitamin stabilizing the cell membranes, possibly by inhibiting the enzyme phospholipase A2 which normally hydrolyses phospholipids.

The time for which supplementation has been used varies. In beef, the critical concentration of α-tocopherol to achieve maximum protection against oxidation in retail-displayed m. longissimus dorsi was about 3.3 μg g^{-1} (Arnold *et al.*, 1993a) which was achieved by feeding the animals 1840 IU day^{-1} for 3 months or 400 IU day^{-1} for 6 months. Arnold *et al.* (1992) found that 300 IU day^{-1} for 266 days, 1140 IU day^{-1} for 67 days or 1200 IU day^{-1} for 38 days were all as effective in extending beef colour stability. Feeding vitamin supplements is relatively easy in intensively reared non-ruminant species and in cattle raised in feedlots. It is more difficult in grass-fed animals. Faustman *et al.* (1998) have reviewed the value of vitamin E supplementation for optimizing the colour of beef.

Because of their different characteristics, including fat, iron and pigment levels, and levels of activity of reducing enzyme systems, different muscles or meat cuts respond differently to antioxidant supplementation. An example comes from the study by Hood (1975) of beef animals injected with vitamin C. There were no benefits to the stability of colour in the m. longissimus dorsi, which is generally good anyway, but considerable benefits in the m. psoas and m. gluteus medius, which are prone to pigment oxidation and discolouration. In the study of

Arnold *et al.* (1992) the colour stability of the m. longissimus dorsi from cattle given supplemental vitamin E was extended by 2.5–4.8 days but that of the m. gluteus medius by only 1.6–3.8 days. The stability of meat from dairy breeds is also less good than that from beef breeds. Vitamin E can benefit the shelf life of ground beef products such as hamburgers (Lavelle *et al.*, 1995) as well as steaks.

There is a synergistic effect between the antioxidant properties of vitamins C and E (Tappel *et al.*, 1961), that is, the benefits of both together are greater than the sum of their individual benefits. This has been demonstrated in beef dipped in solutions of the two vitamins in alcohol (Okayama *et al.*, 1987) and in beef steaks from animals fed supplemental vitamin E and subsequently dipped in vitamin C solution (Mitsumoto *et al.*, 1991). Generally, however, of the two, vitamin E is the more effective antioxidant.

Tenderizing by Marinading and Injection

Tenderizing with salts and acids

Meat can be tenderized by the action of salt solutions or acids. Traditionally, meat is marinaded in vinegar (acetic acid) or wine. The action of the acid is to break the muscle structure down, possibly by encouraging the action of collagenases and cathepsins which work best at low pH. It also makes the myofibrils swell and hold water better, increasing tenderness and juiciness. An extension of marinading is to infuse or inject solutions into pieces of meat. Koohmaraie and his co-workers have shown the benefits of injecting calcium chloride solution (0.3 M) in tenderizing lamb (Koohmaraie *et al.*, 1988) and beef (Koohmaraie *et al.*, 1990). This tenderizing was thought to be through activation of the proteolytic calpain system by the calcium. However, there is a possibility that the mechanism may be a direct effect of the salt on the muscle proteins since sodium chloride seems to work as well, and calcium chloride also seems to work even if the calpain system is inhibited. Calcium may also improve other characteristics besides texture and there is some evidence of a greater effect with higher concentrations (Table 8.5).

Calcium chloride injection has also been shown to improve the tenderness of pork whether chilled normally or blast chilled using air at −25°C for 1 h (McFarlane and Unruh, 1996). A slight problem with the use of calcium chloride in beef is that there may be undesirable effects on taste and flavour if high concentrations are used. Also, it promotes faster oxidation of the haem pigments so that the surface of the meat turns brown sooner and therefore it has a shorter shelf life. However, this effect can be overcome by combining the calcium

Table 8.5. Effect of calcium chloride injection on beef quality (based on Kerth *et al.*, 1995).

	$CaCl_2$ (mM)		
	0	200	250
Shear force (kg)	5.6	4.7	4.4
Tenderness	5.0	5.6	5.8
Juiciness	5.4	5.9	5.7
Flavour intensity	5.9	6.2	6.3
Beef flavour	5.7	5.9	6.0

M. longissimus dorsi muscles were removed 48 h *post mortem* and injected with $CaCl_2$ at 5% of their weight. Shear force was measured instrumentally. The other values are mean scores from a trained taste panel using eight-point scales (8 = extremely tender, 1 = extremely tough, etc.).

chloride with vitamin C (ascorbic acid) as an antioxidant (Wheeler *et al.*, 1996). It is important to inject calcium post-rigor to avoid stimulating contractions. Under commercial conditions, the injection of calcium chloride is carried out 1 or 2 days *post mortem* but delayed injection to up to 2 weeks after slaughter still improves tenderness in beef. The use of calcium chloride injection to improve meat tenderness has been reviewed by Wheeler *et al.* (1994).

Tenderizing with enzymes

Naturally occurring enzymes can be added to meat. A system was developed in which the enzyme papain, derived from the papaya plant, was administered to animals just before slaughter. The enzyme was injected into the blood system in an inactivated form. It became activated during the acidification of the muscles *post mortem* and also when the meat was subsequently cooked. Papain is proteolytic and results in more tender meat. However, there are potential practical problems with its use, particularly ensuring even distribution throughout the body and its effects on organs such as the liver. Also there are some animal welfare concerns associated with the procedure.

Processed Meat Products

Comminution

Texture is one of the most important palatability characteristics of meat. Generally, beef with the best texture characteristics is associated with the highest value parts of the carcass. This is the meat of the loin, sirloin, forerib, topside and fillet from young, rapidly grown animals. However, it forms less than a third of the carcass. Meat from the remaining parts, and that from older animals, which is inherently tougher, can be comminuted. This is particularly appropriate for meat from the forequarter where the amounts of connective tissue are relatively high. At its simplest, the process consists of mincing or grinding the meat into small pieces, which can then be sold as ground beef or hamburger meat, or reformed by being compressed into convenient shaped products. By reducing particle size, comminution breaks up connective tissue and fat. The small pieces of meat are held together by exudate – a solution of the muscle proteins which is sticky. Binding between the meat particles can be improved by incorporating salts or other additives. By controlling the size of the meat pieces or particles, and the degree of adhesion, different textures and mouth feel can be produced. The size of the portion can also be chosen exactly and standardized to produce a consistent product.

There are other advantages to comminution. As well as enabling the modification and control of texture of meat, and increasing the economic value of lower quality parts of the carcass and trimmings from high value cuts, it leads to the potential development of meat products with similar added value. Potential problems are that, as well as as having relatively high loads of microorganisms, comminuted meat tends to lose beneficial vitamins. Comminuted meat products include burgers, reformed and restructured steaks, and sausages. They are often characterized by a relatively high fat content (Table 8.6).

Comminution methods

Comminution can be achieved by mincing (grinding), bowl chopping or flaking. The type of process affects particle size and shape, and so influences other properties. In mincing, a screw auger forces the meat through a plate against which operates a rotating knife. The size of the perforations in the plate determines the size of the particles of minced

Table 8.6. The composition of some comminuted meat products in the UK (derived from Chan *et al.*, 1996).

Product	Percentage water	Percentage protein	Percentage fat	Percentage carbohydrate
Beefburger	56	17	25	0.1
Beef grill steak	57	17	24	0.2
Beef sausage	55	10	24	9.4
Pork sausage	52	12	23	9.2

meat. The meat is subjected to high pressures in the auger and large shearing forces between the knife and plate. If the contact between the knife and plate is poor, or the blade is not sharp, connective tissue is not cut cleanly and can become trapped, therefore remaining unminced.

In bowl-chopping, a circular, slowly rotating bowl carries the meat into a set of rapidly rotating knives operating in a vertical plane. This can break the meat down into very fine particles, depending on the number of passes made past the blades. Bowl-chopping is also a very effective way of mixing added ingredients into the comminuted meat. Both mincing and bowl-chopping increase the meat temperature. In bowl-chopping this can be controlled by introducing the meat at a temperature just below 0°C. In flaking, the temperature of the meat is very important and is maintained between −2°C and −4°C. A blade is used to cut flakes off the end of the frozen block of meat. The flakes have a good shape for sticking together.

Burgers

Traditionally, hamburgers are made of minced or flaked beef but nowadays other meats can also be used. Sometimes salt (sodium chloride) and 'extenders' such as soya protein are added to improve the cohesiveness of the burgers after cooking and reduce the cost of the product. They can also be used to reduce the fat content. In the UK the minimum allowed meat content is 80% but in the USA extenders are not permitted and hamburger meat must consist only of minced beef together with beef fat. The total fat content must also not exceed 30% but is generally lower (15–20%). The best burgers are made from meat with a small connective tissue content. Too much connective tissue produces an undesirable texture. The minced meat is pressed or extruded into moulds to form round patties. Care is necessary not to subject it to too high shear stresses or the burgers will shrink unevenly and lose their shape on cooking.

Concern about eating large amounts of saturated fat has led to the development of low-fat burgers. These contain less than 10% fat, some fat being replaced by vegetable 'binders' such as soya protein, starches or carrageenan, derived from red seaweeds. These improve the WHC of the lean meat and retain some of the desirable organoleptic properties associated with fat, such as juiciness.

Reformed and restructured steaks

In reformed products, the comminuted meat is moulded into a shape resembling a natural steak. The process is a good way of upgrading the value of beef forequarter meat. Flaked meat is used, rather than minced meat, because the particles bind together better and produce a better texture. Adhesion is promoted by the large surface area of the flakes, and the protein exuded from them. Binding is sometimes improved by incorporating salts, such as polyphosphates, or other additives.

Rather than rely on the natural adhesive properties of the meat proteins, systems have been developed in which sodium alginate is used to form a gel that binds the product together. Alginates are derived from brown seaweeds and are used as thickening agents in various foods. The gel is formed by reaction of the sodium alginate with calcium ions. Much of the success of a product depends on how closely this reaction can be controlled to produce the desired gel properties. Larger pieces of meat can also be formed into blocks of tissue using this technique. Reviews of many aspects of restructuring meat can be found in Pearson and Dutson (1987).

Sausages

Sausages are made from chopped or comminuted lean meat and fat, mixed with salt, spices and other ingredients, then filled into a container. The latter is often a casing, made from the cleaned intestines of cattle, sheep or pigs. In cleaning, much of the layered wall of the intestine is removed, leaving mainly just collagen. Artificial casings are now often used. These are made from reconstituted collagen derived from other parts of the animal, particularly the skin of cattle, and have the obvious benefit of uniformity of the product.

Fresh sausages

There are essentially three types of sausage: fresh, cooked and dry. Fresh and cooked sausages are perishable unless refrigerated. A fresh pork sausage in the UK might be made from a mixture of lean meat (45–60%), fat (15–20%), rusk and water, together with salt and spices. Rusk is a cereal filler, essentially made from bread dough, baked and crushed into granules, which binds together the other ingredients. The comminuted meat used to make sausages tends to carry a relatively high level of microbial contamination. To control this, sulphite or metabisulphite may sometimes be added in the UK. Many countries, however, do not allow this. The active agent is sulphur dioxide, which is particularly effective against *Pseudomonas*. Better-quality fresh sausages tend to contain a higher percentage of lean meat. Fresh sausages must be cooked before consumption – often by frying or grilling.

Cooked sausages

Cooked sausages, such as frankfurters and Bologna, as sold require no cooking by the consumer but can be eaten directly. Frankfurters may contain beef or veal as well as pork, and the meat is usually cured by the addition of nitrite or nitrate. Curing is described in Chapter 9. The amount of cereal used, if any, is relatively low (5% or less) and the product may be smoked before cooking. In blood sausage (black puddings), a mixture of pigs' blood, fat and oatmeal, with salt and seasoning, is cooked in casings.

Dry sausages

Dry sausages are not normally cooked before eating but are preserved by the meat being cured with relatively large amounts of salt and by having a very low water content, and hence a low a_w value (see Chapter 9). Examples are salamis and chorizos. In the case of salamis, some types are hot-smoked. Dry sausages are held for relatively long periods to develop their characteristic flavours. This is partly through the growth of various beneficial bacteria, especially lactic acid-producing types such as *Lactobacillus*. The lactic acid is produced during the ripening process. Lactic acid-producing bacteria are always present on meat to some degree. However, the bacteria are nowadays usually introduced as starter cultures inoculated into the sausage mix, which is held initially at quite high temperatures to promote fermentation. Various additives may also be incorporated to increase the acidity of the meat, for example glucono-lactone, which is hydrolysed to gluconic acid, or lactic acid. The acidity inhibits the growth of undesirable microorganisms and reduces the WHC of the meat. The loss of water facilitates drying. In modern production systems the fermentation and drying are carefully controlled by regulating temperature and humidity. A good series of papers relating to modern technologies used for producing cured and fermented meat products can be found in Smulders *et al.* (1992). The science of fermented meats is covered in Campbell-Platt and Cook (1995). An excellent source of information on all aspects of meat products is Varnum and Sutherland (1995).

Mechanically Recovered Meat (MRM)

After normal boning of carcasses to produce boneless joints some meat is still left attached to the bones. This meat can be recovered by grinding the bones into a paste and forcing it through very small holes in a stainless steel drum. The soft meat passes through the holes but the hard bone particles are retained. Another procedure is to use very high pressures to force the meat off the bones prior to separation. Very high standards of hygiene in the original handling of the raw bones are essential but the product can be used in meat products, albeit with care as it is prone to the development of rancidity. The technologies available for the mechanical recovery of meat have been reviewed by Newman (1980–81).

Pressure Treatment

A process has been described (Solomon *et al.*, 1997) in which meat is subjected to a shock wave generated while it is submerged under water. The 'Hydrodyne' process was very effective at tenderizing beef muscles, including ones that had been cold shortened, and could be a potentially useful way of processing meat to make it more palatable.

Chapter 9

Meat Hygiene, Spoilage and Preservation

Meat can be, or become, unacceptable for human consumption either because the living animal has a disease or condition, or because the meat becomes spoiled. Spoilage occurs *post mortem* either by chemical breakdown, for instance the oxidation of fats to produce rancidity, or by the growth of microorganisms. An example of a condition that may make meat unacceptable is the occurrence of extreme boar taint. Disease can make the meat aesthetically unacceptable or, more importantly, can lead to transmission of infection to humans.

Disease and the Contamination of Meat

Transmission of disease

Transmission may be by contact, or inhalation of spores, for example in anthrax, bovine tuberculosis and brucellosis, or by ingestion of infected meat. Examples of the latter are salmonellosis, trichinosis or tapeworm infections (taeniasis). The modes of transmission are illustrated in Table 9.1. Anthrax, bovine tuberculosis, brucellosis and food poisoning are caused by bacteria. *Taenia* is a platyhelminth or tapeworm (cestode). *Trichinella* is a nematode worm and trichinosis is caused by eating raw or inadequately cooked pork from pigs that have been fed uncooked waste food containing *Trichinella* larvae. A temperature of 58°C kills *Trichinella* larvae so normal cooking usually renders infected meat safe. The condition is extremely rare in the UK, the last outbreak being in the 1950s. In the USA the incidence of trichinosis in humans decreased from about 12% in 1940 to about 2% by 1970. The larval stage of the worm lives in the muscles of the pig (and other animals).

Table 9.1. Transmission modes of various types of disease from meat animals.

Disease	Responsible organism	Transmission
Anthrax	*Bacillus anthracis*	Hides and hair
Tuberculosis	*Mycobacterium tuberculosis*	Carcasses and milk
Brucellosis	*Brucella abortus*	Skin surfaces
Food poisoning	*Salmonella* spp. etc	Ingestion of meat
Trichinosis	*Trichinella spiralis* (nematode)	Ingestion of pork
Taeniasis	*Taenia saginata* (beef tapeworm) = *Cysticercus bovis*	Ingestion of beef
	Taenia solium (pork tapeworm) = *Cysticercus celullosae*	Ingestion of pork

Tapeworms are picked up by eating raw, or inadequately cooked, beef or pork infected with the larval stages of the worms (*Cysticercus bovis* or *C. cellulosae*). These are easily visible to the naked eye and give rise to the common description of the meat. It is referred to as 'measly' (see Chapter 4). The host animals become infected through eating grass or other food contaminated with human faeces containing the tapeworm eggs. The adult tapeworm is flattened and ribbon-like, consisting of a head-like scolex provided with hooks and suckers used to attach it to the gut wall of the host, behind which is a chain of segment-like proglottides. The chain of proglottides may be 3 m or more in length. The most mature proglottides are filled with eggs and break off from the main chain, eventually being passed out with the host's faeces. Details of the various parasites potentially occurring in meat can be found in standard textbooks of meat hygiene, for example Gracey and Collins (1992).

Sources of contamination

Spoilage microorganisms can come either from outside the animal, or from the gut, or by being introduced at slaughter on the bolt of the captive bolt stunning pistol or on the blade of the sticking knife. In living, healthy animals, bacteria in the gut are usually prevented from invading the surrounding tissues and the blood system, or their growth is controlled, by the mucous lining of the gut wall, by antibodies in the blood and by phagocytosis by reticulo-endothelial cells especially in the lymph nodes. Normally therefore, the tissues of healthy animals are sterile. Some organisms, such as *Salmonella enteritidis*, can nevertheless sometimes pass into the bloodstream and tissues and cause systemic infection.

Particular sources of contamination from outside the animals are the surface of the skin, hide or fleece, and the feet, and soil and faecal material contaminating them, and the gut contents. The problem of dirty cattle arriving at abattoirs, and the implications for hygiene, were highlighted by Taylor (1993) and the significance of fleece soiling for the microbiological contamination of sheep carcasses was investigated by Hadley *et al.* (1997). Contamination of the carcass from the gut contents can occur by faecal evacuation, by regurgitation of the contents of the stomach during exsanguination, so leading to contamination of the neck and head, and by accidental puncture of the gut wall during evisceration. Contamination and cross-contamination can also come from slaughtermen's hands, arms and clothing, and equipment used in the carcass dressing process. As mentioned in Chapter 4, the high degree of mechanization of poultry processing can lead to cross-contamination of carcasses by the processing equipment. So, if a gut is ruptured during evisceration, there is potential to spread any contamination with gut contents to the carcasses behind it on the line. To a lesser degree contamination can come from the air via aerosols, and from carcass washing water. There is little evidence that greater or smaller amounts of residual blood are important in promoting microbiological deterioration of carcasses although this is implied in much of the older literature (Warriss, 1984a).

Prevention of contamination

'Clean' and 'dirty' areas of the slaughter plant must be kept separate and personnel not be allowed to move between them. Dirty areas include the lairage and the raceways leading to the stunning point, and the stunning pen or stunning box in the case of cattle. Scalding tanks for pigs and poultry can become very dirty and are an obvious source of contamination, particularly via the sticking wound and the mouth. In some pig slaughter plants the bodies of the animals are washed and scrubbed with revolving nylon brushes before entry to the scalding tank. Systems of handling animals *ante mortem* should be directed at reducing skin, fleece, hide or feather soiling, and cross-contamination between animals.

The risks of contamination, by whatever routes, are likely to be higher with fuller guts. The amount of gut contents will be determined by several factors but especially important is likely to be the time for which the animal has been without access to food pre-slaughter. It is therefore generally accepted that animals should not have full stomachs at slaughter and that some period of fasting is desirable (Gracey, 1981). So, for pigs, an ideal total food withdrawal period pre-slaughter of 8–18 h has been suggested (Warriss, 1994). Much shorter times, ranging from 4 to 10 h, have been advocated for poultry (Anon, 1965; Wabeck, 1972). Ruminants have proportionally larger guts than pigs and longer fasting times may be appropriate. However, most of the loss in gut contents still appears to occur in the initial 24 h of fasting in these species (Table 9.2).

Care in skinning and dressing carcasses will reduce the chances of carcass contamination from any soiling, and enclosing pig dehairing and poultry plucking machinery will reduce the production of contaminating aerosols. Personal hygiene is important. Hands, arms, boots and aprons need to be cleaned frequently. All equipment, such as knives and saws, must be washed and sterilized with hot water (≥85°C) frequently.

Carcass decontamination

To prolong shelf life it is obviously beneficial to reduce microbiological contamination of the carcass before further butchery and processing. While the best policy is complete prevention of contamination in the first place, this is unrealistic and various methods of decontamination have been tried. The essential purpose of decontamination is extension of shelf life by a reduction in initial bacterial load. Some techniques may reduce pathogens but this is not generally the main objective except in poultry. Three types of decontamination procedures can be identified: water sprays, chemical methods and physical methods. Chemical methods are permitted in North America but not in Europe.

Water sprays need to be operated at high pressures to be effective since bacteria stick to carcass surfaces. Hot water is better but there is a danger of cooking the surface tissues if temperatures above about 75°C are used. A further danger is the formation of aerosols that may spread contamination rather than controlling it. Very brief steam treatment can overcome this. Chemical methods include use of chlorine and hydrogen peroxide, organic acids such as acetic and lactic acids, and trisodium phosphate. Chlorine is particularly useful in water immersion chilling systems where contact time is prolonged. Unfortunately it is rapidly inactivated by organic material. Acetic and lactic acids benefit from being naturally occurring. Of the two, lactic

Table 9.2. Gut contents weight as a percentage of the initial live weight after different times of food withdrawal in sheep and cattle.

	Food withdrawal period (h)				
	0	24	48	72	96
Sheep[a]	14.1	11.2	11.3	10.2	–
Cattle	14.5	10.7	11.6	9.0	11.7

[a] From Warriss *et al.*, 1987.

acid is the more useful. It can be combined with sodium lactate to buffer the pH since it is the undissociated lactic acid molecule that is effective, rather than the lactate ion. Trisodium phosphate works by dislodging bacteria from the skin, so allowing them to be washed away. Its effectiveness is attributable to its high alkalinity (pH = 12).

Physical decontamination methods comprise ultraviolet light, ionizing radiation such as gamma and X-rays, and ultrasound. Ultraviolet light has very poor penetration and parts of the carcass may 'shadow' other areas. Ionizing radiations can be very effective, particularly against pathogens, but suffer from consumer resistance to the idea of irradiated food. There is also the danger that their effectiveness might lead to less care being taken in preventing contamination in the first place. Ultrasound may be less useful for carcasses than for equipment such as poultry shackles. An excellent review of decontamination procedures that have been used, or proposed, for beef carcasses is that of Dorsa (1997).

Microbial Contamination

Food poisoning bacteria

Microbial contamination can be divided into two sorts: that caused by pathogenic bacteria and that by microbes that cause spoilage. Important pathogens are *Salmonella, Staphylococcus, Clostridium, Campylobacter, Listeria, Yersinia* and *Escherichia coli* O157 (Table 9.3). These can mostly be controlled by good hygiene and ensuring adequate cooking of meat immediately before consumption. *Campylobacter jejuni* and *C. coli, Listeria monocytogenes* and *E. coli* O157 are sometimes differentiated from the other bacteria because they cause a food-borne disease rather than just food poisoning. The difference is that for a person to suffer illness caused by a food poisoning bacterium, millions of bacterial cells must usually, but not always, be ingested. This leads to infection of the gastrointestinal tract and enteric symptoms. In the case of a food-borne disease, only relatively small numbers of bacteria need to be taken in; the food acts only as a vehicle for transmission of the pathogen, rather than as a growth medium. Because of this the incubation period is also much longer. The infective organism sometimes enters the blood stream and the symptoms may not always include vomiting and diarrhoea.

Food poisoning bacteria grow best at 37°C (body temperature) but will multiply at other temperatures. At higher temperatures they multiply more slowly and eventually stop dividing and may be killed. They also stop dividing at temperatures below 5°C. However, under adverse conditions some bacteria form spores which are much more

Table 9.3. Food poisoning bacteria and source of contamination.

Bacterium	Source
Salmonella spp.	Gut of animals
Staphylococcus aureus	Skin, nose, cuts in man and animals
Clostridium perfringens	Gut of animals
Clostridium botulinum	Soil
Campylobacter jejuni	Gut of animals
Listeria monocytogenes	Gut of animals
Escherichia coli O157	Gut of animals
Yersinia enterocolytica	Gut of animals

resistant than the vegetative cells. For example, some spores may resist 100°C for several hours. Of the food poisoning bacteria, *Clostridium* forms spores but *Salmonella* and *Staphylococcus* do not. The spores of *Clostridium* are not destroyed by normal cooking methods. In the UK, the Food Safety (Temperature Control) Regulations 1995 (SI 1995 No 1763) specify that, in general, food likely to support the growth of pathogenic bacteria must be stored below 8°C. If the food is to be served cold it can be kept at a higher temperature but only for a maximum of 4 h. Food to be served hot must be kept at 63°C or above, and for a maximum of 2 h.

Pathogenic bacteria may cause disease through infection, such as *Salmonella* and *Yersinia,* or through producing toxins, such as *Clostridium* and *Staphylococcus,* or may be both infectious and produce toxins, such as *Streptococcus.* The importance of toxin formation is that the toxin can be present even after the bacteria have been killed. Also, the effects of the toxin may occur very rapidly after ingestion since bacterial proliferation need not take place. *Clostridium perfringens* produces a toxin that irritates the gut wall causing diarrhoea. The bacterium is a common cause of food poisoning. Typically this might be through consumption of meat dishes prepared on one day but eaten the next. Cooking does not kill the bacterial spores. Reheating the food on the second day makes the spores germinate and grow. The related species *Clostridium botulinum* causes very severe, often fatal, food poisoning (botulism). In this case the toxin (a neurotoxin) is extremely poisonous, only a small quantity leading to severe illness. Because it is a strict anaerobe, multiplying only in the absence of oxygen, it can grow in tins of meat if these have not been sterilized adequately.

The germination of spores and growth of *Clostridium* is inhibited by the nitrite used in the production of cured meat. A concentration of nitrite of at least 120–200 mg kg^{-1} seems to be necessary – much higher than the concentrations needed to develop the characteristic colour and flavour of cured products. However, when meat is heated in the presence of nitrite to about 70°C or more, a chemical agent is formed, the 'Perigo factor', named after its discoverer. Fortunately, this agent is very much more (×10) inhibitory to Clostridial growth than nitrite alone. Information on methods to eliminate or counteract pathogens in meat is given in Smulders (1997).

Spoilage microbes

Microbes that cause spoilage can be bacteria, yeasts or other fungi (moulds). The bacteria can be those that thrive only in the presence of oxygen or those that grow under conditions where oxygen is absent. Offensive putrefaction is generally associated with the growth of bacteria growing in the absence of oxygen and producing indole, methylamine and hydrogen sulphide from decomposition of proteins and amino acids. Sour odours are produced by the decomposition of sugars. An excellent account of the bacteria found on meat and of the effects of different storage procedures on their growth and control is given in Dainty and Mackey (1992). Whitfield (1998) describes the types of taints produced by microbial spoilage. Methods for the measurement of microbial contamination of meat are described by Fung (1994).

Bacteria are classed as Gram-negative or Gram-positive, based on their reaction with various dyes. Gram-positive bacteria retain the stain, crystal violet, while Gram-negatives do not. Examples of Gram-negative spoilage bacteria often found on carcasses are *Pseudomonas, Acinetobacter* and *Psychrobacter*, as well as *Salmonella* and *Campylobacter*. Examples of Gram-positive bacteria are *Micrococcus, Bacillus* and *Brochothrix*.

Pseudomonas is one of the commonest and most important spoilage bacteria found on both red meat and poultry. Pseudomonads may form up to 90% of the flora on the surface of carcasses stored in chill rooms because many species will still grow at refrigerated temperatures. They are a large and varied group of rod-shaped bacteria, often motile with one or more flagella, and found ubiquitously. Many species cause plant and animal diseases. *Pseudomonas* can metabolize glucose to gluconate and 2-oxo-gluconate. Unlike other bacteria it can also break these compounds down further, giving it a competitive advantage. Where the pH of the meat is high, as in DFD (dark, firm, dry) meat, *Brochothrix thermosphacter*, which grows best at pH values above 6.5, may be important, especially at temperatures above 5°C. Under anaerobic conditions, and where the carbon dioxide concentration increases to perhaps 20%, for example in vacuum packages, the normal aerobic flora is suppressed and lactic acid-producing bacteria, such as *Lactobacillus*, are favoured. These tolerate high carbon dioxide levels.

Fungi (moulds) are considerably less important than bacteria as spoilage organisms. They can cause surface stickiness, or 'whiskers' –

the hyphae that form the threadlike vegetative parts of the fungus. Fungi will grow where too little water is available for the proliferation of bacteria. They may therefore be a problem on frozen meat where the storage temperature is too high. Bacon can be prone to spoilage by moulds because of its low water activity and high fat content.

The growth of bacteria

Four phases are recognized in the growth of bacterial colonies. In the initial *lag phase* the bacteria adjust to the environment. There follows an *exponential phase* where the numbers of bacteria multiply rapidly. Then comes a *stationary phase* when the rates of growth and multiplication are balanced by the number of bacterial cells dying. Finally, in the *reduction phase* there is a progressively greater death of cells because the substrate is depleted. As we have already seen for *Clostridium*, under unfavourable conditions some bacteria can produce spores. These are often very resistant to, for example, high temperatures or dry conditions. Bacteria grow by each cell dividing into two daughter cells. In exponential growth, the number of cells doubles at progressive equal time intervals. Because bacterial growth is exponential it is therefore often defined in terms of the time needed for the doubling of cell numbers. Under optimal conditions for growth the doubling time can be as short as 20 min. After 1 h, eight daughter cells will have been produced and after 4 h more than 8000. Unless limited, for example by exhaustion of nutrients, by 6 h the number will have increased to more than a quarter of a million. Because of the very large numbers involved in describing bacterial populations they are often expressed using a logarithmic scale.

On the surface of carefully handled carcasses the numbers of bacteria (the total viable count) may be up to 10^3 to 10^4 organisms cm^{-2}. With poor hygiene this could rise to more than 10^6 organisms cm^{-2} and off-odours often start to develop at approximately 10^7–10^8 organisms cm^{-2}. Slime may form if adjacent bacterial colonies coalesce.

Factors affecting bacterial growth

An overview of the growth requirements of microbes in relation to their growth on food, and the preservation of food, is given in Boddy and Wimpenny (1992). Important factors are temperature, oxygen availability, pH, redox potential, competition with other bacteria and moisture availability of the substrate. The availability of water is more correctly described in terms of water activity (a_w). The water activity of a solution is the ratio of its vapour pressure to that of pure water at the same temperature. Water activities therefore range from 0 (no water) to 1 (pure water). Solutions containing high concentrations of salt therefore have lower water activity values. Bacteria will not grow below water activities of about 0.75, and most will not grow below 0.91. Because of this, bacteria will not grow in solutions with high osmotic pressure (having a high concentration of low molecular weight soluble substances). Similarly, when water freezes into ice it becomes unavailable to bacteria. Drying the surfaces of carcasses therefore inhibits bacterial spoilage, although yeasts and moulds will tolerate lower water activities and may still grow.

Of all the factors, temperature is the most important with growth rate generally being higher at higher temperatures. However, different types of bacteria will grow best in different temperature ranges and microbiologists group them accordingly (Table 9.4). The temperature ranges for the different groups vary a little between different authorities, and those given in Table 9.4 are mainly for illustration. Some authors use the terms 'psychrotroph' and 'psychrophile' almost interchangeably. However, psychrophiles have lower optimum growth temperatures while psychrotrophs are simply cold tolerant but grow better at higher temperatures. Some thermophiles will grow at 80°C or more. *Listeria monocytogenes* and *Yersinia enterocolytica* can both grow at refrigeration temperatures (≤4°C). *Escherichia coli* will not grow at 5°C or less, and grows only slowly at 10°C. Many *Pseudomonas* will grow slowly at refrigeration temperatures and will continue to grow up to 30°C, but not above 35°C.

Bacteria will grow better at neutral pH values (around pH 7) than at lower or higher values. The acidification that occurs in normal meat *post mortem* therefore tends to inhibit growth. The high ultimate pH of DFD meat is one reason why it is prone to spoilage. Rey *et al.* (1976) studied the growth of bacteria on PSE (pale, soft, exudative), normal and DFD pork. The three meat types had different ultimate pH values, with, as would be expected, that in the DFD meat highest and that in the PSE meat lowest. The initial numbers of bacteria were similar on the three sorts of pork. However, during storage for up to 3 days in packs overwrapped with oxygen-permeable film the shortest lag phase and the most rapid bacterial growth occurred on the DFD meat and the slowest growth on the PSE meat. This was in spite of the large amount

Table 9.4. The temperature ranges in which psychrophiles, psychrotrophs, mesophiles and thermophiles will in general grow.

Psychrophiles	−8 to +25°C
Psychrotrophs	−2 to +25°C
Mesophiles	+10 to +40°C
Thermophiles	+43 to +66°C

of exudate associated with the PSE pork, which might have been thought to provide an ideal medium for bacterial growth. The meat pH also selectively influenced the types of bacteria found. For example, a particular strain of *Pseudomonas* hardly grew on PSE pork but proliferated on the DFD meat.

Redox potential defines whether a system is oxidizing or reducing in character. High redox potentials inhibit the growth of most bacteria.

Bacteria can be divided into those that grow only in the *presence* of oxygen (strict or obligate aerobes), those that only grow in the *absence* of oxygen (strict or obligate anaerobes) and those that will grow in the presence or absence of oxygen (facultative anaerobes). Meat surfaces tend to favour the growth of aerobes, while internally anaerobes are more likely. Packaging meat with over-wrapped films can influence spoilage by modifying the surface oxygen tension. For example, oxygen-impermeable films encourage growth of anaerobes either directly or by encouraging build up of carbon dioxide which inhibits aerobe growth.

Clostridium is an anaerobe so tends to grow only deep within meat where oxygen from the air cannot penetrate. 'Bone taint' in pork, and sometimes beef, is caused by, amongst other bacteria, *Clostridium putrefaciens*, which multiplies in the deep tissues in the region of the bones even at refrigerated temperatures (<5°C). Growth is encouraged by higher than normal ultimate pH in the muscle and poor chilling which allows the innermost parts of the carcass, especially the parts surrounding the deeper bones, to remain at a relatively high temperature for a prolonged time after slaughter. Proliferation of the bacteria leads to the development of very unpleasant putrid smells. The condition is rather rare nowadays because of closer control of refrigeration practices.

The Preservation of Meat

Because it is high in protein and moisture, meat is potentially an ideal medium for bacterial growth. Many techniques have been evolved to reduce or eliminate this growth and so preserve the meat longer. Much information on meat preservation is given in Varnum and Sutherland (1995).

Drying

Drying reduces the water activity. It is a very old technique and one that is still used. Examples of dried meats are biltong in South Africa, pemmican and jerky in North America, and charqui in South America.

In the case of biltong and charqui, the meat may also be salted. A modern technique is freeze drying (lyophilization). In this, water is sublimated from the meat. It passes directly from ice to vapour without an intervening liquid phase. This leaves the meat structure relatively undamaged providing the original freezing is rapid enough.

Curing and smoking

The chemistry of curing

Like drying, salting was discovered a long time ago. As well as preserving the meat the product develops the characteristic desirable taste and flavour. In addition to common salt (sodium chloride, NaCl), potassium or sodium nitrate (KNO_3, $NaNO_3$) and sodium nitrite ($NaNO_2$) are now used in the curing process. In fact, it is the sodium chloride and sodium nitrite which are important in the curing reaction. The nitrate acts only as a potential reservoir of nitrite, some being reduced to nitrite by inherent reducing systems in the meat or often by bacteria present in the curing brine. Sebranek and Fox (1985) give a comprehensive review of the reactions of nitrite and chloride that are important in the production of cured meat products, and an overview of the chemistry of curing can be found in Skibsted (1992).

The nitrite reacts with the haem pigments in the meat to give the attractive pink colour typical of hams and other cured products, and, as mentioned previously, it is very important in inhibiting the growth of bacteria, in particular *Clostridium botulinum*. The sodium chloride inhibits the growth of microorganisms in two ways. First, it lowers the water activity of the meat. Second, the sodium ion (Na^+) has a specific inhibitory effect. The series of reactions leading to the formation of the cured meat colour is complex. However, in essence the nitrite, which has strong oxidizing properties, first oxidizes myoglobin to metmyoglobin. Nitrite is also converted to nitric oxide by the naturally occurring enzyme systems in the muscle, and by any reducing agents, such as ascorbic acid, that may have been included in the curing brine. The nitric oxide molecule is very reactive and reacts with the oxidized metmyoglobin, eventually to form nitrosylmyoglobin. This is pink in colour. It is relatively unstable, particularly when exposed to light. If the meat is cooked the globin part of the nitrosylmyoglobin molecule is denatured to form pink/brown nitric oxide haemochromogen.

Modern cured meats have much lower salt contents than those produced traditionally. For example, traditional bacon might contain over 5% salt but some modern products have only 2%. This is partly because of changes in preferred saltiness and partly because of a desire to reduce sodium levels in foods for health reasons. Indeed, in some cases sodium chloride is replaced by potassium chloride, or other potassium salts. This reduces sodium to minimal amounts but results in a much less stable product that needs to be stored at refrigeration temperatures.

Reduction in the use of nitrite

Nitrite also has an important role in the development of flavour in cured meats. MacDougall *et al.* (1975) discussed the contribution of nitrite to colour and flavour development. A nitrite concentration of 25 mg kg^{-1} of meat was adequate for normal colour development but four times this level was needed for optimal flavour. However, there has been considerable interest in developing technologies to produce cured meat products without the use of nitrite at all. This is because of the involvement of nitrite in the formation of nitrosamines from amines such as amino acids, and the fact that some nitrosamines have been found to be carcinogenic. These new technologies aim to replace the flavour and colour forming, and antimicrobial properties of nitrite with other ingredients of the cure (Shahidi and Pegg, 1991).

Other curing ingredients

In normal curing processes various other substances may be included in the salt mixture. Polyphosphates improve water-holding capacity (WHC) and so increase the amount of curing brine that can be taken up by the meat and improve product yield. Sugars (sucrose or glucose) impart flavour. Ascorbic acid (vitamin C) may be added. As mentioned previously, this acts as a reducing agent and inhibits the breakdown of the nitrosylmyoglobin so preventing discoloration, particularly when cured products are displayed under artificial light. Ascorbic acid also tends to inhibit nitrosamine formation. In the USA, isoascorbic acid is used instead.

The curing process

There are very many types of cured products and curing processes. In dry curing, the salts are added as a solid by being rubbed into the surface of the meat. The process may be repeated and the joints may be held in the salt mixture to allow permeation of the salt through the tissues. Dry curing is rarely used commercially to make bacon but is employed for Spanish hams and Parma ham manufacture. In Parma hams only common salt (sodium chloride) is used. More commonly, meat is cured by immersion in a solution of the salts (brine). Usually, when meat is cured by immersion it is also first injected with brine. Particularly for boneless hams, tumbling or massaging in rotating drums, sometimes under vacuum, may be used to help even distribution of the brine after injection. This can shorten the time needed for curing. After a period, when the curing salts have diffused through the mass of the meat, the product is 'matured'. During this time excess fluid can drain away, and the characteristic flavour and colour develop fully. The product may also be smoked. Originally, smoking helped preservation by drying the meat surface and through the action of antimicrobial substances naturally present in the smoke. It may also inhibit fat oxidation. Its main use now is in contributing to the flavour. Traditionally, the smoke was produced by burning hardwood sawdust (from trees such as oak and beech) but nowadays liquid smokes, containing the active ingredients of actual smoke, but in a liquid extract, are often used.

The penetration of the brine during curing is controlled by osmotic factors. There is first a flow of water out of the meat into the brine, which has a higher osmotic pressure because of its salt content. Then, as salt diffuses into the meat, the difference in osmotic pressure favours flow of brine back into the meat. Because it affects WHC, the curing qualities of meat are influenced by characteristics such as its pH. The relation of WHC to pH is curvilinear with minimum water-holding at between pH 5 and 5.5. At pH values above and below this the water-holding improves progressively. Therefore, meat marinaded in vinegar (acetic acid) has a high WHC and so has meat with a high ultimate pH. If the pH is increased artificially, for example by adding alkaline phosphates, particularly polyphosphates, the WHC also improves (polyphosphates may also improve WHC by mimicking the action of ATP on actomyosin).

In PSE meat, the myofibrillar proteins may have denatured somewhat and WHC is poor. PSE pork therefore takes up less brine and the yield of the cured product is reduced. In contrast, DFD meat, with a high ultimate pH, has a high WHC. However, the relatively closed texture may inhibit salt uptake leading to uneven curing. Moreover, the high pH encourages bacterial conversion of nitrate to nitrite so nitrite levels may be unacceptably high. Salt penetration is faster in meat that has been frozen compared with unfrozen meat. It is also faster at higher temperatures but the potential benefits of high temperature curing are outweighed by the need to maintain low temperatures to prevent the growth of spoilage bacteria.

Bacon

The main cured meat is pork, but beef and, to a lesser degree, sheep meat, are also cured. Originally beef was cured using a granulated form of salt called 'corn', hence the name 'corned beef'. Pork is cured into bacon or ham. Ham is made from the legs and bacon mainly from the back and belly. In traditional Wiltshire curing, named after the county in the south west of England which was originally the major bacon curing region of the country, the trimmed half carcass (side) of a pig is cured as a whole. The major steps in the process are shown in Box 9.1. After trimming the sides and removal of various bones, including the vertebral column, the head, feet and the fillet muscle (m. psoas), the meat is injected with brine containing about 20% sodium chloride. To inject the brine a multi-needle injector is used. This has several rows of hollow needles that penetrate the soft tissues of the side as it is moved forwards by a conveyor belt. The sides are pumped to increase their weight by about 10% or so. After pumping, they are held immersed in tanks for 3–5 days in brine containing up to 25% sodium chloride to complete the curing process. The sides are then removed, drained and stacked on pallets for about 5–7 days. During this time the concentration of the curing salts equilibrates through the meat and a certain amount of drying occurs.

Processing starts with the chilled carcasses and the temperature is maintained at 5°C or below throughout curing to minimize the risk of spoilage. The immersion brines are recycled, with salt being added periodically to maintain the salinity, and they develop a deep red colour from dissolved haem pigments, and a beneficial bacterial population. The bacteria are important in reducing the nitrate to nitrite, and probably in flavour development. Traditional Wiltshire curing of whole sides is becoming less common nowadays and has been replaced by curing boneless primal joints. In 'sweetcure' curing methods the product generally has a lower salt content than traditional Wiltshire style bacon. The name derives from the inclusion of about 2% sugar (sucrose or glucose) in the brine. A modern development is 'slice curing' where slices of pork are dipped in brine for a short period then packed, the curing process continuing in the bag so ensuring a very rapid manufacture time.

Hams

Cured hind legs and shoulders from pigs may be cooked to produce hams. These can be dry-cured or, more commonly now, produced by

Box 9.1. An outline of the major steps involved in the traditional curing of pork carcasses by the 'Wiltshire' process.

- The half carcasses (sides) are prepared by removal of head, feet, backbone and other bones, and psoas muscle.
- Sides are injected with brine (20% NaCl, 0.2% $NaNO_3$, 0.1% $NaNO_2$), increasing their weight by about 10%.
- The pumped sides are stacked in tanks and covered with brine for up to 5 days.
- They are removed from the brine and stacked for up to 7 days to mature (when normal bacon flavour and colour develop). This is 'green' bacon.
- The green bacon is smoked if desired (using wood smoke).

immersion in brine. Traditionally, like bacon, these would have had a fairly high salt content but there has been a general trend to reducing both salt and flavour. After cooking, the skin is removed from the ham (derinding).

Some rindless, boneless hams, produced mainly for slicing, are cooked slowly at a relatively low temperature in cans. The low temperature is necessary to ensure that the ham's structure, which is rather fragile because of the action of the salt on the muscle proteins, is not damaged by over-cooking. The canned meat is pasteurized. The mild cooking does not sterilize the can contents so the product must be held at refrigerated temperatures for storage. In contrast to sterilization, which kills all bacteria, pasteurization kills only non-spore-forming bacteria and some spores. However, many spores are heat resistant. Prevention of the germination and growth of these relies on the nitrite present in the curing brine. As mentioned previously, the effect of the nitrite is magnified by development of the 'Perigo factor' when the cured meat is heated during pasteurization. Even so, particularly if not stored correctly, bacterial growth can sometimes occur, resulting in 'blown' cans caused by the evolution of gas by the metabolism of the bacteria. The pasteurization process is analagous to that used for milk. Milk is held between 62.8°C (145°F) and 65.6°C (150°F) for 30 min, or alternatively for 71.7°C (161°F) for 15 s, then cooled rapidly to below 10°C for storage. Boiling the milk would sterilize it but would also cause undesirable changes in its structure and flavour.

Dry cured hams and sausages

In continental Europe a number of hams are made for eating without cooking. Italian Parma hams are cured with sodium chloride (but not nitrite) and air-dried. Spanish hams are traditionally made from a special breed of black Iberian pig that is allowed to feed on acorns from cork oaks. Spanish hams are dry-cured with sodium chloride and potassium nitrate. After salting, the hams are characteristically matured for many months. During this time the salt distributes evenly through the ham and complex chemical changes occur, leading to the development of the very characteristic flavours associated with the products.

Dry sausages like salamis are cured with relatively large amounts of salt and may also be smoked to preserve them. They can be eaten raw. Their production was outlined in Chapter 8.

Irradiation

Meat can be rendered sterile, and therefore preserved, by exposing it to ionizing radiation (X-rays, gamma rays). The advantage is that very large pieces of meat can be processed, practically all vegetative cells (but not all spores) of microorganisms are killed, and there is effectively no change in the physical or chemical composition of the meat. Disadvantages include some destruction of vitamins, and the potential production of off flavours (Sudarmadji and Urbain, 1972) and also carcinogens from other chemicals. Off flavours can be caused by the promotion of fat oxidation through generating free radicals. There is also considerable public distrust of irradiation. Various sources of radiation are possible. For example, cobalt 60 and caesium 137 emit gamma rays. Electron accelerators produce X-rays. The preservation of meat by irradiation has been reviewed by Elias (1985) and Stevenson (1992).

Refrigeration

Benefits of chilling and freezing

Because lower temperatures reduce or prevent microbial growth, cooling carcasses as soon as possible after dressing, and keeping meat at low temperatures, can considerably reduce the rate of spoilage and the growth of pathogenic bacteria. Fresh meat can normally be stored for 5–7 days at refrigerated temperatures. An important point is that it is the outside surfaces of carcasses that it is most important to cool rapidly because these are where the bacterial contamination is likely to be. Apart from very small numbers of microorganisms potentially introduced at sticking, the interior parts of the carcass tissues will generally be sterile if they have not been contaminated during the dressing procedures. Chilling has other benefits. It reduces evaporative weight loss and makes the fat firmer, so contributing to the 'setting' of the carcass and making it easier to handle. Freezing can be a very effective way of storing meat. Mammoths have been preserved for thousands of years in the ice of Siberia. Meat freezes at about −1.5°C but the lower the temperature of storage the more stable will be the product. This is mainly because low temperatures inhibit chemical as well as microbial spoilage. For example, changes associated with oxidative rancidity will be delayed if meat is held at lower frozen temperatures. Beef and lamb can be stored at −18°C for at least 6–12 months, pork can be stored for 6 months and poultry for 3 months. Freezing will kill some microorganism vegetative cells by thermal shock, ice formation, dehydration or solute concentration, more dying with longer storage, and some cells will be damaged, but sublethally. Spores are generally resistant to freezing. Slow freezing is likely to kill more bacteria than fast freezing.

The thermophysical properties of meat

Understanding and predicting the process of refrigeration of carcasses and joints depends on a knowledge of the thermophysical properties of meat. Two important properties are its specific heat and thermal conductivity. The specific heat of a substance defines the amount of energy required to raise its temperature by 1°C at any particular temperature. It also therefore determines the amount of energy required to lower its temperature. Water has a value of 1. At room temperature, the specific heats of lean, fat and bone are approximately 0.85, 0.95 and 0.60. However, the value for fat varies considerably with temperature, the specific heat being minimal at 15–20°C and increasing at both lower and higher temperatures. This is because the fat may be liquid or solid, the change in phase having an important influence. The specific heat of bone depends on what sort it is, in particular its density. Because carcasses consist of lean, fat and bone, their specific heat is approximately 0.75 but this can obviously vary depending on the actual composition of the carcass.

Thermal conductivity defines the rate of flow of heat through a substance. In cooling carcasses the flow is from the centre of the tissues to the surface. Fats have a lower thermal conductivity than lean meat, the value for bone depending on whether it is solid or spongy. The thermal conductivity of lean depends on the fibre direction to a small degree – it is greater along the axis of the muscle fibres.

Predicting the loss of heat from carcasses is complicated by their complex shape as well as by variation in their composition. The situation is further complicated during freezing. Ice has a significantly higher thermal conductivity than water, so, when a layer of ice forms at the surface, this improves flow of heat out from the sub-surface tissue. Therefore, the rate of freezing increases as freezing progresses. In contrast, when meat or carcasses are thawed, conversion of ice to water in the surface layers reduces the subsequent rate of heat flow. Thawing a particular carcass or piece of meat therefore always takes longer than freezing given the same rates of external heat transport. The situation is complicated by the need to keep the surface layers of the carcass/meat at low enough temperatures to prevent microbial growth. An interesting account of the thawing of beef is given in James *et al.* (1977) and a comparison of different thawing methods in Bailey *et al.* (1974).

Practical considerations

Heat is lost from carcasses or meat through four mechanisms. The most important is convection. Air (or a liquid) passing over the surface takes heat from that surface and carries it away. Increasing the rate at which the air flows, or decreasing its temperature, increases the rate of cooling. So, to chill carcasses rapidly, high air speeds at low temperatures are most effective. However, an average chill room might have an air speed of only 0.5 m s^{-1}, and, at an air temperature of 0°C, a beef carcass will take more than 24 h to reach 10°C in the deep leg tissues. Achieving 7°C throughout the carcass before distribution or further processing may take place, as required by EU legislation, might take up to 48 h in practice.

The other mechanisms of heat transfer from carcasses are radiation, evaporative cooling and conduction. Radiation is not normally significant because the temperature difference between the carcass and its surroundings is too small. Evaporative cooling produces only a very small effect. Conduction requires physical contact with the cooling surface and is generally impracticable.

Because the specific heat varies with temperature the amount of heat that needs to be removed to chill a carcass depends on its actual temperature. At higher temperatures proportionally more heat needs removal. The best way of using refrigeration is therefore to chill carcasses initially in a 'pre-chiller' running at a higher rate of heat exchange. This removes much of the heat in the carcass relatively rapidly. Then the carcasses are transferred to the chiller proper, which runs at a lower rate of heat exchange to carry out the final cooling. The rate at which carcasses need to be cooled is determined by the requirement for the process to fit in with normal slaughter operations – often killing one day and cutting or despatch the next after overnight chilling, the legislative requirements, and the need to prevent undesirable changes to quality. So, chilling needs to be slow enough to prevent cold shortening while still controlling microbial growth. As mentioned above, within the EU there is a legislative requirement to chill carcasses to 7°C before further processing or transport. This is possible to attain in lamb and pork carcasses but not so in sides of beef within the constraint of a 24 h cycle. Mallikarjunan and Mittal (1995) gave a description of methodology for predicting the optimum conditions for chilling beef carcasses given certain constraints such as the need to avoid cold shortening, the need to avoid surface freezing and the time scale required. Chilling in red meat species is almost invariably using cold air. However, poultry are often chilled by immersion in ice water. The process is very effective and in fact leads to an increase in carcass weight rather than the loss associated with air chilling. Examples of the pattern of temperature fall measured in beef, pork and lamb carcasses are shown in Fig. 9.1. Note the different rates of cooling of the m. longissimus dorsi (near the surface of the carcass) and the m. semimembranosus (which lies deeper), particularly in the larger beef and pig carcasses.

Carcasses are often transported chilled. In this case it is important that there is good airflow within the containers, so that all carcasses and parts of them are maintained at a uniform temperature, and that carcasses are prevented from touching the container walls which may be relatively warm.

Freezing methods

Industrial freezing methods are designed to remove heat from the meat as rapidly as possible. In blast freezers, very cold air (down to −40°C) is blown over the meat in a 'tunnel'. Belt freezers, in which the meat is

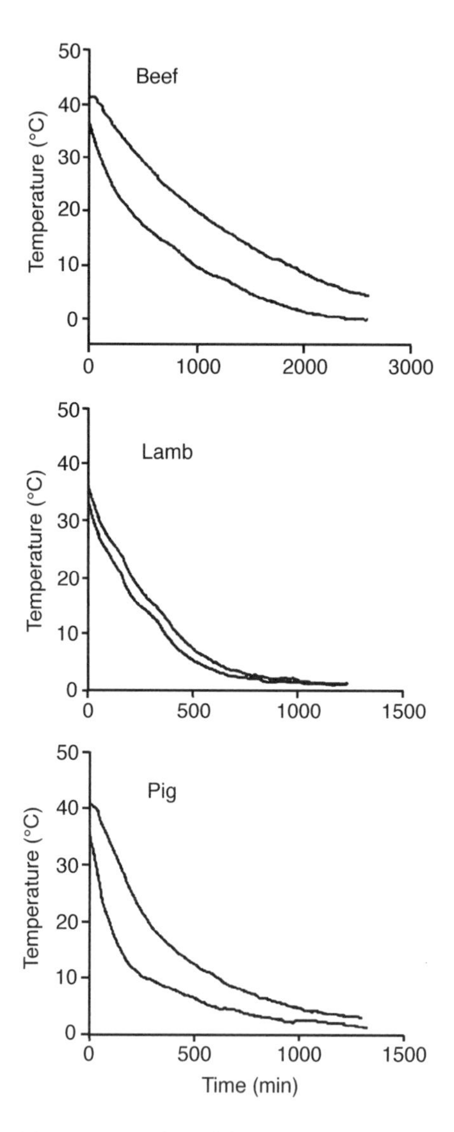

Fig. 9.1. Examples of the patterns of the fall in temperature in the muscles of beef, lamb and pig carcasses held in a chiller set to run at +2°C (in each species the upper lines show the temperature measured in the m. semimembranosus of the hind leg, and the lower lines the temperature in the m. longissimus dorsi of the loin).

supported on a conveyor belt, are used for small items like burgers and chicken parts. Burgers can also be frozen using plate freezers. In these, metal plates cooled to very low temperatures are pressed onto the surface of the meat. Cryogenic freezing uses liquid nitrogen (at −196°C) in which the items are immersed.

Potential effects of chilling and freezing on quality

Chilling and freezing can have some effects on meat colour, WHC and other aspects of quality. Chilling influences the rate of penetration of oxygen from the surface of lean meat, and the rate at which the enzymic reducing activity in the muscle combats metmyoglobin formation. Because of the greater decrease in reducing activity than the rate of oxygen diffusion into the meat when it is stored at lower temperatures, the oxymyoglobin layer is thicker, and the meat colour brighter. Rapid chilling *post mortem* tends to reduce drip formation, probably by limiting protein denaturation. Depending on the particular conditions the effect may be to approximately halve drip formation, with the size of the reduction being greater in pork from more susceptible breeds where WHC is inherently poorer and drip loss greater. Storage at lower chill temperatures also tends to reduce drip formation.

Jakobsson and Bengtsson (1969a) reviewed much of the literature on the effects of freezing rate on the quality of beef. They also studied (Jakobsson and Bengtsson, 1969b) the effects of ageing time, freezing rate and cooking method, amongst other things, on the eating quality, appearance and thawing losses of beef m. longissimus dorsi. A notable finding was the large number of significant interactions between the effects of the different factors. Generally, compared with rapid freezing, slow freezing damages the muscle structure resulting in decreased myofibrillar protein solubility and WHC, and increased weight losses on thawing (Petrovic *et al.*, 1993). Faster freezing, usually obtained by freezing at lower temperatures, can lead to a lighter lean meat colour. At very low temperatures the colour may be too pale. The effect is attributed to the different sizes of ice crystals formed. The smaller crystals formed by fast freezing scatter more light and the meat surface therefore appears paler.

Freezing reduces WHC. Water outside the muscle fibres freezes first. The remaining liquid is concentrated by osmotic effects, which tend to draw water out of the fibres. This water is not reabsorbed on thawing and results in the relatively large amounts of exudate lost in the process. The rate of freezing may influence the degree of the reduction in water-holding capacity by changing the balance of freezing of the free water in different muscle ‘compartments’ – that is, whether it is extracellular, intracellular and, if the latter, whether within or outside the myofibrils. The portion of water chemically bound to the muscle proteins may never freeze. Generally, faster freezing seems to reduce subsequent drip loss on thawing. The full effects of fast and slow freezing are still unclear. Indeed, some authors have found no effects. Sakata *et al.* (1995) froze pork in air at temperatures of −20°C or −80°C. The slower freezing at −20°C produced larger ice crystals but there were no effects on WHC, colour or lipid oxidation. An excellent concise review of the chilling and freezing of red meat is that of James (1996).

Cooking

The main reason we cook meat now is to make it palatable. Very little meat is eaten raw. However, a very important additional benefit of cooking is to make meat safer to eat. Cooking kills bacteria, especially important in the case of pathogens. To do this the temperature needs to be high enough for long enough. The centre of the meat must reach at least 70°C for 2 min, or an equivalent combination of temperature and time. Cooking also improves sensory characteristics by developing flavour from, for example, the Maillard reaction and fat oxidation. Particularly for meat from old animals containing lots of cross-linked connective tissue, it improves tenderness. Meat from old animals, or cuts with much connective tissue, are usually cooked at lower temperature by wet heat, that is in water (e.g. stewing), for longer times. This breaks down the connective tissue. Meat with small amounts of connective tissue is usually cooked at high temperature with dry heat (e.g. roasting) for a shorter time.

Changes caused by cooking

Various changes occur as the temperature of meat increases. Between 30 and 50°C the myofibrillar proteins start to denature, leading to loss of WHC and protein solubility. At 55°C there is considerable protein denaturation and coagulation causing shrinkage of the myofilament lattice and toughening. Between 60 and 63°C collagen shrinks and the collagen sheaths in the muscle contract, producing considerable extra toughening. As the temperature increases and the cooking time is prolonged more of the collagen is converted into gelatin with corresponding tenderization of the connective tissue component. At 65°C most of the myofibrillar and sarcoplasmic proteins have coagulated and much of the water originally contained in the muscle has been lost. Between 65 and 70°C the collagen denatures, and between 70 and 90°C disulphide bonds form in actomyosin resulting in toughening of the myofibrillar component. The effects of heating on the structure and ultrastructure of meat have been described by Hostetler and Landmann (1968), Cheng and Parrish (1976) and Sims and Bailey (1992).

Flavour develops on heating with characteristic flavours produced by different cooking methods, partly because of the differences in the intensity of heating. So, roasting leads to drying of the meat surface and production of many more volatile flavour components than boiling. Temperature also affects appearance. 'Doneness' is attributable to denaturation of the haem pigments to give a progressively more brown appearance. Beef cooked to 60°C (rare) is quite red inside, at 70°C (medium) it becomes pink–brown and at 80°C (well-done) brown. At higher temperatures the surface brown colour is enhanced by dehydration and the products of Maillard browning reactions.

Effect of cooking temperature

Temperature achieved during cooking has important influences on palatability characteristics. Because heat has to flow from the outside of the meat to the inside, the temperature achieved will vary throughout the joint or cut unless cooking is prolonged. The important figure is the endpoint temperature in the centre of the joint. How this can influence sensory characteristics is illustrated by the results of a study by Wood *et al.* (1995), which confirmed the findings of an earlier North American study (Simmons *et al.*, 1985). Pork loin steaks were grilled to three internal temperatures and the eating quality was assessed by a trained taste panel (Table 9.5).

As temperature increased, tenderness and juiciness decreased but flavour improved. Seemingly, the flavour improvement was partly attributable to a more intense pork flavour but also because of reduced abnormal flavour scores. These effects were also seen in roasted pork legs but the size of the effects on tenderness and juiciness was smaller. The authors recommended that steaks were cooked to the intermediate temperature of 72.5°C but that roasts could be taken to higher temperatures. They speculated that the reductions in tenderness and juiciness were caused by myofibrillar protein denaturation leading to loss of water from the meat. This was evidenced by differences in cooking losses. At higher cooking temperatures greater cooking loss was seen, increasing from about 30% at 65°C to over 40% at 80°C.

Changes in composition caused by cooking

Cooking loss reflects loss of mainly water, but also some other components. Based on data in McCance and Widdowson (1997), cooking by grilling reduces the water content of rump steak from 66.7 to 59.3% and the fat content from 13.5 to 12.1%. This has the effect of concentrating the protein content (from 18.9 to 27.3%) and increasing the relative energy content (from 821 to 912 kJ 100 g^{-1}). Of particular

Table 9.5. Eating quality[a] and cooking loss of pork loin steaks (m. longissimus dorsi) grilled to three internal temperatures (from Wood *et al.*, 1995).

	Final internal temperature (°C)		
	65	72.5	80
Texture	5.1	4.5	4.2
Juiciness	5.0	4.3	3.5
Pork flavour	3.4	3.5	4.1
Abnormal flavour	3.3	3.1	2.7
Cooking loss (%)	29.5	35.0	41.9

[a] Pork from female pigs assessed using eight-point category scales. Higher scores for texture, juiciness and pork flavour indicate greater 'liking'. Higher scores for abnormal flavour indicate higher perception of the flavour component.

interest is loss of fat since this has implications for consumer health. Cooking melts fat and some of this is likely to be lost in methods such as grilling, frying and roasting.

Sheard *et al.* (1998b) found that, after grilling to 80°C, pork loin chops lost 48% of their water, 34% of their fat and 2% of their protein. The loss of fat can be greater in comminuted meat products like mince (ground meat), sausages, burgers and restructured steaks. These contain relatively large amounts of fat. The effect was investigated by Sheard *et al.* (1998a). Some of their results are shown in Table 9.6. The greatest reduction occurred in minced (ground) beef, where fat content was reduced to less than half of that in the raw product, but even in restructured steaks, which showed the least effect, the amount of fat was reduced by 19%. Different cooking methods had little effect on the size of the losses.

The contribution made to the palatability of meat by the external fat covering of the joints during cooking is unclear. There is some evidence that removal of external fat may reduce the eating quality of some beef joints after certain cooking methods (Coleman *et al.*, 1988). This could be because part of the external fat melts into the lean tissues. However, some studies suggest that, at least in pork, removal of the external (subcutaneous) fat does not reduce the final lipid content of the lean after cooking (Novakofski *et al.*, 1989).

Canning

In canning the meat is cooked to sterilize it after being sealed in a container. The container is now made of sheet steel that has been coated with a very thin layer of tin (hence 'tin cans'). The tin prevents the steel from corroding. In *sterilizing* the contents it is important to kill the spores of *Clostridium botulinum* which can grow under anaerobic conditions. This is usually ensured by heating in steam at 116°C or higher, in contrast to the much lower temperatures used to *pasteurize* some hams (see above), which are therefore not sterile.

Table 9.6. The effect of cooking on loss of fat from comminuted products (from Sheard *et al.*, 1998a).

	Fat (g) in		
Product	Raw product	Cooked product	% Reduction
Minced (ground) beef	18.9	7.1	62
Burgers	25.1	15.7	37
Restructured steaks	17.5	14.1	19
Sausages	21.8	16.6	24

Ensuring Meat is Safe to Eat

Traditional systems

Traditional meat inspection is based on examination of live animals *ante mortem* and carcasses *post mortem* to identify pathological and other conditions that might make the meat unwholesome. This enables abnormal or infected meat to be prevented from entering the food chain. Additionally, feedback to farmers may help to eradicate some diseases. The system operates at the end of the meat production chain rather than concerning itself with the hygienic acceptability or otherwise of particular procedures in the overall process of slaughtering an animal and dressing its carcass. This does not mean that the individual procedures are of no concern, just that the process is monitored at the end. So, for example, the meat inspector may reject a carcass because it is soiled with faeces. He is not primarily concerned with how the faeces got on to the carcass but with the fact that they are there and that their presence makes the carcass unacceptable.

This inspection process is analogous to traditional methods of quality control in the food industry as a whole. In these methods, quality control staff are employed to inspect production systems and check that good manufacturing practices (GMPs) are being used so that quality, particularly hygiene, is maintained. The GMPs are defined by codes of practice, which specify how things should be done. Samples of the end product are tested to check they meet acceptability criteria. In the case of hygienic quality this would probably entail measuring the presence and numbers of bacteria. This process is inherently retrospective. It only identifies unacceptable products after production. Moreover, the results are often too late to do anything about the problem (particularly if the testing involves culturing bacteria) and do not identify where the process has gone wrong. Unless very large numbers of samples are tested it also often fails to detect substandard products at all.

Hazard Analysis and Critical Control Points (HACCP) systems

HACCP systems, in contrast to traditional quality control systems, are designed to assure food safety by monitoring and control of the whole production process, rather than by just making measurements on quality control samples taken at the end of the process. The essence of HACCP systems is therefore that they are preventive. They prevent the production of poor quality product, rather than just identifying when a production system has failed. They can be applied to whole systems, from animal production through to the final stages of preparation for consumption, but their major impact so far has been in the meat processing sector where the control of processes such as heating, cooling, cleaning and sterilization is very amenable to this kind of quality assurance system.

HACCP systems were originally conceived for use in the chemical industry and became associated with food production in the quest by the US space programme to produce foods for astronauts that would be absolutely free from hazards such as pathogens. An excellent historical introduction to HACCP is that of Bauman (1990) and overviews of the potential use of HACCP systems in the control of hygiene and chemical safety in the meat and poultry industries are given by Adams (1990) and Tompkin (1990). The National Advisory Committee on Microbiological Criteria for Foods of the US Department of Agriculture has recently produced a very useful summary of the principles of HACCP and guidelines for its application (NACMCF, 1998) in the food industry. This gives examples of operation of the seven principles (see below). It is now generally acknowledged that HACCP is the best system available for promoting food safety.

Hazards and risks

There will inevitably be hazards associated with food production. A hazard is any property that could cause an unacceptable consumer health risk; it is a potential source of harm. The likelihood or probability that a hazard will actually occur is assessed as a risk and risk assessment tries to estimate how significant the risk is. The possibility of suffering from a transmissable spongiform encephalopathy (CJD) after eating beef from cattle that may have been infected with BSE is a hazard. The risk associated with this hazard seems, however, to be very low (based on the number of recorded cases of CJD). Suffering from food poisoning caused by eating meat contaminated with *Salmonella* and inadequately cooked is also a hazard. In this case, evidence suggests that the risk is much higher (because a large number of cases of food poisoning are recorded). The seriousness of the consequences of a hazard is assessed as its severity. The consequences of contracting CJD are very severe in that recovery seems extremely unlikely and the almost inevitable outcome is death. The consequences of contracting food poisoning are unpleasant but not as severe, at least for the majority of the adult population who will generally survive the episode.

Setting up a HACCP system

Seven steps or stages are involved in setting up and instituting a HACCP system (Box 9.2).

1. *Conduct a hazard analysis*: A *hazard analysis* is carried out by listing where hazards might occur in the production process and describing how they could be prevented. Significant hazards are those that are

Box 9.2. The seven stages involved in instituting a HACCP system.

1. Identify hazards.
2. Identify critical control points.
3. Establish critical limits for preventive measures.
4. Devise system to monitor critical control points.
5. Establish corrective actions to take if critical limits exceeded.
6. Establish record keeping system.
7. Establish verification procedures.

likely to cause illness or injury if not controlled. Examples of hazards are contamination with pathogens, the presence of chemical residues such as those from pesticides or hormones, and the presence of physical hazards such as pieces of bone in supposedly boneless products, or other foreign bodies. A good way of identifying hazards is by preparing a flow diagram of the process. The flow diagram is a clear outline of all the steps in the production process, an obvious requisite being that it is complete and accurate.

2. *Determine the critical control points*: *Critical control points* are identified. A critical control point is a point in the production process where control can be exercised over the factors that can cause or prevent a hazard. The hazard can therefore be prevented, eliminated or reduced to an acceptable level. For example, in a meat processing system a critical control point might be where the product is held at a particular high temperature for a certain length of time to destroy pathogenic bacteria. In this case, if the product is held at too low a temperature, or for too short a time, the bacteria will survive and are likely to cause illness in anyone eating the product. Identification of critical control points is often helped by using 'decision trees' in which the process is broken down into a series of questions each requiring a yes or no answer. The corresponding answer leads to another question, eventually identifying points in the production process as critical control points or not. Good examples of decision trees are given in NACMCF (1998).

3. *Establish critical limits*: *Critical limits* are established for the preventive measures associated with each critical control point. Critical limits could relate to measurements like temperature, humidity, time, pH, moisture level or salt content. They are minimum or maximum values within which a parameter must be controlled to prevent, eliminate or reduce the hazard to an acceptable level. Outside these limits the product is potentially unsafe. In the example above, critical limits would be for the temperature achieved and the holding time. The critical limits must be met to ensure that each critical control point is under control. If the temperature were too low, or the time for which the temperature was maintained were too short, any pathogens would not be destroyed and the hazard would not be under control.

4. *Establish monitoring procedures*: A system is devised to *monitor* the critical control points and record the observations. The monitoring is carried out in a planned way to ensure that the critical control points are under control. Recording the observations enables people to follow the operation of the HACCP system and check the control is working. Ideally, monitoring is carried out continuously, and this is feasible with measurements such as temperature. If this was not possible then discrete monitoring would be carried out at set intervals. In the example, the temperature and exposure times would be monitored continuously and a permanent record kept of the observations. Monitoring may show that, while the critical limits have not yet been exceeded, there is nevertheless a trend toward loss of control of the process. This might allow the process to be brought back under complete control before the critical limits were exceeded.
5. *Establish corrective actions*: The *corrective actions* that need to be taken when there is a deviation from the critical limit are established. The deviations would indicate that a critical control point was not in control. The corrective actions might include discarding potentially unsafe product produced when the critical limit was exceeded, rectifying the cause of the deviation from the critical limit and keeping a record of the corrective action.
6. *Establish record-keeping and documentation procedures*: Effective *record keeping* procedures are established to document the whole HACCP system. These will include such things as a summary of the hazard analysis, the HACCP plan, the flow diagram of the process, the critical control points and their limits, the monitoring and the corrective actions that may need to be taken.
7. *Establish verification procedures*: Procedures are established to *verify* that the HACCP system is working correctly. These could include inspection schedules and regular reviews of the whole system. They could also include periodic testing of the end product, for example microbiological surveys to check for the absence of pathogens, or chemical tests of the attainment of specified processing temperatures. Verification may be by internal staff, or by external experts to ensure completely unbiased, independent assessment.

The HACCP system of quality assurance is inherently more efficient than the traditional end point quality control scheme. The quality of all the product is assured. Potential deviations from quality are detected rapidly by monitoring each stage of the production process and this rapid detection prevents unnecessary wastage of product since the material that needs to be discarded is more closely and precisely identified. A very important benefit from HACCP systems is that, once set up, they involve participation by the whole production personnel so that quality assurance involves everybody rather than just a restricted number of quality control staff.

Chapter 10

Animal Welfare

One component of meat quality recognized by many people is ethical quality. This has two main elements. One is producing meat in agricultural systems that are sustainable and environmentally friendly, the other is producing it in ways sympathetic to animal welfare. Different individuals have widely varying views of the importance of these concepts. This is especially true of animal welfare where our viewpoint largely reflects how we see animals in relation to ourselves. It is therefore an emotive subject. Those who have greatest empathy with animals are most concerned about their welfare. At the other extreme are people who look on animals with detachment and are comfortable with exploiting them as in the case of any other agricultural crop. However, it is important to realize that the consideration we individually attach to animal welfare does not inherently influence whether a specific animal's welfare is good or bad. Only the conditions the animal finds itself in, and its response to these conditions, do this. A full and stimulating consideration of animal welfare is that of Webster (1995). A recent compilation of papers that address many current concerns and areas of interest in welfare research can be found in Appleby and Hughes (1997), and Gregory (1998) gives an extensive and detailed consideration of the relation between animal welfare and meat science.

Welfare and its Measurement

Defining animal welfare

Welfare is hard to define precisely. It obviously relates to an animal's mental and physical well-being. Physical well-being implies that an animal is fit and healthy, but mental well-being is harder to define because it is difficult to know whether an animal is content or not with its environment. This implies that just because an animal is healthy does not mean that its welfare is necessarily good. Neither does productivity, for example fast growth or high milk production, alone imply good welfare. Broom (1986) defined welfare in a useful way as the 'welfare of an individual is its state as regards its attempts to cope with its environment'. The implication is that welfare is compromised if an animal cannot cope with its environment or can only cope with difficulty. In this sense the environment means anything outside the animal, whether the physical environment or, for example, other animals.

This concept of welfare leads to the recognition of two types of welfare indicator. The first type is one that shows that an animal has *failed* to cope with its environment. Examples are increased mortality, reduced reproductive capacity, greater disease and reduced growth. The second type shows the *amount of effort* required to cope. Examples of this type are indices of distress or *stress*, such as increased heart rate, and behavioural changes. The welfare of a man being chased by a lion is likely to be low. If the lion catches and eats the man, the man has failed to cope with his environment. The man's death is an indicator of the first type. If the lion doesn't quite succeed in catching the man then, although the man survives, he is still likely to be very distressed by the experience and we could assess this by his behaviour and probably by noting the rise in his heart rate. These are examples of the second type of welfare indicator.

Numerous indicators of poor welfare can be imagined and used. The presence of any of these may show that welfare is poor. However, the absence of a particular indicator of poor welfare does not necessarily indicate that there is no welfare problem. When assessing welfare therefore, and particularly when trying to establish that an animal's welfare is good, a range of indicators needs to be used (Broom, 1994). Sometimes, indices of production efficiency like growth rate are used as evidence of good or bad welfare. Animals that are not growing well may be suffering from poor welfare. However, great care needs to be taken in interpretation – just because an animal is growing well does not necessarily mean its welfare is good.

Types of welfare concern in meat animals

The various concerns that people have about the welfare of meat animals can be considered under several headings. Some relate to breeding, some to rearing conditions, some to management practices during rearing and some to potential fear and pain at slaughter. Obviously they have different time scales and this may be important in helping to decide how serious a concern they are to us. Things that are of greatest concern operate over a long time or are severe. To a degree, a third factor, the number of individuals affected, seems intuitively important. Something that affects large numbers of animals appears to be more important than something that affects only a few. However, welfare must really be considered at the level of the individual. A system that fails even a few individuals is unacceptable from a welfare point of view.

Some examples of welfare concerns

Concerns with production methods

In the UK a large amount of beef is produced as a by-product from the dairy herd. To produce beef carcasses with good conformation and well-defined muscling from dairy cows, which do not have these characteristics, the sire breed may be chosen such that the calves are too large for easy birth. An extreme example is the use of bulls of the Belgian Blue breed which are large, muscular cattle. The calves may need to be delivered by Caesarean section because they are too large for normal delivery through the cow's pelvic opening. Caesarean section is likely to be traumatic for the cow. Some of the cows also suffer from inflammation and infection of the abdominal cavity.

Broiler chickens have been selected to grow meat very fast. A bird may reach slaughter weight in 40 days or even less. Food conversion rate is very efficient and therefore poultry meat is produced cheaply. Unfortunately, the body tends to develop faster than the ability of the legs, and particularly the leg joints, to support the bird's weight. This leads to a range of skeletal deformities and joint problems which together result in lameness. This condition is often referred to as 'leg weakness'. In the UK, some flocks of broilers may show very high frequencies of leg weakness (Kestin *et al.*, 1992), and it is likely that the problem is worldwide. There is good evidence that the condition is painful. Affected birds modify their behaviour so they stand and walk less, and spend more time sitting. Long periods sitting on soiled litter, on which they are reared, particularly if it is damp, may also lead to a lesion called hock burn developing on the legs. Giving the lame birds analgesic agents, which reduce or eliminate pain, improves their walking ability and changes their behaviour to resemble that of normal birds that do not suffer the condition (Mc Geown *et al.*, 1999). The walking ability of severely affected birds may be so poor that they cannot stand to reach the drinkers and may die from dehydration if they are not culled beforehand. There are two main causes of leg weakness. These are those caused by infections of the leg joints and those attributable to skeletal abnormality. The latter are probably more important. Husbandry factors, such as hygiene, stocking density in the rearing sheds, lighting regimen and feeding, particularly feed restriction in the young bird, have some beneficial influence on the condition but the essential factor is genetic. The only real cure may be to select for reduced growth rates although this goes against current commercial logic. Whatever the causes, the selection pressures put on modern broilers to grow fast have led to the welfare of many birds being severely compromised.

There is also some concern about aspects of husbandry of the parent stock used to produce broilers (the broiler breeders). Broiler breeder hens produce eggs from about 18 to 60 weeks of age. Broiler strains have been bred to grow fast and convert food into meat very efficiently when fed to appetite. The breeding birds would grow too fast if fed in this way, compromising their later egg-laying ability, so their food intake is considerably restricted. They are therefore allowed to grow only about a third as fast as the table broilers. However, the severe food restriction necessary to achieve this probably results in extreme hunger and sometimes leads to abnormal behaviour.

There has been a gradual intensification of animal production, especially for pigs and poultry. Animals are housed in relatively barren environments at high stocking densities. These rearing conditions may not provide adequate stimulation for the animals' psychological needs and frustrate normal behaviour patterns. The wild ancestors of pigs and poultry spent a large part of their time foraging for food and this behaviour has been retained by domestic stock. Foraging is unnecessary and impossible in animals reared intensively. The frustration of not being able to perform the behaviour probably leads to stress and may result in redirected and inappropriate behaviours such as tail biting in pigs and feather pecking in poultry. Both of these behaviours, or 'vices' as they are sometimes described, may lead to cannibalism although the exact aetiology of the problem is unclear. High stocking densities may restrict normal movement and can promote competition for resources such as food, leading to increased aggression. In the wild, sows build a nest prior to giving birth (farrowing). This is not possible in intensive rearing systems. Moreover, the sow may be closely confined in a stall, or tethered, to control her movement during pregnancy and held in a 'farrowing' crate to reduce the chances of her lying on her piglets in the first few days of life. Segregating individual sows also prevents the bullying that may occur when they are kept in groups. Although this protects some aspects of the sow's, and the piglets', welfare (and reduces economic losses) it is probably undesirable from the point of view of the sow's overall welfare.

Ruminants are generally reared less intensively than pigs and poultry. However, consumers in some countries like veal to be extremely pale in colour. To produce this pale meat the calves were confined in small crates to restrict movement, and fed a milk-substitute diet inadequate in iron. Hay, straw or other fibre was not fed and resulted in animals that were potentially, or actually, anaemic. The confinement in individual crates prevented normal social interactions and the calves often showed abnormal behaviour patterns.

Castration, tail docking and de-beaking

Some practices used in normal husbandry may be cause for concern. Many male animals are castrated, often just after birth. This reduces the aggressive behaviour frequently associated with entire males and may prevent undesirable odours in the meat, such as boar taint. The techniques used to do this, particularly as they do not usually involve anaesthesia or analgesia, may be painful (Kent *et al.*, 1995). Lambs' tails are often cut short by use of a tight-fitting rubber ring that prevents blood flow to the distal part of the tail. This subsequently dies and falls off. Pig's tails are sometimes cut short (docked) to prevent or discourage other pigs from biting them. Tail biting can lead to severe damage to the hindquarters of the pig and infection may spread along the spinal cord. Piglets' teeth can damage the sow's udder when they suckle. They may be clipped to prevent this. The clipping could be painful and lead to infection of the tooth dentine.

Poultry may peck one another. Feather pecking is probably just 'misdirected' ground pecking but can lead to considerable damage to the pecked bird. In the worst situations birds may eventually be killed. To prevent or reduce this damage, newly hatched chicks are sometimes 'debeaked'. The operation as performed routinely has various degrees of severity but in all cases a lesser or greater part of the upper beak is cut off, often with a hot knife, which automatically cauterizes the wound. Sometimes only the very tip of the beak is removed but very much more can be removed. The beak is a very sensitive organ provided with nerve endings and the operation is probably painful. Additionally, the ends of the cut nerves can form neuromas that may continue to produce pain sensations. Beak trimming is often used in broiler breeders to reduce the effects of aggressive pecking. In the males 'dubbing', or removal of part of the comb to prevent damage to it, may be practised. The males may also be de-spurred and de-clawed to prevent damage to the females during mating.

These 'mutilations', as they are often referred to, are usually justified by the farming industry with the argument that they are necessary to prevent even worse welfare problems developing. In effect they are the lesser of two evils. Nevertheless, it should be remembered that these very problems are often largely the result of modern intensive farming practices. They are the price paid for cheap and easily available human food. The price is paid by the animals, and the balance between it and the benefits to humans is eventually the responsibility of society, not just farmers and producers.

Concerns during marketing and slaughter

The processes involved in the marketing and slaughter of animals sometimes also give cause for concern. Removal from their home environments, mixing with unfamiliar animals and transport over sometimes long distances is potentially distressing to animals (Warriss, 1992; Hall and Bradshaw, 1998). The tendency to centralization of the slaughter industry in many countries, with fewer, larger slaughter plants operating at faster line speeds, is likely to make the situation worse. Animals will tend to be transported further and will often be subjected to greater coercion to move them to the point of slaughter more quickly. The killing of animals is an emotive subject and many people place considerable importance on the need to carry out the process in the most humane way possible. Animals should be free from fear and should be killed painlessly. It is generally believed that this requires effective stunning before exsanguination. Ideally, stunning should render the animal instantaneously insensible. If not instantaneous, for example when gaseous anaesthesia is used, it needs to be carried out in a stress-free manner. Inaccurate shooting positions with a captive bolt pistol, inappropriate cartridge size, or air pressure in pneumatically operated percussion systems, inadequate current flow or poor electrode placement in electrical stunning and delayed induction of anaesthesia in gas stunning all compromise animal welfare.

Other examples of where the welfare of meat animals is of concern are ascites in broilers, circulatory insufficiency in modern breeds of pig and lameness in sheep. Lameness is also a considerable problem in dairy cows (which we eventually eat) and breeding sows (which produce the slaughter pigs we eat).

Measuring animal welfare

Some indicators of welfare appear self-evident. It seems incontrovertible that an animal that dies because of some failure or inadequacy of a husbandry or handling system has had its welfare compromised totally. Moreover, systems that result in higher mortalities are also likely to be detrimental to the welfare of all animals, not just those that die, since the conditions that result in the death of some individuals often affect all. Mortality rates are therefore a very objective, albeit crude, indicator of welfare. Warriss *et al.* (1992) showed that longer journeys spent by broiler chickens going to a processing plant were associated with higher mortality. For journeys lasting less than 4 h the incidence of dead birds was 0.156%; for longer journeys the incidence was 0.283%. In other words, mortality was about 80% higher in the longer journeys. This is good evidence that the welfare of all birds subjected to longer journeys is likely to be worse than that of birds transported for less time.

Physical injury, resulting in broken bones or bruising, is, by analogy with human experience, painful. The prevalence of bruises or the number of broken bones can therefore, like mortality, be used as a welfare indicator. The prevalence of bruises is greater in the carcasses of cattle and sheep that have passed through live auction markets than in those from animals sold direct from the farm (see Table 7.2). Because of this we may infer that the welfare of animals sold through markets is in general likely to be poorer. Gregory and Wilkins (1989b) studied broken bones in culled hens sent to slaughter. The overall level was very high (29%) suggesting that the welfare of these birds pre-slaughter was poor. In a trial in which individual removal of birds from the battery cages was compared with the normal commercial method of 'depopulation' the prevalence of broken bones was reduced from 24 to 14%. Although still unacceptably high, the reduction in broken bones in the more careful handling system is a good measure of the potential improvement in bird welfare. Similar types of welfare indicator could be the prevalence of lameness in flocks of sheep and the amount of feather pecking damage in hens.

Poor welfare may be indicated by changes in the behaviour of the animal. Two questions can be asked. Does the animal perform normal behaviour and does it show abnormal behaviour? A problem is often to know what the normal behavioural repertoire is. Webster and Saville (1981) recorded the behaviour of calves reared in different ways. In particular they were interested in the effect of rearing calves in veal crates, which potentially limit the calves' behavioural repertoire. Amongst other differences, calves reared in crates spent 17% of their time either self-grooming, or licking or chewing their pen, compared with only 3% in calves suckled by their mothers at pasture and 10% in calves reared in straw yards. The extra time spent in these oral activities by the calves in crates suggested that this was some kind of compensation for the lack of stimulation they received in comparison with a more 'natural' rearing system. The calves were trying to satisfy their motivation to eat roughage where insufficient was available. Veal crates also obviously restrict movement. Webster and Saville found that the size of the crate prevented bigger calves sleeping in the normal position – with the head tucked into the calf's side.

Behavioural observations can be very helpful in deciding the minimum space requirements for animals. To reduce costs, farmers would like to house animals in the least possible space. For example, Edwards *et al.* (1987) found that pigs reared on fully-slatted floors needed a minimum space allocation equivalent to 0.59 m^2 100 kg^{-1} live weight to maintain growth rate and food conversion efficiency. This space is more than that (about 0.4 m^2) required for sternal recumbency (where the pig lies on its front) but, rather surprisingly perhaps, less than the space required (about 1 m^2) for full lateral recumbency (where the pig lies on its side). In the UK, 'The Welfare of Livestock Regulations 1994', implementing an EU Directive, specify that groups of pigs with an average weight of >85 kg, but ≤110 kg, must have a space allowance of 0.65 m^2 per pig.

The space needed by an average hen to stand is about 475 cm^2. However, groups of four or more hens reared in battery cages may be allocated as little as 450 cm^2 per bird to live in. This figure is prescribed as the minimum area under UK legislation (The Welfare of Livestock Regulations 1994). The legislation, however, recognizes that this space would be inappropriate for a single bird on its own. In this case, 1000 cm^2 are prescribed. An area of 450 cm^2 is not large enough to allow uninhibited feather ruffling, wing stretching, preening, turning around or wing flapping (Dawkins and Hardie, 1989). All these are normal behaviours of hens allowed sufficient room to exhibit them. In order to flap its wings a hen needs nearly four times the floor area required simply to stand. The relation of the space allowed for animals to live in to that needed to perform normal behaviour patterns therefore provides an indicator of welfare, although not a very quantitative one. Intuitively, most people would imagine the bird's welfare to be compromised with so little space available. Even if productivity is not reduced, the bird's mental well-being might well suffer by the restriction in space for normal behaviour.

These concerns have been recognized by proposed changes in legislation within the EU. The present type of battery cages will be banned from the start of the year 2012. From 2003 cages will need to provide each bird with 550 cm^2 of floor area rather than the current 450 cm^2. For new installations, alternative non-cage systems or 'enriched' cages offering 750 cm^2 per hen will be the only systems allowed from 2002. The enriched cages will have to have a nest, floor litter and perches.

Abnormal behaviours are those not normally seen under natural conditions. Additionally, animals can show changes in the levels of behaviour, for example reduced activity and responsiveness. Tail biting in pigs, and feather pecking in poultry, are probably abnormal behaviours caused by inadequacies (from the animal's point of view) in the rearing environment. A particular kind of abnormal behaviour characteristic of animals kept in barren, and often small, cages or pens are stereotypies. These take many forms. However, all are characterized by being repetitive, unvarying and without any obvious purpose. Stereotypies are often seen in carnivores such as large cats and polar bears kept in zoo cages. The animals pace relentlessly along the same route seemingly oblivious to outside stimuli. In sows housed in farrowing crates, a recognized stereotypy is 'bar-biting'. The animal bites and chews the bars of the crate for no apparent reason and with no obvious purpose. It is slightly unclear how stereotypies should be interpreted in welfare terms since they may be a mechanism by which animals 'cope' with their environment. However, spending excessive amounts of time in the activity – up to 40% of their active time in some individuals – is generally considered to reflect poor welfare and sometimes the behaviour is linked with physiological signs of 'stress'.

Abnormal behaviour patterns often reflect inadequacies of the animal's environment. Although the animal's physical needs are being met, its mental needs are not. Defining exactly what these needs are is often very difficult because we are trying to understand what the animal is thinking. The significance of animal cognition to animal welfare is discussed in Curtis and Stricklin (1991) and Duncan and Petherick (1991).

Simple behavioural observations, particularly those related to feeding, drinking or resting, can give valuable insights into the animal's feelings, allowing some assessment to be made of how fatigued, hungry or thirsty animals are. Sound levels, reflecting pigs' vocalizations, were used by Warriss *et al.* (1994) as an index of distress in pigs during handling. It might be possible to test whether different times or conditions of transport were more or less aversive to animals by measuring whether they showed greater reluctance to enter the vehicle with repeated exposures to the treatment. This could be done by, for example, monitoring the time taken to load them, but from a practical point of view this is a difficult experimental approach and it does not appear to have been tried yet. A good overview of welfare assessment techniques is given by Broom (1996).

Stress

The concept of stress

We have seen that an animal's welfare is compromised where it cannot cope with its 'environment' or can only cope with difficulty. The environment effect is often referred to as a 'stress' or 'stressor'. A stress may overtax the animal's ability to cope and reduce its 'fitness'. In this sense fitness means lack of disease, injury, death or ability to reproduce. An animal normally responds to stress with physiological and behavioural changes that are designed to be adaptive or to promote survival. In our example of the man chased by the lion, the behavioural response was running away, and the probable increase in his heart rate a physiological response to improve the flow of oxygenated blood to his muscles to facilitate the running. Rather confusingly, the words 'stress' and 'stressor' are used to mean either the same thing, or different things, by different people. Where they are used to mean different things, 'stressor' refers to the environmental pressure or stimulus, and 'stress' is reserved for the animal's response to it. In the second sense we talk of an animal being in a stressed state as well as referring to the stimulus as a stress. Definitions of 'stress' in animals have been discussed by Scott (1981) and Moberg (1987).

The nature of the stress response

Animals respond physiologically to stresses in a characteristic way. This stress response has two components. The first is a rapid short-term 'alarm' response. This was studied by the American physiologist W.B. Cannon in the 1930s who referred to it as the Emergency Syndrome. The animal's response to a threat, for example the sudden arrival of a predator, is to prepare its body for 'flight or fight'. The preparations largely involve the activity of the sympatho-adrenal system and the secretion of the catecholamine hormones, adrenaline and noradrenaline (epinephrine and norepinephrine).

The second component of the stress response occurs after the 'alarm' response and over a longer time period. Its role is to allow the animal to recover from the alarm response or to 'adapt' to the new situation. It was first recognized by Hans Selye working in the 1950s who referred to it as the General Adaptation Syndrome when considered along with the alarm response. This component of the animal's response to stress mainly involves the hypophyseal-adrenal axis.

The sympatho-adrenal system

The nervous system of an animal such as man or the pig consists functionally of two parts (Fig. 10.1). As well as the brain, spinal cord and sensory and motor nerves that comprise the central and peripheral nervous systems, there is the autonomic nervous system. The principal role of the autonomic nervous system is to maintain the body's homeostasis. In other words, it controls the internal environment of the animal's body. The autonomic system itself has two components. The parasympathetic nervous system, characterized by having acetylcholine as its neurotransmitter, is associated with the cranial and sacral parts of the spinal cord. The sympathetic system, in which the neurotransmitter is noradrenaline, is associated with the thoracic and lumbar parts of the spinal cord. Neurotransmitters are substances that transmit information between nerve cells – specifically at synapses. The neurotransmitter is secreted by one cell, passes across the small gap between the cells and stimulates receptors in the second cell's membrane. The stimulation promotes the generation of an electrical impulse.

The sympathetic nervous system innervates the adrenal glands. These are situated anterior to the kidneys and are therefore sometimes

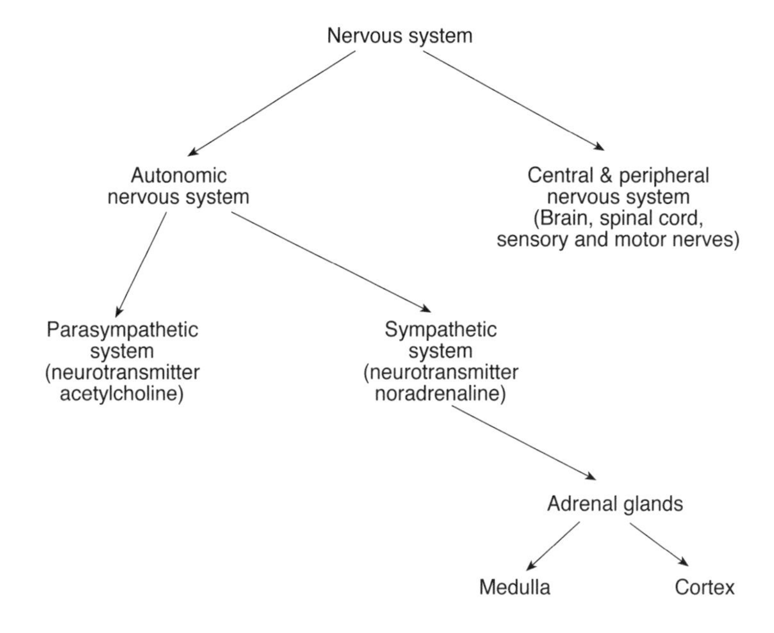

Fig. 10.1. The sympatho-adrenal system.

called the suprarenal glands. Each consists of two parts, the central medulla and the surrounding cortex. There is also sympathetic innervation to the eye, salivary glands, hair follicles, sweat glands and the viscera.

When an animal is subjected to a stressful stimulus, the sympatho-adrenal system is stimulated. Noradrenaline is secreted into the blood stream and the adrenal medulla is stimulated directly via the nerves. This causes the adrenal medulla to release both noradrenaline and adrenaline in the blood. These two hormones prepare the animal for 'fight' or 'flight'. Amongst these preparations are an increase in heart rate and a rise in blood glucose levels from the rapid breakdown of glycogen in the liver. The result is that the circulation of nutrient-rich, oxygenated blood is increased to the body, blood flow is switched away from the viscera to the muscles and the spleen contracts. The spleen acts as a reservoir of red blood cells. On contraction these are released into the circulatory system increasing its oxygen-carrying capacity. Other effects of stimulation of the sympathetic nervous system are dilation of the pupils of the eyes, reduced salivation, pilo-erection, secretion of more sweat and constriction of the blood vessels of the skin. In human experience these effects are manifested if we are stressed as a dry mouth, the hair on the back of our neck standing up, sweaty hands and pallor of our faces.

The hypophyseal–adrenal axis

An outgrowth from the base or ventral surface of the brain below the hypothalamus forms the pituitary gland. During stressful episodes the hypothalamus secretes a hormone – corticotrophin-releasing factor (CRF). This stimulates the pituitary gland to secrete adrenocorticotrophic hormone (ACTH) into the blood (Fig. 10.2). ACTH in the blood stimulates the cortex of the adrenal gland to secrete corticosteroid hormones. The release of the corticosteroid hormones, cortisol (hydrocortisone) and corticosterone, is a characteristic response of an animal to stressors. Most animals produce both hormones but cortisol predominates in primates such as man, and in dogs, cats, pigs, sheep and cattle, while corticosterone predominates in rodents and chickens. When administered to animals, cortisol increases blood glucose levels and promotes deposition of glycogen in the liver. The increase in blood glucose comes partly from a decrease in the rate of its breakdown and partly from increased synthesis from protein (gluconeogenesis).

The effects of the corticosteroids are, in fact, complex and extensive but it is apparent that they tend to counteract many of those of the catecholamines (adrenaline and noradrenaline). So, catecholamines promote the breakdown of liver glycogen to increase the amounts of glucose available to the muscles at a time when they are likely to be very active in escape or defence. During the recovery or adaptive phase of the stress response, the corticosteroids promote resynthesis of liver glycogen from circulatory glucose while maintaining the levels by gluconeogenesis. The function and regulation of the sympatho-adrenal and hypophyseal-adrenal systems in farm animals have been reviewed by Minton (1994).

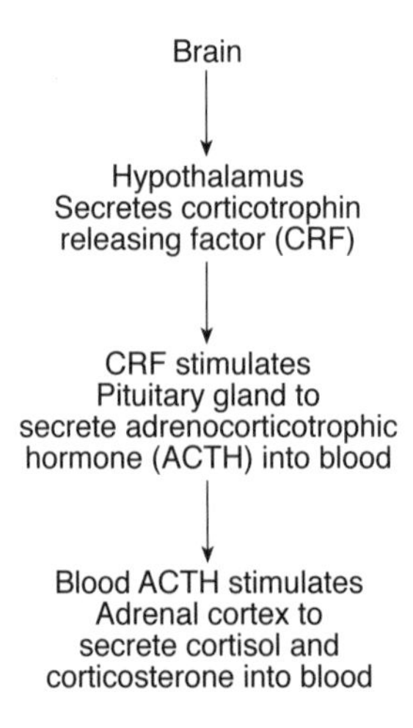

Fig. 10.2. The hypophyseal-adrenal system.

Endorphins

As well as secretion of ACTH, CRF promotes release of various peptides from the pituitary gland. These have effects similar to the drug opium. The opioid peptides include β-endorphin, Met-enkephalin and β-lipotrophin. All, together with ACTH, are formed from the same pro-opiomelanocortin precursor molecule. β-Endorphin, particularly, has analgesic properties. A reduced perception of pain has obvious importance to an animal that needs to escape from a predator.

Monitoring the stress response

The effects of stressors in animals can be monitored using changes in the levels of hormones produced in response to the stress, secondary responses in the biochemistry and physiology of the animal's body and long-term changes occasioned by these responses.

Hormonal changes

As we have seen, stimulation of the sympatho- and hypophyseal-adrenal systems is characteristic of psychological stress. Corresponding increases in the concentrations of catecholamines (adrenaline, noradrenaline) and, later, corticosteroids (cortisol, corticosterone) will be seen. Because they have a very short half-life in blood (less than 5 min), the catecholamines are really only useful as indices of acute stress where samples can be taken very soon after the stress. Troeger (1989) used blood adrenaline levels to measure the stress response in pigs in the period immediately before stunning. From this he could show, for example, that moving the pigs through a restraining conveyor elevated concentrations 12-fold compared with resting levels. Despite having such a short half-life, catecholamines were also used by Pearson *et al.* (1977) to monitor the stress involved in transporting sheep.

Corticosteroids have a much longer half-life in the circulation (15–30 min) and have been used in many investigations of handling and transport stress, for example in broiler chickens (Freeman *et al.*, 1984), in pigs (Moss and Robb, 1978) and in sheep (Reid and Mills, 1962). Interpretation of levels of corticosteroids is sometimes complicated by the response time in relation to the stimulus. Warriss *et al.* (1995b) found that, somewhat paradoxically, the largest increase (200%) in cortisol concentration in transported cattle occurred in animals transported for 5 h followed by that in animals after a journey of 10 h (88%) and then for 15 h (42%). These results suggested that cortisol levels were elevated by the stresses associated with loading and the initial stages of transport but then recovered as journey time was prolonged. Another complicating factor in the interpretation of changes in corticosteroid concentrations in the blood is that there is usually diurnal variation in the basal levels. However, one advantage is that, as well as from concentrations in the blood, useful information can be derived from measurements of salivary cortisol. Saliva is considerably easier to collect from animals than blood, and the sampling procedure is less likely to confound the findings by itself being somewhat stressful.

Secondary responses

Secondary responses to stressors that can be monitored are heart rate and blood pressure, and ventilation (respiratory) rate. Heart rate provides a very rapid response and can be recorded by telemetry. Baldock and Sibly (1990) measured heart rate in sheep subjected to various stressors. Spatial isolation from the flock produced no increase in rate over 'resting' values but visual isolation increased rate by 28 beats per minute (bpm). Mixing with a new flock of unfamiliar animals increased rate by 49 bpm and driving with a dog 83 bpm. Blood pressure is difficult to measure but ventilation rate can often be observed directly. Packed cell volume (PCV), sometimes referred to as haematocrit, increases during stressful episodes because of splenic contraction. Glucose and free fatty acid (non-esterified fatty acid) levels in the blood rise in response to catecholamine-induced glycogenolysis and lipolysis. Increased frequency of urination and defaecation is sometimes seen.

Long-term responses

Over the longer term suppression of the immune response can occur. For example, sows that are tethered, a practice that is probably stressful to them, show a reduced antibody production when they are injected with sheep red blood cells. There can be changes in the ratio of heterophil cells to lymphocytes in the blood. Long-term changes are recognizable as pathological changes. Examples are stomach ulcers, thickening of the walls of blood vessels, enlargement of the adrenal glands and reductions in the size of the spleen and thymus gland.

Measurement of physical and metabolic stressors

Physical stressors, such as exertion or exercise, may fatigue animals. Stress-related changes in the permeability of muscle cell membranes lead to increased blood levels of the enzyme creatine kinase (CK). Plasma CK activities increased progressively in cattle with longer transport (Warriss *et al.*, 1994). Circulating levels of other enzymes, such as lactate dehydrogenase, also increase after activity. In pigs, circulating lactate levels are rapidly elevated by physical stress. Pigs killed in slaughter plants subjectively judged to have poor pre-slaughter handling systems, producing apparent high levels of stress in the animals, had significantly higher levels of CK and lactate in their blood at exsanguination than those killed in plants subjectively assessed to have well-designed systems (Warriss *et al.*, 1994). In man, the feeling of fatigue is associated with the depletion of muscle glycogen reserves and the lowering of blood glucose levels (Newsholme and Start, 1973). There is evidence of muscle glycogen depletion in broiler chickens, caused both by food deprivation (Warriss *et al.*, 1988) and transport (Warriss *et al.*, 1993b).

Long periods of food deprivation reduce liver glycogen reserves and liver weight in broilers (Warriss *et al.*, 1993b), pigs (Warriss and Brown, 1983) and sheep (Warriss *et al.*, 1987). There are also rises in the blood concentrations of free fatty acids (non-esterified fatty acids) and ketone bodies such as beta-hydroxybutyrate (Warriss *et al.*, 1989a). In ruminants a disruption in normal eating patterns, leading to inadequate nutrition, can increase blood urea concentrations (Hileman *et al.*, 1990).

Dehydration, which can be caused by insufficient water intake, will increase the concentrations of plasma constituents, particularly proteins, and increase osmolarity of the blood. Warriss *et al.* (1983) found higher concentrations of plasma total protein in pigs subjected to a 6-h journey than in those transported for 1 h or not at all. Transported pigs drank correspondingly larger amounts of water when given access to it in lairage after transport. Plasma total protein concentrations increased progressively with longer transport in broilers, with corresponding increases in plasma osmolarity (Warriss *et al.*, 1993b) and both plasma total protein and albumin concentrations increased in sheep exported to southern France in journeys lasting 18 or 24 h (Knowles *et al.*, 1994c).

While physiological measurements can help us understand how animals are responding to imposed stresses, and sometimes allow identification of the specific nature of the stress (whether inanition, fear etc.), their value in deciding whether particular treatments are acceptable from a welfare standpoint may be limited. This is because there is often a lack of information on normal variation and an inability to relate particular levels of substances in the blood to the feelings of the animal. An exception is possibly body temperature which must be maintained within a close range for survival. Studies on the environment inside the containers in which poultry are transported have suggested that at certain locations on the vehicle the ability of the birds to thermoregulate is likely to be compromised (Kettlewell *et al.*, 1993). This is because the thermal load on the birds is too high and there is consequently a risk of severe heat stress.

Physiological measurements can, however, be very useful in defining the necessary duration of recovery periods providing basal or resting levels are known. For example, they can be used as an indication of how long an animal must be rested after an episode of transport before it can be considered acceptable for it to be subjected to another journey or how long it takes to re-aliment an animal after a period without food.

Pain

Pain is a special kind of stress. It is not easy to define concisely. The International Society for the Study of Pain defines it as: 'Pain is an unpleasant sensory and emotional experience associated with actual or potential tissue damage or described in terms of such damage'. The key points are that it is aversive, and that in general it is associated with tissue damage. Bruises and broken bones have already been described as examples of likely painful experiences. Because pain is a subjective perception it is very hard to measure objectively. Most animals in pain show a stress response but this is not specific. They usually exhibit behavioural changes, particularly in posture and gait. They may rest in a hunched-up posture. Animals that have injured feet or legs show obvious signs of lameness. Animals in pain may vocalize. A particularly powerful tool in investigating whether animals are in pain is to observe changes in their behaviour after administration of analgesics. A return to 'normal' behaviour implies that the animals were previously in pain. A good review of the assessment of pain in farm animals is given in Malony and Kent (1997).

Ways to Promote an Improvement in Animal Welfare

Changing public opinion

It is the goal of many people to improve the welfare of meat animals. Strategies for doing this have been outlined by McInerney (1991). There are three main ways in which it can be done. The first is to appeal to people's better nature. People are actively informed of cases of perceived poor welfare and encouraged to empathize with the animals' condition to the extent that they are motivated to try and improve it. They might do this by pressuring governments to change the situation or simply by not buying products associated with the poor welfare.

A problem with this approach is that different people have quite different views on what is acceptable or not in regard to welfare. A person's position will be influenced by factors such as cultural background, standard of living, and the type of animal in question. People in northern European countries generally appear to have a different perception of welfare than those in southern Europe where, for example, spectacles such as bull fighting are accepted. People with a very low standard of living may find it difficult to afford the standards of animal welfare demanded by more affluent individuals and cultures. Many countries are poor enough for the welfare of their human population to be of greater concern than that of animals.

Lastly, even in affluent cultures with a history of high concern for animal welfare, this concern may be different for different types of animals. Concern is greatest for species kept as pets, such as cats and dogs, less for meat animals such as pigs and cattle, and least for pest species such as rats. Even within the meat species there may be variation in concern, with non-mammalian species such as poultry, and especially fish, ranking lower than cattle, sheep or pigs. Many people who show the utmost concern for the welfare of cattle are happy to kill pest species such as rats in very welfare-unfriendly ways. There is little logic in this distinction.

Nevertheless, in the UK, considerable concern for animal welfare is apparent. Bennett (1996) found that 89% of people questioned were somewhat, or very concerned, that farm animals might be mistreated or suffer in the process of producing our food. Sixty-two per cent had altered their purchasing of veal and battery eggs because of these concerns. In order of importance, their concerns centred around housing and confined living conditions, feed and medicines, livestock transport and selling through live auction markets and slaughter.

In trying to promote animal welfare, a constraint can be ignorance and uncertainty as to exactly what is good welfare. A frame of reference is helpful here. In the UK, the results of the investigations of a committee chaired by F.W.R. Brambell in the early 1960s led eventually to proposals by what in 1979 became the Farm Animal Welfare Council that welfare could be thought of in terms of five 'Freedoms' that all animals should have. These are:

1. Freedom from hunger and thirst.
2. Freedom from discomfort.
3. Freedom from pain, injury or disease.
4. Freedom to express normal behaviour
5. Freedom from fear and distress.

Later (FAWC, 1993), these statements were amplified to clarify what was meant. So, freedom from hunger and thirst would be achieved by ready access to fresh water and a diet to maintain full health and vigour. Freedom from discomfort would be produced by providing an appropriate environment, including shelter and a comfortable resting area. Freedom from pain, injury or disease was ensured by prevention, or rapid diagnosis and treatment. Providing sufficient space, proper facilities and the company of the animal's own kind allowed the freedom to express normal behaviour. Freedom from fear and distress would be provided by ensuring conditions and treatment that avoided mental suffering.

The first three freedoms are generally consistent with good husbandry to ensure profitability. Everyone wants healthy animals that grow profitably. The last two freedoms are slightly more difficult. Often we don't want animals to express *all* their normal behaviour – we want for example to control their mating and breeding – and often to prevent it, and who is confident that they know exactly what mental suffering for an animal is. A positive approach is to ensure that people responsible for animals have the knowledge to ensure their welfare. This can be achieved by education, training and clear guidelines.

Legislation and codes of practice

People can be forced to maintain certain welfare standards by enshrining them in law. In the UK, 'The Protection of Animals Act (1911)' makes it an offence to cause cruelty or unnecessary suffering to an animal. More recent UK legislation that specifically protects the welfare of farm animals during rearing is particularly found in 'The Welfare of Livestock Regulations 1994' (and its amendment). In livestock auction markets, it is 'The Welfare of Animals in Markets Order (1990)' (and amendment). During transport, the welfare of all animals in the UK is protected by 'The Welfare of Animals (Transport) Order 1997'. At slaughter, it is protected by the 'The Welfare of Animals (Slaughter or Killing) Regulations 1995' and to some degree is also provided for in the 'Fresh Meat (Hygiene and Inspection) Regulations 1995'.

One problem with legislation is that it generally applies only in the country in which it is enacted. A situation may arise where differences in legislation give unfair commercial advantages to the producers in some countries but to the detriment of animal welfare. Other countries, where welfare legislation is more stringent, and production costs higher, may still import meat from places where it is less stringent and costs lower. To prevent this in the European Union, national legislation in the constituent countries is to a large degree harmonized. This is done through Directives that are legally binding on all the member states once they have been unanimously approved by a council made up of representatives from each country. For Directives concerning farm animals these are the Ministers for Agriculture for each EU country. The requirements in a Directive are incorporated into each country's national legislation. In the UK, legislation on animal welfare is often supplemented by codes of practice published by the Government. It is not illegal not to abide by these, but failing to do so can tend to establish a person's guilt if animal welfare is compromised and they are subsequently prosecuted.

Modern retailers, if they are large and economically powerful, such as supermarket chains often are, may impose codes of practice on their suppliers. They may therefore specify welfare standards for livestock which cover every aspect of meat production from breeding and rearing through to transportation, handling and slaughter. Often, these codes are more stringent than legislation. Large retailers can therefore be powerful vehicles for the improvement of animal welfare.

The relation between welfare and profit

Profit is usually related to productivity. The relation of productivity to welfare is complex (McInerney, 1991). With domestication of animals their productivity and welfare often improves over that in the natural state. They are ensured food and given protection from predators. However, as the pressure to improve productivity increases through intensification, apparent welfare can decrease. So, in very intensive systems, productivity and profit are high but aspects of welfare may be poor. Poultry, whether reared for meat or to produce eggs, can be kept under intensive or extensive systems. The intensive systems (broilers reared in sheds of 10,000–30,000 birds or more, and hens in battery cages) are more efficient than the extensive systems (free range birds). Use of true extensive systems may double the cost of production and therefore the price of the final product to the consumer.

If we accept that extensive systems are generally more welfare-friendly than intensive ones, although this is a dangerous generalization because it is not always true, then good welfare costs money to achieve. However, people may well be willing to pay this in terms of the extra price they must be charged for the product. In the UK, Bennett (1996) found that, on average, people would be willing to pay an extra 43 pence per dozen eggs for them to come from non-battery cage systems. Interestingly, this was more than the actual extra cost of producing non-battery eggs.

In production terms therefore, greater perceived animal welfare often costs money, although many consumers are willing to pay this. Nevertheless, there are some examples of where good welfare may actually save money, although the economics usually do not appear to have been worked out fully. Broiler chickens housed on litter that becomes moist sometimes develop foot-pad dermatitis. In this condition, lesions form on the bottom of the birds' feet, sometimes producing erosion of the skin and ulcers. These are likely to be painful and therefore compromise the birds' welfare. However, affected birds also grow more slowly, so there is a financial loss associated with the condition as well. Ekstrand *et al.* (1998) showed that the costs of reducing the prevalence of foot-pad dermatitis in Swedish broilers would be easily offset by the economic gains resulting from the improved growth rate of the affected birds. In this case therefore, improved animal welfare would also lead to higher economic returns.

In a similar manner, careful handling of animals pre-slaughter generally leads to lower carcass and meat quality losses as well as better welfare, and this can be an important stimulus to people to take greater care in handling. So, as well as being better from the animals' point of view, reduced transport mortality, lower levels of bruising, and reduced stress leading to smaller amounts of PSE and DFD meat also result in economic savings and greater profitability. Improved handling *may* cost more money than 'normal' handling. For example, lower stocking densities might reduce mortality rates in transported pigs, but this would increase the cost of transport per pig. Levels of PSE pork might be reduced by decreasing the speed at which the pigs were killed and increasing the time available to move them to the stunning point but, unfortunately, this would reduce line speeds and so increase costs. There are few, if any, figures comparing the overall economics of these alternatives. However, it seems that the net effect of greater care could often be greater profitability.

Chapter 11

Measuring the Composition and Physical Characteristics of Meat

There are various reasons for wanting to measure meat quality. One is in breeding programmes where we want to select animals that have desirable quality characteristics. Animals are chosen by monitoring these characteristics in siblings or progeny that are slaughtered for this purpose. An example might be the monitoring of lean pork colour in pig breeding schemes to try and reduce the levels of PSE (pale, soft, exudative) meat. When new animal husbandry or meat production methods are developed, it is important to know what the effects on quality will be, particularly if there are likely to be improvements or reductions in quality. Before introducing new procedures like electrical stimulation of carcasses or rapid chilling it is essential to carry out research to ensure quality will not be adversely influenced.

Because of the relatively small scale of breeding programmes and research and development, and the value of the potential benefits to be gained from them, the quality assessment methods can often afford to be sophisticated and necessarily expensive. This may not be true for quality measurements made for the purposes of quality control or payment, or for marketing reasons. In these cases, rapid and cheap assessments are usually required. Major goals in marketing are to achieve uniformity of product and to specify quality. Batches of meat of uniform quality can be produced by sorting samples based on some measurement of quality, for example colour. By continual sampling for the presence of residues or high microbiological loads, or compliance with some other specification of quality, the product can be marketed at a premium. To maintain or improve quality in a product, better quality needs to be rewarded by paying the producer more. To do this, a simple, reliable, cheap and generally accepted assessment method is required. The fatness of pigs in many European countries was progressively reduced by paying producers more for leaner carcasses. This was based on simple measurements of backfat thickness. The context of the quality measurement will therefore determine the time and resources that can be devoted to it.

Chemical Composition

This includes the composition in terms of the major chemical components – proteins, fats, carbohydrates, minerals and water (moisture) – and the levels of added substances like nitrite and sodium chloride in cured products, or residues of agents such as antibiotics, growth promoters, pesticides and heavy metals (lead, mercury, cadmium). It can also include measurements of 'spoilage' indicators such as ammonia or thiobarbituric acid. Proximate composition refers to composition described in terms of the percentages of protein, lipid, water (moisture) and ash only. A particularly good source of information about analytical methods dealing with the composition of meat is Kirk and Sawyer (1991). The chemical analysis of meat is reviewed in Ellis (1994).

Sample preparation and moisture content

In determining chemical composition it is essential to ensure that the sample is homogeneous. This is done by mincing, grinding and macerating, taking care not to allow overheating of the sample. Modern food processors are very effective for this. Water (moisture) is determined by drying to 103–105°C but inevitably this causes the loss of some other volatile substances. The term 'moisture' as used in the context of chemical composition includes these volatiles. Lyophilization, or freeze-drying, may overcome this. Comparison of the determined water content with the water content expected in normal meat allows the determination of 'added water'. The amount of added water allowed in processed products like hams is often prescribed by legislation. It may amount to 10–20%.

Protein determination

Protein is determined as nitrogen. Non-protein nitrogen, for example that in amino acids or nitrate, is therefore included. On average, meat proteins contain about 16% nitrogen. Multiplying the nitrogen content of a sample by 6.25 therefore gives an estimate of its protein content. To estimate nitrogen, the sample is often digested in hot sulphuric acid with the aid of a catalyst – usually containing copper sulphate and sometimes selenium – and the ammonia (NH_3) formed on adding excess alkali distilled off and titrated against acid. This is the classical Kjeldahl method.

Nitrogen factors are often mentioned in the analysis of the meat content of meat products. The nitrogen factor is equivalent to the percentage nitrogen content of fat-free meat. For example, 100 g of fat-free meat might contain 75 g of water and 25 g of protein. On average, this protein would contain 16% nitrogen, or a total of 4 g. Therefore the 100 g of fat-free meat would contain 4 g of nitrogen and the nitrogen factor would be 4.00. In fact there is some variation in composition throughout a carcass and the appropriate nitrogen factor varies correspondingly. Figures between about 3.3 and 3.8 are typical.

Collagen determination is valuable as an index of connective tissue content. Use is made of its unusually high (12–13%) hydroxyproline concentration. The sample is hydrolysed with hot hydrochloric acid to liberate the hydroxyproline, which is then determined colorimetrically.

Fat extraction

Fat (lipid) is extracted from a dried sample, and preferably a freeze-dried sample, using an organic solvent. Diethyl ether, hexane or petroleum ether (boiling point 40–60°C) extracts triglycerides but not phospholipids. To extract these as well, an initial acid hydrolysis must be used or very polar solvents, such as a 2:1 mixture of chloroform and methanol, employed. Chloroform/methanol extraction is used in the classic method for the isolation of lipids from animal tissues (Folch *et al.*, 1957). Whether the phospholipid component is included in the total fat measurement may be very important when assessing intramuscular fat concentration if the triglyceride levels are low. In this situation the phospholipid can make a sizeable contribution to the total fat. Extraction with solvents like ether is usually carried out in a clever device (the Soxhlet apparatus) which facilitates exhaustive extraction of the sample (Fig. 11.1). After evaporation of the solvent the fat is determined gravimetrically.

Other components

The inorganic mineral content of a meat sample is determined by incineration (ashing) at about 550°C when all the organic matter is burnt off. Specific salts such as sodium chloride, nitrate and nitrite can be assayed separately by standard chemical methods: precipitation with silver nitrate to give silver chloride for sodium chloride and photometrically for nitrite (and nitrate, after reduction to nitrite).

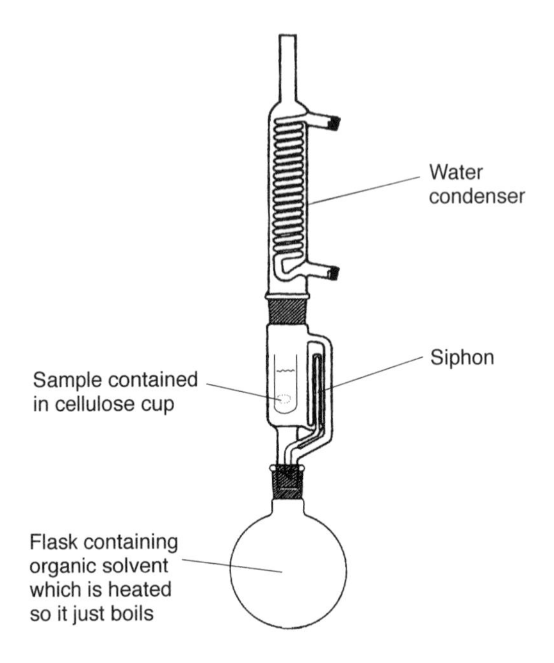

Fig. 11.1. The Soxhlet apparatus used for extracting fat from meat samples with low boiling point organic solvents.

Knowing this mineral content, together with the concentration of water (moisture), protein and fat, enables any carbohydrate to be determined by difference:

$$\% \text{ Carbohydrate} = 100 - (\% \text{ water} + \% \text{ protein} + \% \text{ fat} + \% \text{ minerals}).$$

Sometimes in processed products, added starch is measured separately. Glycogen in fresh muscle can be determined by extraction, precipitation by addition of ethanol, and hydrolysis with dilute acid to glucose. The glucose is measured colorimetrically. Accurate determination of the major chemical components of meat is especially important to comply with legislative requirements for the composition of food products. This is reflected in standard methods for them. In the UK these methods are published by the British Standards Institution, and in North America by the Association of Official Analytical Chemists (Table 11.1). Many British standard methods are identical to those of the International Standards Organisation (ISO).

The determination of residues in meat from substances administered to animals such as antibiotics, growth promoters and tranquillizers is described in Heitzman (1996). Maximum Residue Limits (MRLs) are often specified in legislation.

Table 11.1. Standard methods for the analysis of moisture, fat, protein, collagen and ash.

Component	British Standards Institution	Association of Official Analytical Chemists
Moisture	BS 4401 : Part 3 : 1970	AOAC 950.46
Total fat	BS 4401 : Part 4 : 1970	–
Free (crude) fat	BS 4401 : Part 5 : 1970	AOAC 960.39
Protein (nitrogen)	BS 4401 : Part 2 : 1980	AOAC 981.10
Collagen (hydroxyproline)	BS 4401 : Part 11 : 1979	–
Ash	BS 4401 : Part 1 : 1980	AOAC 920.153

Characteristics of fats

The degree of unsaturation of the fatty acids in fats can be measured by the amount of iodine with which the fat will combine. The *iodine value* is the weight of iodine absorbed by 100 parts of the sample. Animal fats like lard have values below 100, and vegetable oils like sunflower oil values above 100. More detailed fatty acid profiles can be obtained by gas liquid chromatography (GLC).

As has been mentioned previously, oxidative rancidity can be assessed using the reaction of the oxidized fatty acids with thiobarbituric acid (TBA). The *peroxide value* measures the amount of peroxides formed during oxidation. The acidity produced by the liberated fatty acids when triglycerides break down gives the *acid value*.

Meat Species Identification

The adulteration of meat of one species with that from another is difficult to detect. For example, beef can be adulterated with horsemeat. Adulteration is of particular concern to certain cultural groups whose religious views preclude the eating of meat from some species. Muslims do not eat pork and Hindus do not eat beef. Adulteration of fats with those of other species can sometimes be detected by the unusual fatty acid composition. Attempts to detect adulteration of lean meat have been made using immuno-diffusion techniques, immuno-electrophoresis, or latterly with enzyme linked immuno-adsorption assays (ELISAs) (Patterson and Jones, 1990). In terms of sensitivity these methods often work better with raw than with cooked meat. Recently, very sensitive methods based on characterizing DNA after amplification with the polymerase chain reaction (PCR) have been developed (Koh *et al.*, 1998).

Colour and Appearance

These characteristics are determined by two main factors. The first is the concentration and state of the haem pigments, myoglobin (Mb) and haemoglobin (Hb); the second is the muscle micro-structure. An excellent account of the factors determining meat colour is that of Cornforth (1994). The measurement of colour is reviewed in MacDougall (1994).

Measuring the concentration of the haem pigments

The overall concentration of pigments determines how red the meat appears. They can be measured by extracting them into solution, converting them into a single suitable form and measuring their absorption using a colorimeter or spectrophotometer. The two pigments have very similar absorption spectra and react similarly with other substances and to factors which influence their chemical state. The spectra are characterized by a very strong peak between 410 and 430 nm, the Sorêt or γ band, and one or two smaller peaks in the green and yellow regions of the spectrum (the α and β bands) depending on the particular form of the pigment (Fig. 11.2).

The pigments are not completely extracted into water but are in dilute buffer solutions such as 0.1 M phosphate at pH 7. The extracts need clarifying by centrifugation or the addition of detergents. It is common then to convert the haemoglobin and myoglobin to the stable cyanmet forms (HbCN and MbCN) by addition of cyanide and to measure the absorption at 540 nm. To overcome the difficulty of clarifying the extracts, and to avoid the use of cyanide, which is extremely toxic, an alternative extraction method uses acidified acetone

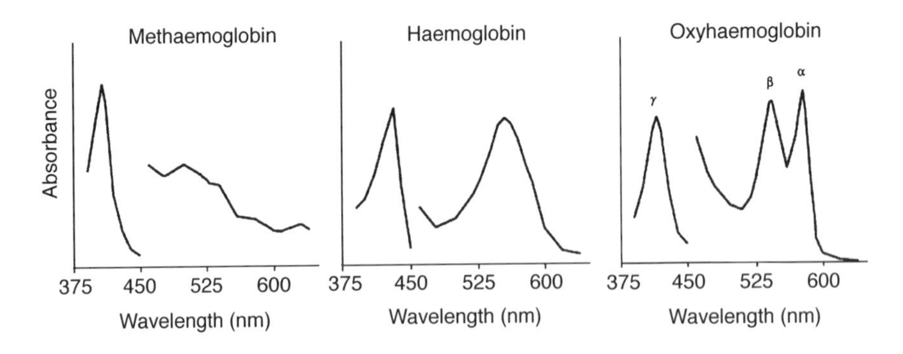

Fig. 11.2. The absorption spectra of methaemoglobin, haemoglobin and oxyhaemoglobin.

(Hornsey, 1956). This converts the pigments to acid haematin, which is measured at 640 nm. The concentrations of combined myoglobin and haemoglobin range from less than 0.1 mg g^{-1} muscle in the breast muscles of broiler chickens, through 1–3 mg g^{-1} in the m. longissimus dorsi (LD) of the pig to 3–6 mg g^{-1} in the LD of cattle. Myoglobin forms between about 50–90% of the total pigments depending on the species and the particular muscle. In very pale muscles, haemoglobin, derived from the residual blood, makes a more important contribution to the total pigment concentration. If necessary, haemoglobin and myoglobin can be differentiated from one another and measured separately by exploiting very small differences in the absorption spectra of the compounds formed when the pigments react with carbon monoxide (the carbonyl compounds), or by chromatographical separation. The quantification of haem pigments is described more fully in Warriss (1996b).

In general, higher myoglobin levels are found in the muscles of more active compared with sedentary animals, free-ranging compared with intensively-reared animals, and older compared with younger animals. A diet low in iron, as may be fed to some veal calves, also leads to pale meat. Diving mammals like whales and seals have very high muscle myoglobin concentrations (~9 mg g^{-1}) as a physiological adaptation to long periods underwater.

Measurement of colour

The colour changes that occur because of oxygenation or oxidation of the haem pigments could also be described directly, either subjectively or objectively. Describing the colour of meat subjectively is rather difficult because our perception of colour depends on the individual, the appearance characteristics of the object and how it is illuminated. So, for example, it is relatively easy to describe something as red or green to enable an observer to distinguish which object is being referred to. It is much harder, if not impossible, to so distinguish between two objects, both of which are red but different shades of red. Even a description of the reds as vermilion or scarlet is open to misinterpretation by different observers and subtle variations in shade are impossible to describe adequately.

Colour cards

The difficulties associated with the subjective evaluation of meat colour have been identified by Hegarty (1969). Reference scales make the subjective description of colour easier. In these, the colour of the sample is matched to the closest of a series of colour 'tiles' on a colour card. For example, a colour card is available for the assessment of the pink/red colour of the flesh of salmonid fish. The colour is due to the orange pigment astaxanthin which occurs naturally in the shells of the tiny shrimps that form part of the diet of wild salmon, or to the synthetic analogue, canthaxanthin, often fed to farmed fish. The card comes with specific instructions regarding the lighting conditions for the samples to be assessed.

Photographic scales

A potential improvement to this kind of system is to use photographs of actual meat samples rather than just colour tiles. An example of such a photographic scale is shown in Fig. 11.3. Scales for pork quality, such as those produced by the University of Wisconsin in the USA and by Agriculture Canada, and which also include an assessment of muscle structural properties, have been in use for a number of years (Murray and Johnson, 1990). The main limitation with these sorts of scales is that it is unlikely that there will be an exact match of the sample colour with a scale point and some interpolation will be necessary. However, subjective scales are cheap and easy to use, requiring no expensive equipment, and are particularly suitable for monitoring colour for the purposes of quality control.

The Munsell system

A refinement of these non-instrumental methods is the Munsell system. In this the colour matching is carried out in two stages. In the first stage the sample colour is matched as closely as possible to one of twenty

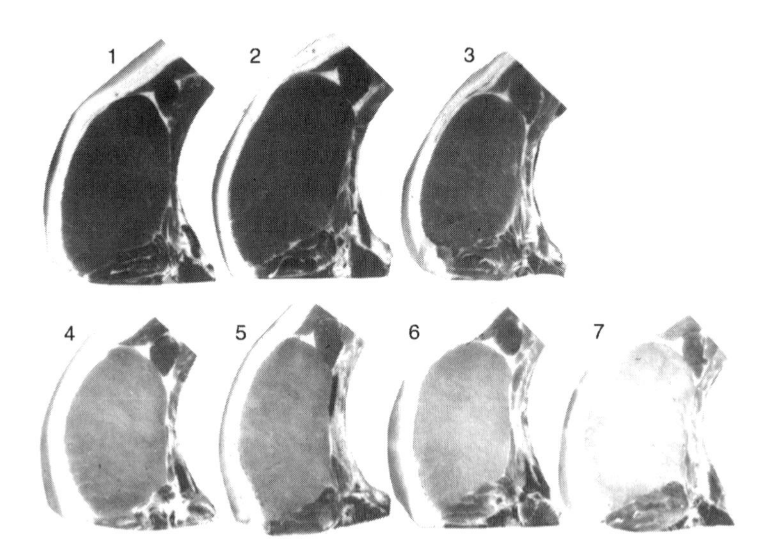

Fig. 11.3. An example of a photographic scale used for assessing the colour of pork.

colours arranged in the form of a wheel. There are five main colours: red, yellow, green, blue and purple. Between these main colours are intermediate ones. After identifying the nearest colour to that of the sample in this first stage the user is referred in the second stage to a two dimensional matrix which offers the choice of a number of shades of the colour. The two dimensions of the matrix show graduations of paleness/darkness and purity/greyness of colour, enabling a close match to the sample.

The reason the Munsell system is so effective is that the colour matching in effect takes place in three dimensions. The first gives hue, the second gives lightness and the third gives saturation, usually now referred to as chroma. These three characteristics define any conceivable colour in what is a colour 'space'. Hue describes what we commonly refer to as colour, that is red, green, yellow or blue for example. The terms saturation and chroma define the purity, colourfulness or lack of dullness of colour. Lightness is often now referred to as value and has as extremes, black and white.

The CIELAB system

The slight disadvantage with the Munsell system is that it is discontinuous; the sample colour has to be matched to a particular colour tile. However, continuous colour spaces are also available. Objectively, any colour can be specified as a combination of different amounts of pure red, pure green and pure blue light. These are 'real primaries'. Systems developed to measure colour transform these into 'imaginary primaries', X, Y and Z. The values of X, Y and Z are tristimulus values that define a colour as a point in space. The tristimulus values can be used to specify various colour spaces. The Commission Internationale de l'Eclairage (CIE) has specified a colour space referred to as CIELAB. This has the shape of a sphere and has the advantage that it closely approaches visual uniformity so that equal distances in the system represent approximately equal visual distances as perceived by human beings. The tristimulus values are used to calculate three coordinates: L^*, a^* and b^*. Any set of L^*, a^* and b^* values defines a colour exactly as a point in the three-dimensional colour sphere. L^* is the *lightness* component or *value*; a^* and b^* are chromaticity coordinates. The a^* coordinate measures red–greenness, the b^* coordinate yellow–blueness (Fig. 11.4).

The a^* and b^* coordinates can be used to calculate saturation (chroma) and hue (Fig. 11.5). Saturation (chroma) is calculated as the square root of $(a^{*2} + b^{*2})$. Hue is calculated as the angle whose tangent is (b^*/a^*), that is, $\tan^{-1}(b^*/a^*)$. This formula works when a^* and b^* are >0 but needs modifying with certain negative values of a^* and b^*. If $a^* < 0$, hue = $180 + \tan^{-1}(b^*/a^*)$. If $a^* > 0$ but $b^* < 0$, hue = $360° - \tan^{-1}(b^*/a^*)$. This is necessary because the system that defines colour in

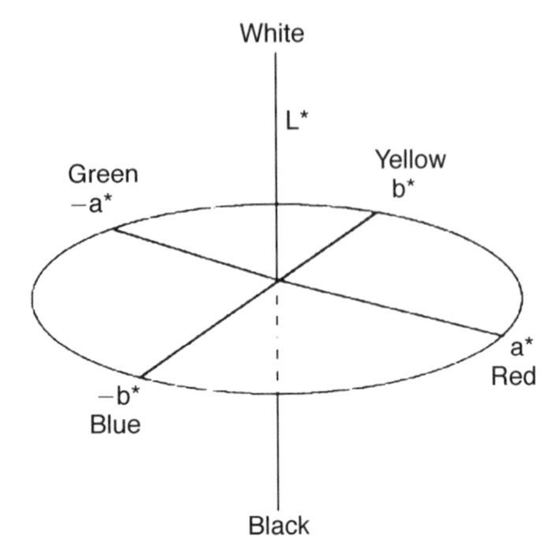

Fig. 11.4. The CIELAB colour space showing the L^*, a^* and b^* coordinates.

terms of lightness, hue and saturation (chroma) uses polar or cylindrical, rather than Cartesian coordinates. 'Brightness' is a function of both lightness and saturation. It can be estimated as the square root of $(L^{*2} + S^{*2})$.

L^*, a^* and b^* values are conveniently measured using portable tristimulus colour analysers such as the Minolta Chroma Meter (Minolta (UK) Limited, Milton Keynes, UK). These instruments will usually also compute hue and saturation values automatically if

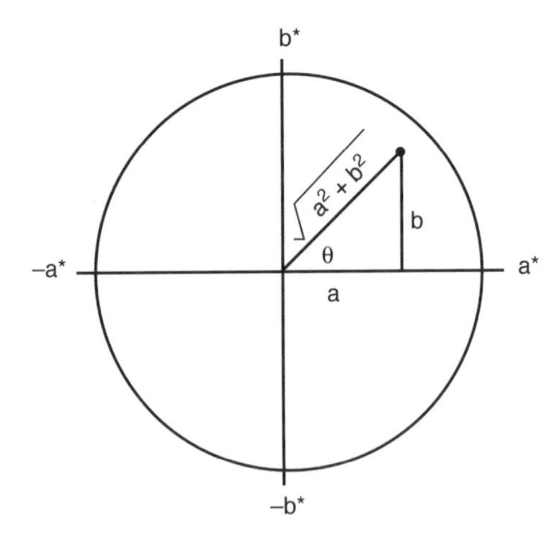

Fig. 11.5. Calculation of hue and saturation. Hue is defined by the angle whose tangent is b^*/a^*. Saturation is defined as the length of the line forming the hypotenuse of the right angled triangle whose other sides are a^* and b^*.

required. There are some practical considerations when measuring the colour of meat. The samples need to be thick enough to prevent light passing through them. In practice this means a minimum depth of at least 1 cm, and preferably 2.5 cm. They need to be exposed to the air for long enough to 'bloom' (the surface pigments to oxygenate) if a fresh surface is cut. This takes a minimum of 15 min, or better, an hour's exposure. Any clear plastic film overwrap will influence the readings slightly and must be allowed for. Tristimulus analysers can operate with different illuminant characteristics. CIELAB specifies two illuminants. Illuminant C is equivalent to natural daylight. Illuminant D_{65} includes part of the ultraviolet. Choice of either illuminant has only very slight effects on the readings made in meat.

Reflectance spectrophotometry

Differences in the degree of oxygenation or oxidation of the haem pigments at the surface of meat can be monitored by recording the changes in their spectra using reflectance spectrophotometry. As the name implies, this measures the reflectance of light from the meat surface, the changes in reflectance at different wavelengths enabling calculation of the relative proportions of myoglobin, oxymyoglobin and metmyoglobin. A method for measuring the relative amounts of the three forms of pigment in beef and pork is described by Franke and Solberg (1971).

Light Scattering and Paleness

The structural properties of the muscle affect the reflectance of light from the meat surface, and therefore its perceived paleness. Materials that appear translucent absorb more light. Those that appear opaque scatter and reflect larger amounts of light. Scattering occurs by structural elements in the surface layers of the meat producing differences in refractive index. The structural properties are very pH-dependent. Offer and Trinick (1983) suggested that the pH-dependent scattering is produced at the boundary between the sarcoplasm and myofibrils because the structures have different refractive indices. The larger the difference in refractive index, the higher the light scattering and the paler the meat appears. Because of the large variation in paleness seen in pork, and its commercial significance, various portable instruments were developed in the 1960s to measure it. These included the German Goefo meter and the EEL smoke stain reflectometer developed by D.B. MacDougall in the UK (MacDougall *et al.*, 1969).

The iridescence sometimes seen on the surface of bacon and ham is caused by light refracted from the surface. The refraction is due to the different refractive indices of water and fat at the surface. The fat forms an emulsion in the water like oil on the surface of a puddle in the road. Light shining on the surface is scattered by the two components, rather than simply being reflected. The scattering produces a spectrum of colours much as a rainbow is formed.

Water-holding Capacity

Approximately three-quarters of meat is water. In the living muscle about 10% is bound to the muscle proteins and another 5–10% is located in the extracellular space – the small channels between parts of adjacent muscle fibres. However, most of the muscle water is probably held in the spaces between the thick and thin filaments of the myofibrils. Lateral expansion or contraction of the filament lattice caused by differences in the state of interaction between the myosin and actin will therefore lead to uptake or expulsion of this water. During the development of rigor mortis the lattice shrinks and the water which is expelled will eventually be lost from the muscle fibres into the extracellular space. If a muscle is cut post-rigor this extracellular water will tend to be at least partially lost and contributes to drip. Drip is a dilute solution of the sarcoplasmic proteins. Drip loss leads to lower meat yield and is unsightly if it collects in the tray or pack containing the meat.

Factors that affect the state of the myofilament lattice, such as the rate and extent of the muscle acidification that occurs *post mortem*, will also affect the amount of drip lost from the meat. A reduced extent of acidification and high ultimate pH results in low drip loss while high rates of initial acidification lead to increased drip loss. The rapid initial pH fall occurs at a time when carcass temperature is still relatively high and may lead to myosin denaturation resulting in greater shrinkage of the myofilament lattice.

Drip formation is a function of the water-holding capacity (WHC) of meat. More drip is formed when WHC is poor and less when it is high. WHC is sometimes referred to as water-binding capacity (WBC), particularly when water is added to meat, for example during the production of cured products by injection of a salt solution into the meat. Salts lead to swelling of the myofilament lattice and greatly improved WBC.

Excellent, comprehensive reviews of WHC are given in Offer and Knight (1988a and 1988b) and Offer *et al.* (1989). There are a very large number of methods that have been used to measure WHC. Unlike colour, WHC is not definable in absolute units since each method measures slightly different things. A working definition of WHC is 'The ability of meat to hold its own or added water during the application of any force' (Hamm, 1986). A good comparison of methods for use in pork was given by Kauffman *et al.* (1986), and a general overview of WHC methods is that of Honikel and Hamm (1994). WHC methods can be divided into three sorts: those in which the only force applied is that of normal gravity, those in which a greater force is applied, and indirect methods.

Gravity methods

The simplest method is where sample joints or steaks are stored for a period of time and the loss of drip measured. It is common to suspend whole 'chops' (slices of the loin) inside polythene bags (to prevent evaporative losses) at 1 to 5°C for 48–72 h. Results for whole chops are affected by the fat:lean:bone ratio but the advantage is comparability with actual practice. An improvement is to use only the muscle (m. longissimus dorsi) or to use defined-geometry samples of it. A related method is to cook a sample of meat and measure the loss in weight, but the correlation between cooking loss and WHC measured on raw samples is poor. Cooking can be considered a *thermal* force. If making measurements on the m. longissimus dorsi it is important to appreciate that WHC can vary in different parts of the muscle.

Enhanced force methods

In the filter paper press method originally developed by Grau and Hamm (1953) a small (0.2 g) piece of meat is pressed on a filter paper between two clear plastic plates to form a thin film. Water is squeezed out and absorbed by the filter paper to form a ring of expressed juice. The area of this ring relative to the area of the meat is an index of WHC. Meat with a high WHC forms a larger area on pressing than meat with a low WHC. In fact, the area of meat is more variable than that of the expressed juice and can be used alone to assess WHC. A major advantage of the press method is that it can be employed with ground or processed meat. The pressure exerted can be controlled with a hydraulic press or tensile testing machine but there appears to be little improvement in precision over that in methods where pressure is exerted manually.

Centrifugation methods involve centrifuging small samples of meat at high speed and under high gravitational forces (60–100,000 *g*) for long periods (Bouton *et al.*, 1971). The exudate forms as a supernatant and can be poured off and weighed. Capillary methods involve the use of absorbent materials such as gypsum ($CaSO_4$) or filter paper. A sample of meat is pressed between a plate and a block of gypsum (Hofmann, 1975). Air is displaced from the block by exudate and rises up a capillary tube, in turn displacing a coloured liquid. The volume of exudate is read off a scale. In another method, a disc of filter paper is applied for 2 s to the meat surface about 15 min after cutting. The paper absorbs juice, the amount being assessed subjectively or by re-weighing the filter paper. The method is quick and easy but not very precise (Kauffman *et al.*, 1986).

Indirect methods

Danish workers have made extensive use of protein solubility methods to assess WHC in pork. The contractile (myofibrillar) proteins are extracted only at high ionic strength, e.g. by 1.1 M potassium iodide in 0.1 M potassium phosphate at pH 7.4. Non-structural (sarcoplasmic) proteins are extracted by low ionic strength buffers, e.g. by 0.04 M potassium phosphate at pH 7.4. The correlations with drip loss measured directly are higher with sarcoplasmic than with myofibrillar or total protein concentrations (Fig. 11.6) and only sarcoplasmic protein concentrations reliably differentiate between normal and DFD pork (Lopez-Bote *et al.*, 1989).

A standard procedure for the measurement of water-holding capacity

This was proposed for pork by Honikel (1987) based on a wide survey of methods. It is a standardized version of the drip loss method that uses 2.5 cm thick slices of loin m. longissimus dorsi from which associated fat and other small muscles are removed. The slice (weighing 70–100 g) is suspended by a thread or in a plastic net and enclosed in a sealed plastic bag. It is re-weighed after storage at 0–4°C for 48 h or longer. The relationship of the drip loss so measured with the total loss of exudate from whole butchered pig carcasses has been established (Fig. 11.7).

Use of On-line Measurements to Predict Pork Quality

Reflectance probes

Electronic grading probes such as the Fat-o-Meater developed in Denmark, the Hennessy Grading Probe designed in New Zealand, and the Destron from Canada measure fat and muscle depth to provide estimates of the lean content of carcasses. They operate by using reflected light to detect the interface between fat and muscle when the probe tip is pushed through the carcass. The light is generated by a

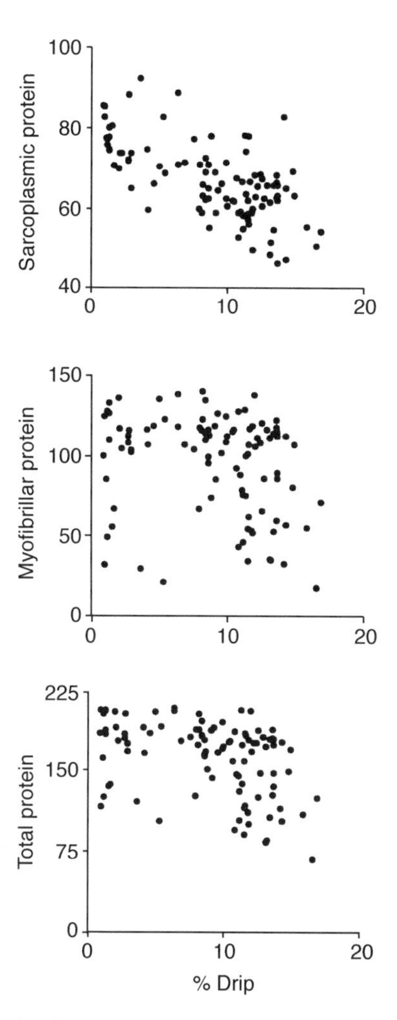

Fig. 11.6. The relationship between sarcoplasmic, myofibrillar and total protein solubility and drip loss from pork. Reprinted from Lopez-Bote *et al.* (1989), with permission from Elsevier Science.

light emitting diode (LED) and is detected by an adjacent detector diode. Because they measure reflected light they can also be used to provide a measure of the reflectance of the muscle tissue itself, and therefore its quality. In this respect they operate in a similar way to the more specialized Fibre Optic Probe (FOP; MacDougall, 1984). In this, light is transmitted into the meat by optical fibres and emitted from a small window at the end of the steel probe. Back-scattered light is returned by another set of optical fibres to the detector. The wavelength of the emitted light (~900 nm) is chosen so that error through absorption

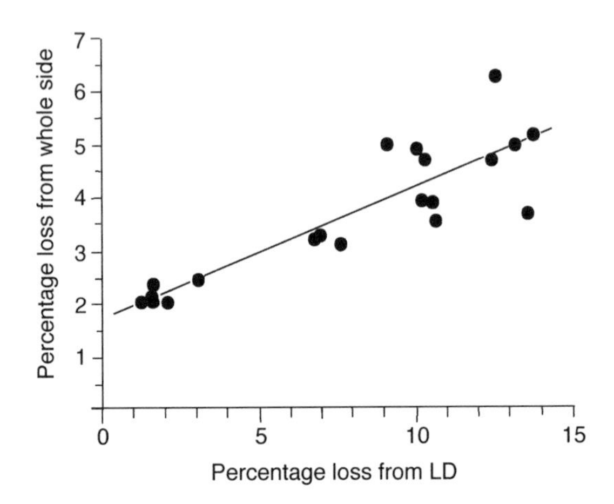

Fig. 11.7. The relationship of drip loss from the LD and total exudate loss from whole butchered carcasses. Reprinted from Lopez-Bote and Warriss (1988), with permission from Elsevier Science.

of light by the red haem pigments is minimized. Inherent in the idea of using reflectance to predict meat quality is that there is a relation between colour and WHC. This relation in pork is complex (Warriss and Brown, 1987; Irie and Swatland, 1993).

An important consideration in the use of on-line reflectance probes is the time when measurements are made. Ideally this should be several hours (~18–20) *post mortem* since only by this time will the characteristics of the meat be sufficiently developed to allow differentiation between PSE (pale, soft, exudative), normal and DFD (dark, firm, dry) conditions. However, measurements made about 45 min after death, just as the carcasses enter the chiller on most modern slaughter lines, can detect a proportion of carcasses showing extreme PSE characteristics. The relationships between FOP readings taken 20 h *post mortem*, reflectance, drip loss and subjective assessments of quality are shown in Fig. 11.8. Reflectance readings made at 45 min *post mortem* do not differentiate between normal and DFD meat (Table 11.2).

Measurements made with the Fat-O-Meater are very similar to those made using the FOP and the same constraints apply (Warriss *et al.*, 1989b). Based on measurements with the Hennessy Grading Probe, Fortin and Raymond (1988) found that correlations with subjectively assessed muscle paleness and structure increased with time *post mortem*, reaching values comparable to those at 24 h by 7 h after death.

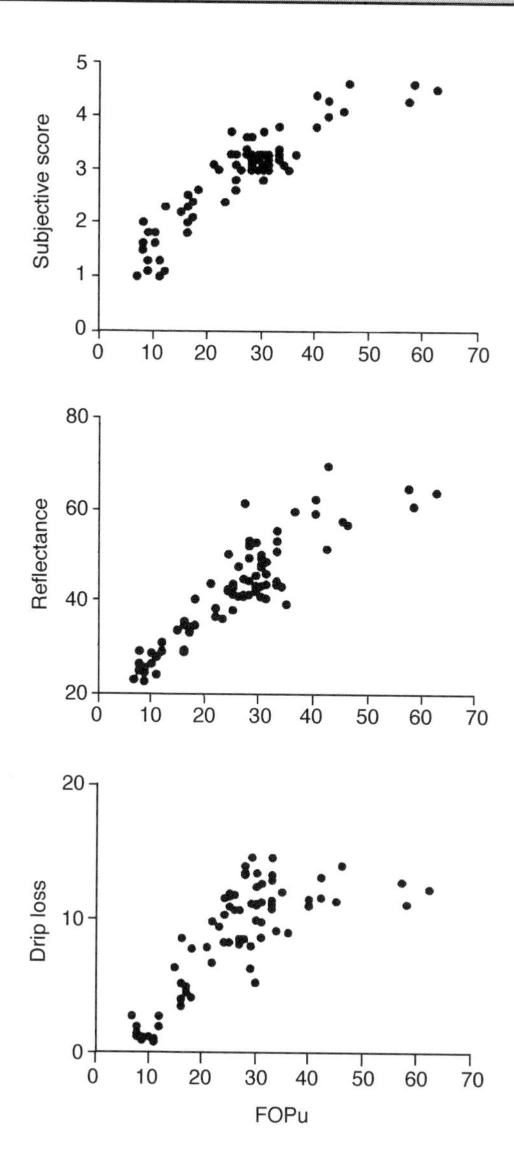

Fig. 11.8. The relationship between Fibre Optic Probe values measured 20 h *post mortem*, reflectance, drip loss and subjective assessment of pork quality. Reprinted from Warriss *et al.* (1989b), with permission from Elsevier Science.

Probes that detect electrical characteristics of muscle

Muscle has certain electrical characteristics, such as capacitance and conductivity, which change with time after slaughter. Several instruments have been developed to exploit these properties and their

Table 11.2. Fibre Optic Probe values (means + SE) measured either 45 min (FOP_{45}) or about 20 h *post mortem* (FOPu) associated with PSE, normal and DFD pork (from Warriss *et al.*, 1989b).

	PSE	Normal	DFD
FOP_{45}	35.9 ± 3.5	10.8 ± 0.4	11.3 ± 0.5
FOPu	45.3 ± 3.0	26.8 ± 0.8	11.0 ± 0.8

variation in meat of different quality. Two commercially available systems are the MS-Tester and the Pork Quality Meter (PQM). The PQM was evaluated by Warriss *et al.* (1991). Measurements made at either 45 min or 20 h *post mortem* were moderately correlated with initial pH but less well correlated with reflectance and drip loss. The instrument could not differentiate between normal and DFD pork, but it does have value for identifying potentially PSE carcasses. The major advantages of the PQM are its robustness, ease of use, and the fact that measurements made 45 min *post mortem* are apparently as good as those made several hours later after chilling. An assessment of the MS-Tester was given by Seidler *et al.* (1984).

Murray *et al.* (1989) compared the Minolta Chroma Meter, the Colormet probe, an instrument which uses a photodiode array to measure light reflectance over the whole visible spectrum, the Fibre Optic Probe and the Pork Quality Meter in terms of their ability to predict pork quality (Table 11.3). Both the Colormet and Fibre Optic Probe were better than the Pork Quality Meter, but none were as good as the Minolta (which of course must be used on a cut surface of muscle) in correctly assessing quality.

Other probes

The development of new probes able to measure various quality characteristics is an active area of research. Currently available reflectance probes can give an estimate of the intramuscular fat content of pork by assessing and integrating the small discontinuities seen in the output from the detector diode since these represent small areas of marbling fat. Swatland (1991) has used the characteristic of collagen to fluoresce in ultraviolet light to develop a prototype connective-tissue probe. Collagen, together with haem pigment concentration and marbling fat can also be measured in the near infrared (at a wavelength of 800–1600 nm; Andersen *et al.*, 1993). Earlier, Andersen *et al.* (1989) described a probe for assessing pigment concentration using the whole spectrum of reflected light. The Danes have also developed automated analytical equipment to measure 'boar taint' on-line. This is based on

Table 11.3. Percentage of pork loins whose quality was assessed correctly by different electronic instruments (from Murray *et al.*, 1989).

	Loins grouped subjectively according to:	
	Colour	Structure
Minolta Chroma Meter	90	82
Colormet probe	71	81
Fibre Optic Probe	74	72
Pork Quality Meter	50	57

All measurements were made 24 h *post mortem.*

the spectrophotometric determination of skatole in fat (Mortensen and Sørensen, 1986).

A trend is towards taking a large number of measurements simultaneously and processing the data using multivariate statistical methods. There is also the potential for on-line data collection using robotics to position and control the probes. An example is the evolution of the Danish MQM probe. Good reviews of these developments are given by Andersen *et al.* (1993) and Swatland *et al.* (1994).

The pH of Meat

The acidification of muscles *post mortem* is one of the fundamental changes in their conversion to meat. As we have seen, variation in the rate and extent of this acidification particularly influences meat colour and WHC. The acidification is measured in terms of the pH value of the muscle. Measuring pH can therefore give valuable information about the potential quality of meat, particularly in situations where more detailed or sophisticated measurements are impossible or inappropriate. The most widely accepted and workable definitions of PSE and DFD meat are in terms of pH values measured 45 min and about 24 h *post mortem.*

The pH scale

The pH is a measure of the amount of hydrogen ions (H^+) in a solution. Pure water dissociates to give equal numbers of hydrogen and hydroxyl (OH^-) ions:

$$H_2O = H^+ + OH^-.$$

Only a very small proportion of the total number of water molecules is dissociated. At 25°C the concentration of hydrogen and hydroxyl ions in solution is 10^{-7} mol l^{-1}:

$$[H^+] = [OH^-] = 10^{-7} \text{ mol l}^{-1}.$$

The pH is defined as the negative logarithm to the base 10 of hydrogen ion activity or concentration:

$$pH = -\log_{10} [H^+]$$

Therefore, the pH of pure water at 25°C is 7 and this is termed neutral because the numbers of hydrogen and hydroxyl ions are exactly equal. Temperature affects the dissociation of water so that more molecules dissociate into ions at higher temperature. At temperatures lower than 25°C, the pH at neutrality is therefore slightly higher and at higher temperatures it is lower. Because of this it is important to take temperature into consideration when making pH measurements.

Acids are defined as substances that are hydrogen ion (or proton) donors. In contrast, bases are hydrogen ion acceptors. When acids are added to water they dissociate to produce large amounts of hydrogen ions and reduce the number of hydroxyl ions. When bases are added to water they dissociate to produce large amounts of hydroxyl ions and reduce the number of hydrogen ions. Substances that liberate hydroxyl ions in water are known as alkalis. When acids are added to bases the hydrogen and hydroxyl ions neutralize one another to form water. The product of the concentration of hydrogen and hydroxyl ions is constant:

$$[H^+] [OH^-] = 10^{-7} \times 10^{-7} = 10^{-14}.$$

This figure is known as the ionic product of water. In acid or alkaline solutions there are unequal numbers of hydrogen and hydroxyl ions but their product must be 10^{-14}. For example, in 0.01 M hydrochloric acid (HCl) the hydrogen ion concentration $[H^+] = 1 \times 10^{-2}$ mol l^{-1}. The hydroxyl ion concentration is therefore $10^{-14} - 10^{-2} = 10^{-12}$ mol l^{-1}.

The pH can be calculated from the hydrogen ion concentration. If $[H^+] = 10^{-x}$ mol l^{-1}, then the pH = x. So, the pH of 0.01 M hydrochloric acid is 2. For 0.001 M sodium hydroxide (NaOH) the hydroxyl ion concentration $[OH^-] = 1 \times 10^{-3}$ mol l^{-1}. The hydrogen ion concentration is therefore $10^{-14} - 10^{-3} = 10^{-11}$ and the pH would be 11. The pH scale extends from 1 (extremely acidic) to 14 (extremely alkaline). It is important to remember that the scale is logarithmic so a pH of 6 represents ten times the number of hydrogen ions in solution as a pH of 7, and a pH of 5 one hundred times as many. This is especially important to be aware of when discussing changes in pH. In living systems the pH is normally maintained very close to 7 (between about 6.8 and 7.4) but, as we have seen, the pH of muscle after death of the animal can fall to below 6.

Measuring pH

The pH of solutions can be measured using indicator dyes or with a glass pH electrode. Indicator dyes change colour with different pH values. A well-known one is litmus, which is red in acid and blue in alkaline solution, the change occurring between pH values of 5 and 8. Indicators are not particularly precise for measuring the small changes in pH that occur in meat. However, special plastic-backed indicator strips have been produced for this purpose by E. Merck of Darmstadt, Germany and could be used for screening out meat with unacceptable very low or very high pH (Yndgaard, 1973).

Glass electrodes are made of a special glass that is sensitive to hydrogen ions. Nowadays they are usually made as 'combination' electrodes that also incorporate a reference electrode. A pH-dependent voltage is generated between the two electrodes, which is amplified and displayed on a meter calibrated to the pH scale. A diagram of a combined pH electrode is shown in Fig. 11.9. The sensitive glass of the electrode is rather fragile and also prone to contamination with substances like proteins and fats. This makes pH measurements in meat quite difficult to carry out accurately. Partly to overcome the disadvantages of glass electrodes, pH electrodes based on the use of ion sensitive field effect transistors (ISFETS) have been designed recently. These are much more robust and show great promise for use on the slaughter line.

In use, pH electrodes are first calibrated using solutions of known pH (buffers) and the meter adjusted accordingly. Usually, two buffers are needed, one to calibrate the position, the other the slope of the line defining the relationship between pH and voltage. It is best to calibrate meters over the range within which they are to be used. Buffers of 7 and 5 would be appropriate for measurements in meat. The pH is affected by temperature so it is important to calibrate the pH electrode at the temperature it will be used at, that is, to the sample temperature.

Practical considerations in measuring pH

The pH of meat can be measured directly by pushing the glass (or ISFET) electrode into the muscle, if necessary after making a suitable hole or incision with a knife, so that the pH sensitive area comes into close contact with the tissue. This technique is quick and accurate because the pH is measured *in situ*. The bulb at the end of the electrode can be made in different shapes. Very small bulbs, or spear-pointed electrodes, are more suitable for making direct measurements in meat. Sometimes, however, there is a danger of contaminating the sensitive glass with fat, or it may not be appropriate to use a probe, for example where there is concern about contaminating human food.

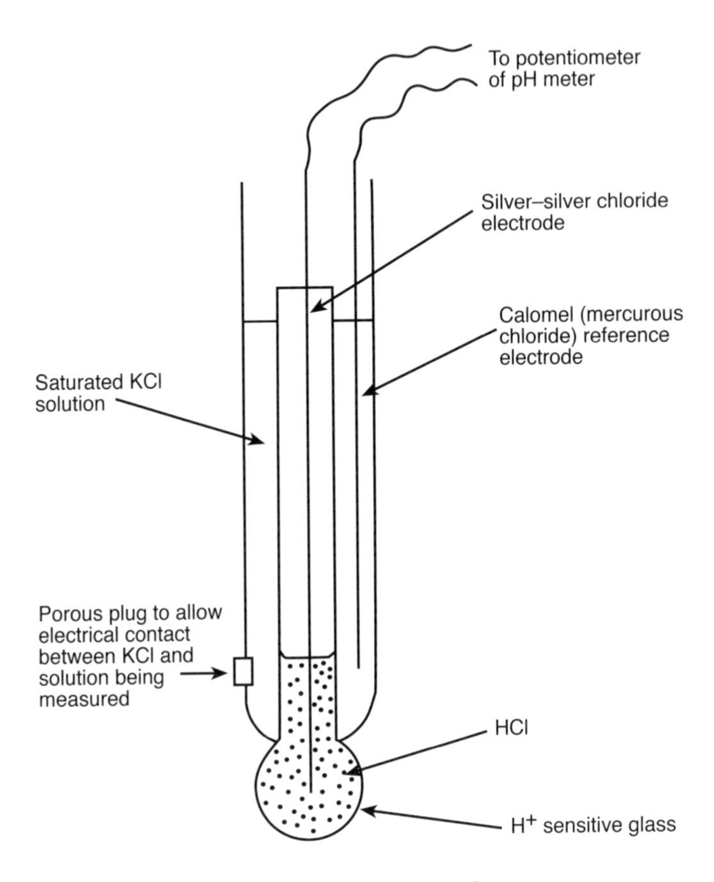

Fig. 11.9. The parts of a combined glass pH electrode.

An alternative to direct probing is to remove a small sample of meat, homogenize it in water and to measure the pH in the homogenate. A ratio of 1 part meat to 10 parts fluid is suitable. Because a larger volume of muscle is being sampled the measured pH may be more representative than a probe value. However, small inaccuracies can arise because of changes that occur during homogenization. In particular, the change in the concentrations of ions surrounding the muscle cells may be important, and there are 'dilution' effects. Homogenizing in 0.15 M potassium chloride, rather than water, will reduce these. If the pH of the muscle is still likely to be changing, for example because the measurement is being made before about 24 h *post mortem*, then it is better to homogenize in sodium iodoacetate which poisons the enzyme, glyceraldehyde-3-phosphate dehydrogenase and therefore stops glycolysis. Normally, a solution of 5 mM sodium iodoacetate in 0.15 M potassium chloride and adjusted to pH 7.0 is used. A useful comparison of the different methods available for pH measurement in meat is given in Dutson (1983). Jeacocke (1977b) described an ingenious system for the continuous measurement of pH in the muscles of intact carcasses.

Describing groups of pH values

It is important to remember that the pH scale is a logarithmic one. Strictly speaking, the arithmetic mean of a set of pH values is incorrect unless they are first transformed to a linear scale. This can be done by converting them back to hydrogen ion concentrations. So, a pH of 6 corresponds to 1×10^{-6} kmol m^{-3} of hydrogen ions and a pH of 7 to 1×10^{-7} kmol m^{-3}. The average of the two pH values, 6 and 7 is equivalent to a hydrogen ion concentration of 5.5×10^{-7} kmol m^{-3}. This has a pH of 6.26 (not 6.5). In fact, in calculations of average pH values, most people treat the scale as linear and use un-transformed pH values since in practice this does not lead to major errors of interpretation.

Rigor Mortis

Because rigor is associated with the breakdown of adenosine triphosphate (ATP) to adenosine diphosphate (ADP), then to adenosine monophosphate (AMP) and inosine monophosphate (IMP), which may degrade further to inosine and hypoxanthine, the ratios of these substances in muscle provide a good index of the progress of rigor in meat. The adenine nucleotides (ATP, ADP and AMP) have different absorption spectra from IMP and inosine. Honikel and Fischer (1977) therefore proposed the ratio of the absorbances of an aqueous extract of muscle at the wavelengths of 250 and 260 nm, the '*R*-value', as a simple index of the progress of ATP breakdown, and therefore rigor, in pig muscle. The method has since been extended to meat from other species (Koh *et al.*, 1993). For use on the slaughter line, a special rigorometer has been developed, based on measurement of the hardness of muscles (Sybesma, 1966). Hardness is assessed by the degree of depression of a spring-loaded probe. A simple method to estimate the development of rigor in pork carcasses was described by Davis *et al.* (1978). In this, the relative position of the foreleg indicates whether it has entered rigor.

Chapter 12

Measuring Eating Quality

As well as the appearance of raw meat, mainly determined by its colour, the important sensory (or organoleptic) characteristics are texture, juiciness, flavour and odour of the cooked product. All these characteristics can obviously be assessed by taste panels. In these, meat samples are tasted and scored subjectively by a group of people under more-or-less controlled conditions. Texture can also be measured instrumentally, some estimation of potential juiciness can be made from chemical analysis of the amount of fat in the meat, and some of the components of flavour can to a degree be identified by sophisticated chemical analysis systems such as gas chromatography (GC).

Meat Texture

Factors affecting meat texture

Three main factors are known to influence inherent meat texture. These are sarcomere length, the amount of connective tissue and its degree of cross-linking, and the extent of the proteolytic changes that occur during conditioning *post mortem*. Additionally, large amounts of intramuscular (marbling) fat will make meat more tender because fat is softer than muscle. Particularly in the initial period *post mortem*, before the changes associated with conditioning have progressed far, there is evidence that the diameter of the muscle fibres influences texture. A higher proportion of smaller fibres, which tend to be slow oxidative fibres, is associated with more tender meat (Tuma *et al.*, 1962; Crouse *et al.*, 1991). In beef, after about 3–6 days of conditioning the importance of fibre size declines substantially. Meat with a high water-holding capacity also tends to be more tender. This effect may reflect an interaction with ultimate pH. High ultimate pH values favour the proteolysis produced by the calpains which have optimal activity near neutral (pH = 7). Despite the concomitant rapid breakdown of the calpains themselves, the meat can be more tender than meat of lower pH. In fact, the toughest meat tends to occur in the middle range of ultimate pH values – between about 5.8 and 6.2. Below pH 5.8 the meat becomes more tender, but not as tender as above 6.5. In other words, there appears to be a curvilinear relationship between texture and ultimate pH.

As well as these inherent factors, cooking can influence meat texture. High cooking temperatures can reduce tenderness; long cooking times, particularly when cooking by 'boiling', can tenderize meat containing large amounts of connective tissue by converting it to gelatin. A very useful introductory overview of the determinants of meat texture is given in Bailey (1972). A more recent and comprehensive one is that of Dransfield (1994b), and the biophysical aspects of tenderness have been reviewed by Tornberg (1996). Methods available for the measurement of texture are reviewed in Chrystall (1994).

Sarcomere length

Muscles that are relaxed or stretched when they enter rigor have longer sarcomeres, and are more tender after cooking, than contracted ones (Locker, 1960). Recent ideas regarding the factors influencing the extent of post-mortem muscle shortening and sarcomere length, and the relation with toughness, can be found in Swartz *et al.* (1993). The sarcomere length determines how many myosin heads of the thick filaments can be attached to the actin of the thin filaments. The larger the number, and therefore the greater the number of cross-bridges that are formed, the tougher the meat. Sarcomere length can be measured directly by examining prepared myofibres under the microscope or by using optical diffraction (Voyle, 1971). This method has been described in detail (Meat Research Institute, 1972).

As mentioned previously, myofibrillar fragmentation often increases with longer conditioning times and has been used to monitor tenderness (Olson and Parrish, 1977; Crouse *et al.*, 1991). The relationship is, however, not always clear cut, although, as seen in Table 12.1, there is often reasonable correlation between the myofibrillar fragmentation index, instrumentally measured shear force and tenderness assessed by a taste panel.

So-called compressive or shear tests

These are instrumental measurements of meat texture and are carried out on cooked meat. The cooking procedure is important and must be

Table 12.1. The relationship between myofibrillar fragmentation index (MFI), instrumentally determined shear force and tenderness assessed by a taste panel, in beef (based on figures in Crouse *et al.*, 1991).

MFI	Shear force (kg)	Panel tenderness[a]
49.7	7.71	4.29
55.4	6.20	4.80
71.2	4.61	5.11
72.4	3.89	5.38

[a] 1 = Extremely tough, 8 = extremely tender.

standardized. In particular, the temperature reached determines whether the collagen starts to be converted to gelatin. This occurs above about 60°C. Normally, samples are cooked by roasting, grilling or by enclosing them in thin-walled plastic bags and immersing them in a water bath closely maintained at a temperature between 80 and 100°C until an internal (meat) temperature of 70 or 80°C is reached. The samples are then cooled quickly and can be stored for a couple of days if necessary until the texture is measured.

The Warner–Bratzler test

Various so-called compressive or shear tests have been described. A very commonly used method is the Warner–Bratzler test. The concept behind the test, and the instrument associated with it, originated with the American workers K.F. Warner and L.J. Bratzler in the early 1930s. The technique was described in its final form by Bratzler (1949). A cylindrical sample of cooked meat of cross-sectional area about 100 mm^2 is removed using a 'cork borer' cutting device with the grain of the muscle running parallel to the long axis. The sample is cut through by a metal blade about 1 mm thick. This is effected by the sample being passed through a triangular-shaped hole in the blade (Fig. 12.1). The blade is pulled through a narrow slot in a plate that supports the sample. The force required to move the blade to shear through the sample is measured, the blade being moved by a geared electric motor and the force measured using a scale.

The Volodkevich method

In the late 1930s, N. Volodkevich, working in Germany, devised an instrument in which the meat was 'squeezed' or compressed and cut between two jaws which mimicked the action of the incisor teeth (Fig. 12.2). The sample is again cut with the grain of the muscle parallel to the long axis. However, the cross-section of the sample is rectangular – in modern methodology, square, usually 10 $\times$ 10 mm. The jaws were originally wedge-shaped with the cutting edge formed with a radius of 2.5 mm. The rounded edge is retained in modern instruments. An

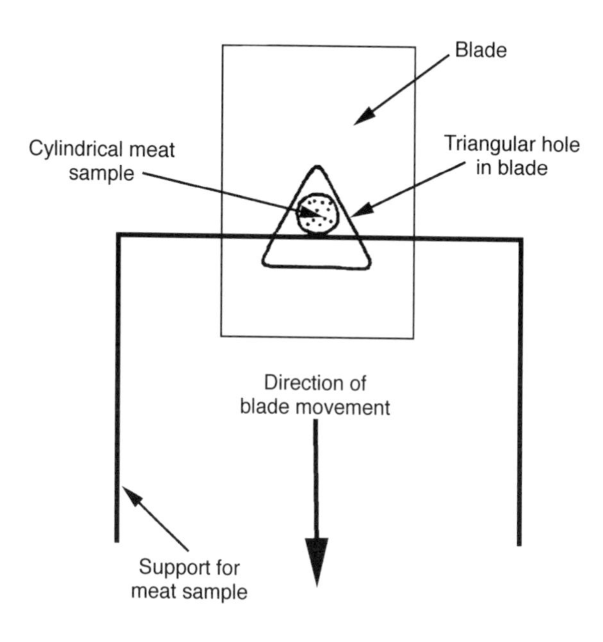

Fig. 12.1. Schematic representation of the Warner–Bratzler shearing blade.

excellent description and figure of a modern version of the system is given in Rhodes *et al.* (1972). To restrict sideways expansion of the sample as it is compressed during the test, it is constrained by side pieces or 'cheeks'.

Modern instruments for measuring texture

In modern instruments the Warner–Bratzler blade or Volodkevich jaws are operated, and the forces measured and recorded, by sophisticated computer-controlled systems which enable different rates of shear to be used. An example is the Instron Universal Testing Machine (Instron Corporation, High Wycombe, UK). The shear rate often ranges from 50 to 100 mm min^{-1}. The shape of the curve obtained by plotting shear force against time, or the amount of sample deformation, as the blade or jaws compress and then pass through the meat can sometimes be interpreted in terms of the different components of the shear (Fig. 12.3). An example of such an interpretation is given in Rhodes *et al.* (1972).

Because even cooked meat is easily deformed, the sample is compressed before any shearing of the muscle takes place. In fact, while the term shear force is generally used, the methods do not necessarily measure just shear. As well as shearing there are likely to be compression and tensile forces involved. Dransfield (1977) found that

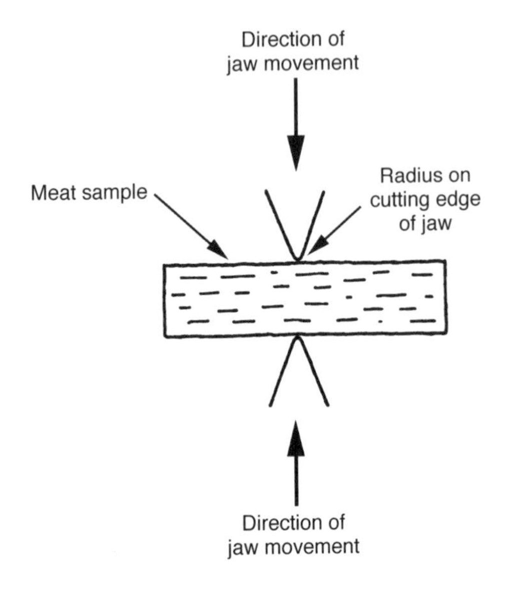

Fig. 12.2. The Volodkevich jaws.

different aspects of the force–deformation curve were associated with different components of cooked beef muscle. The compressive force was related to the collagen content, and fat, moisture, sarcomere length and pH were related to yield force.

Because foods like meat have such a complex structure of fibres enclosed in connective tissue sheaths and including fat deposits, and because the way humans chew meat is very complex, various other methods have been devised to try to better assess meat texture. Perhaps one of the most interesting instruments was that developed by Proctor *et al.* (1955, 1956) in which a full set of false teeth (dentures) were mechanically operated in such a way as to imitate the action of chewing. The forces generated were measured by strain gauges. A photograph of the instrument is given in Proctor *et al.* (1955).

Among the other techniques and systems that have been developed is the Texture Test System which was originally developed in the 1950s as the Kramer Shear Test and which is effectively a multiple blade shear test. Various penetrometer and punch tests can be used and some interest has been shown in measuring tensile strength directly, especially to investigate the cohesion between fibre bundles attributable to the connective tissue component (Lewis and Purslow, 1990). An excellent and comprehensive review of the instrumentation for measuring meat texture is that of Voisey (1976).

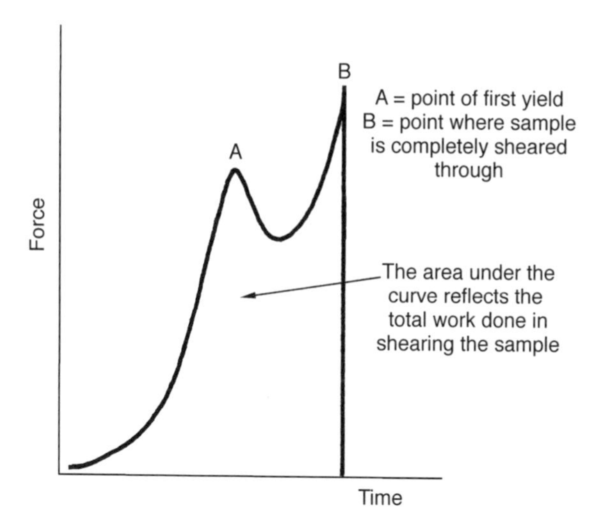

Fig. 12.3. Schematic representation of a possible compression–shear curve.

Practical considerations

Samples must be selected from as wide a range of sites within the muscle as possible. The muscle fibres must be at right angles to the plane of the shear and the samples must be cut accurately to the defined cross-sectional dimensions – to within 0.5 mm – using a very sharp knife or borer. The rate of shear must be defined since this will probably influence the actual forces recorded. At testing, the samples should all be at the same temperature. Normally this is chosen as room temperature (about 20°C) as it is impracticable to shear hot samples. Cold samples are slightly (5%) tougher than hot samples. Recommendations for a standardized methodology for measuring the texture (amongst other quality characteristics) of beef have been published by Boccard *et al.* (1981). For the m. longissimus dorsi, and based on estimates of total work done in the Volodkevich compressive test, Dransfield and MacFie (1980) recommended ten replicate determinations (shear or compressions) for samples of beef and lamb and seven for pork. There was slightly less variation between replicates for hindquarter muscles, so fewer determinations would be acceptable for a reliable estimate of texture in these. The variability between measurements made with the Warner–Bratzler shear and Volodkevich compressive test are about the same. An example of a suitable protocol for measuring instrumental texture of pig m. longissimus dorsi using Volodkevich jaws is given in Box 12.1.

The variation in texture measurements seen in practice is illustrated in Fig. 12.4. The data were derived from instrumental assessments of

Box 12.1. Example of suitable protocol for measuring instrumental texture of pig m. longissimus dorsi using Volodkevich jaws.

- Remove muscle samples at 24 h *post mortem* and blast freeze.
- Store at −20°C.
- Thaw at +1°C and age for 3 days at +1°C (i.e. total of 4 days at +1°C).
- Trim samples of fat and bone and cut to similar geometry and size (length about 10 cm).
- Vacuum-pack and cook samples in waterbath at 80°C until internal temperature reaches 78°C.
- Cool samples under running water for 45 min, remove from bags and drain.
- Store overnight at 4°C in a plastic bag to prevent evaporation.
- Cut samples 1 × 1 × 2.5 cm (± 0.5 mm) with long axis accurately aligned with muscle fibre direction.
- Shear eight (or more) samples per muscle.

texture made using Volodkevich-type jaws on 20 pork loins (m. longissimus dorsi). Two samples were taken from each loin, one immediately anterior (F) and one immediately posterior (H) to the head of the last rib. The texture of each was assessed independently. The loins represented a wide range of texture. The variation, reflected in the correlation between the two values for each loin, is attributable both to measurement error and the variation within the muscle itself.

Units of measurement

Compression and shearing create forces. A force is produced by a mass being accelerated. The force of 1 kg being accelerated at the rate of 1 metre per second per second (m s^{-2}) is referred to as a Newton (N):

$$1\ \mathrm{N} = 1\ \mathrm{kg\ m\ s^{-2}}.$$

Often, instead of describing the forces generated by compression or shearing in terms of Newtons they are quoted in kg. Because the acceleration due to gravity is 9.8 m s^{-2}, 1 kg is 'equivalent' to 9.8 (or approximately 10) N. An average-sized apple weighs about 150 g. It therefore generates a force of about 1.5 N when resting on the hand. The yield force of an average piece of pork might be about 5 kg or 50 N. A piece with a yield force of 10 kg or 100 N would be considered rather tough. If desired, the total work done in compressing or shearing a meat sample can be calculated from the area under the curve obtained by plotting force against time. This is expressed in joules (J).

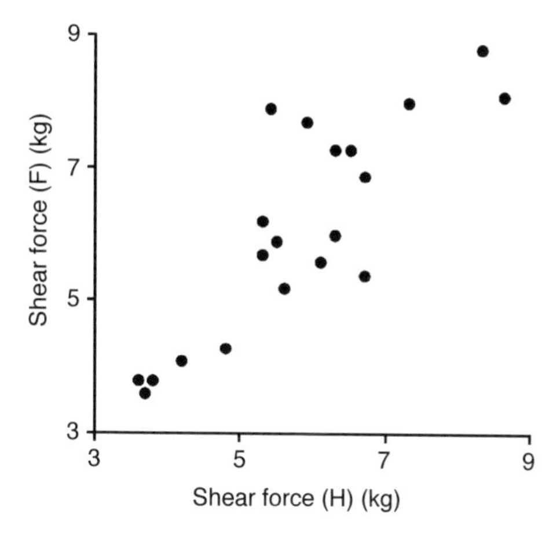

Fig. 12.4. An example of the variation in shear force measurements in pork muscles (the texture measurements are recorded in kilograms).

Predicting cooked meat texture from measurements soon after slaughter

It would be very useful to be able to predict eventual meat texture on the slaughter line. This would, for example, enable carcasses with tough meat to be diverted into further processing. An instrument called the Armour Tenderometer (Hansen, 1972) was developed which, it was claimed, enabled prediction of cooked beef texture from measurements on the raw muscle. The machine measured the force required to push ten needles into the cut surface of the m. longissimus dorsi where it was exposed at the quartering point. An important point is that the needles are pushed into the meat in line with the approximate direction of the fibres and, of course, before cooking. The measurement is therefore completely different from the usual system where fibres are cut *across* and after cooking. While it did seem to be able to differentiate between extremes of texture its predictive precision was poor. Its real usefulness in practice is unclear (Parrish *et al.*, 1973). Unfortunately too, a more recent trial carried out in The Netherlands on pork loins (Van der Wal *et al.*, 1988) found no relationship between tenderometer values and toughness.

The Tendertex Beef Grading Instrument (US Patent No. 4939927) is also an electromechanical penetrometer designed to assess meat tenderness by measurements made on-line soon after slaughter. Studies (George *et al.*, 1997) have shown a correlation with subsequent taste panel assessments, particularly for the amount of connective tissue in meat, but these are very low and the instrument appears to be no more useful for predicting meat tenderness than the United State Department of Agriculture (USDA) quality grades given by expert graders.

The apparent lack of success in finding a way of predicting tenderness might of course be expected because of the importance of post-mortem handling factors such as temperature and conditioning time. Any predictive ability is therefore likely to reflect gross differences in connective tissue or intramuscular fat content rather than differences in the myofibrillar component. Unfortunately it is also likely that this myofibrillar component will be the most important for a particular muscle from animals of a limited age and maturity range.

Meat Flavour

There are two components to flavour: taste, and aroma or smell. It is generally accepted that there are only four taste perceptions: sweet, sour, salt and bitter, caused by a relatively few non-volatile, water soluble components and detected on the tongue. Aroma or smell is produced by volatile substances that are detected by olfactory receptors in the passages at the back of the nose. The information from the tongue and nose is integrated and interpreted by the brain. Overviews of the science of meat flavour are those of Farmer (1992) and Shahidi (1998). The methods available to measure flavour and odour are reviewed in Bett and Grimm (1994).

Origins of meat flavour

Raw meat has little flavour. Only on heating during cooking do the characteristic flavours associated with meat develop. These flavours have two aspects. There is a non-species-specific component common to all meat, and there is a species-specific component that determines the differences between beef, lamb, pork and chicken, etc. The non-species-specific meat flavour is derived from heating low molecular weight water-soluble compounds. The main precursors are free sugars, sugar phosphates, nucleotide bound sugars, free amino acids, peptides, nucleotides and other nitrogenous compounds (Mottram, 1992). The myofibrillar and sarcoplasmic proteins are not thought to be important. The species-specific flavour comes from heating the fats present in meat, especially the phospholipids and to a lesser degree the triglycerides. The fat component in meat is also important because many of the volatile compounds produced on heating are fat-soluble.

A very large number of compounds (about a thousand) have been identified as potential or actual contributors to meat flavour. However, it is probable that only a relative few of these (20–30) are important. A compound's contribution to flavour depends on two things: first, how much is produced, and second, the odour threshold, that is, the minimum concentration at which it is detectable by the nose. Some compounds are present only at concentrations of parts per million (mg per kg) or parts per billion (μg per kg).

Two main processes contribute to the generation of these flavours on cooking meat. The first is the reaction between reducing sugars and amino acids, or other amino compounds such as peptides, and referred to as the Maillard reaction after the Frenchman, L.C. Maillard, who described the reaction between glucose and glycine in 1912. This is the most important flavour-producing reaction when meat is cooked. Its products contribute directly to flavour and are themselves reactants for further flavour-producing reactions. The second important contributor to flavour is the effect of heating on the lipid components of the meat. These undergo oxidative degradation. The flavours produced in this way can be both good and bad. We have already seen in Chapter 3 that lipid oxidation can lead to undesirable warmed-over flavour (WOF). Desirable flavour compounds are produced by very similar chains of reactions. Aliphatic aldehydes (compounds containing the –CHO group and derived from open chain hydrocarbons) are thought to be especially important. Unsaturated fatty acids give rise to more unsaturated aldehydes and therefore different flavour notes. This probably contributes to the differences in flavour seen between beef (with a low concentration of unsaturated fatty acids) and pork (with a high concentration of unsaturated fatty acids). Sheep meat contains methyl-branched saturated fatty acids, particularly 4-methyloctanoic and 4-methylnonanoic acids, which give the characteristic 'mutton' flavour.

Sugars present in meat also caramelize at higher cooking temperatures – for example, when grilling or frying meat, to produce flavour components. The compounds produced by fat oxidation can also react with those arising from the Maillard reaction.

The Maillard reaction

In the Maillard reaction the carbonyl group (CO) of a reducing sugar like glucose reacts with the amino group (NH_2) of the amino acid or peptide. The reaction (known as the 'browning' reaction) is a condensation and a molecule of water is lost to give what is referred to as an Amadori product. This is then dehydrated and deaminated to give furfurals, furanones and dicarbonyl compounds. The latter may then react with an amino acid, especially cysteine, to give an aldehyde (a reaction known as the Strecker degradation). The aldehydes, hydrogen sulphide (H_2S), and ammonia (NH_3) that are produced may then take part in further inter-reactions to produce numerous flavour-producing substances. Examples are pyrazines, thiazoles and thiazolines. These are all heterocyclic compounds. Heterocyclic compounds contain ring systems made up of more than one kind of atom. In the pyrazines it is carbon and nitrogen, in the thiazoles carbon, nitrogen and sulphur and in the oxazolines it is carbon, nitrogen and ozygen.

Particular effects on flavours

Clover and other legumes may give lamb meat a particular flavour. Both lamb and beef produced from animals fed on grass have more flavour than corn-fed animals. DFD (dark, firm, dry) meat has lower concentrations of carbohydrates than meat of normal pH. This may reduce the Maillard reactions and consequently lead to poorer flavour. Nucleotides such as adenosine triphosphate (ATP) and nicotine adenine dinucleotide (NAD) may act as flavour enhancers, rather than themselves producing flavours. Inosine monophosphate (IMP) especially has been implicated in this role. IMP breaks down to inosine and then hypoxanthine. Hypoxanthine has a bitter taste. Naturally occurring antioxidants such as vitamin E and vitamin C may improve meat flavour by reducing lipid oxidation and the production of WOF. The problem of 'boar taint' associated with the presence of high levels of androstenone and skatole in pork has already been mentioned. Meat from male reindeer in the mating season may also be tainted. Occasionally, 'fishy' taints can occur in pork if the pigs have been fed too high a concentration of fish meal in their diet as a source of protein.

Measuring the components of flavour

An example of the approach that can be adopted is seen in the work of Wasserman and Gray (1965). To identify what substances might contribute to beef flavour they extracted the meat exhaustively with water and, after clarification, fractionated the extract using a combination of dialysis, gel filtration chromatography and chromatography on ion exchange resin. This produced a total of 11 different fractions. Each fraction could then be analysed in regard to its composition, particularly the presence of sugars like glucose and deoxyribose, organic acids like succinic acid, amino acids, and hypoxanthine and inosine, and whether it produced a meat aroma when heated to dryness. This procedure identified the likely most important precursors of meat flavour.

In investigations of the individual components of flavour in meat, the volatile compounds produced during 'heating' are collected, concentrated and then separated using techniques such as gas chromatography (GC). By connecting the outlet of the chromatograph to a mass spectrometer the different compounds can be identified by comparing their mass spectra with published values. The combination of gas chromatography and mass spectrometry is often referred to as GC-MS. An example of this kind of approach is given in Madruga and Mottram (1995). These workers were interested in the effect of pH on the formation of flavour compounds in beef. They cooked finely minced beef that had been mixed with hydrochloric acid to adjust its pH to the required value. Cooking was done by autoclaving the mixtures in sealed bottles at 140°C for 30 min. The volatile compounds that collected in the headspace above the cooked meat slurry were adsorbed onto a collecting column. They were subsequently analysed by GC-MS. The authors identified 85 aliphatic compounds and 52 heterocyclic compounds. Dropping the pH from the normal value of 5.6 to 4.0 resulted in changes in the amounts of the compounds detected.

To match the compounds detected using gas chromatography with specific aromas, part of the effluent from the GC column can be diverted to an odour port so the substances can be smelt by a human observer as they are separated and detected. The technique is referred to as olfactometry.

Particular analytical techniques are available for some substances known to cause taints. For example, skatole is frequently determined colorimetrically by coupling it with dimethylamino benzaldehyde using a procedure described by Mortensen and Sørensen (1984). A colorimetric method has also been described for the other compound implicated in boar taint, androstenone (Squires, 1990), although GC methods (Garcia-Regueiro and Diaz, 1989) are more common. The relationships between the levels of boar taint-causing compounds and the sensory perception of taint have been described (Squires *et al.*, 1991; Xue *et al.*, 1996). Mottram (1998) gives an excellent overview of chemical taints in foods, including meat.

The 'Electronic Nose'

Recently, analytical instruments have been designed to mimic the operation of the human nose. An example is the 'Electronic Nose' developed by Neotronics Scientific Limited (Stanstead Mountfitchet, Essex, UK). This is able to analyse smell through an array of individual sensors that respond to various aroma-producing substances, the overall response of all the sensors resulting in a 'fingerprint' characteristic of the aroma. Sophisticated computer software enables these fingerprints to be remembered and analysed. An Electronic Nose has been used to discriminate between different levels of boar taint in pork (Annor-Frempong *et al.*, 1998).

Taste Panelling and Sensory Evaluation

Instrumental assessments of the components of eating quality can only be approximations to the true measure of particular attributes. This is because no machine can measure the range of interacting characteristics that contribute to eating quality and palatability. We do not perceive tenderness in isolation, we perceive it in relation to juiciness and 'mouth feel' and perhaps even apparently unrelated attributes such as flavour and odour. For some assessments there is therefore no real alternative to use of a taste panel.

Trained panels

There are different sorts of panel and different types of sensory test. A trained panel can be used to taste meat under closely controlled conditions of sample preparation, cooking and assessment. Normally a panel would consist of eight to ten individuals, screened and trained for their tasting acuity and carefully monitored over time to detect drift in scoring baselines. Testing needs to be carried out under conditions of controlled lighting and ventilation with individual panellists unable to be influenced by their colleagues.

Consumer panels

Consumer panels, in which selected members of the general public cook and assess the meat in their own homes, offer less controlled conditions and require larger numbers of individuals – usually more than 100. Preparation and cooking procedures will inevitably vary and people are likely to be influenced by other members of their family in making assessments. To overcome some of the variation in preparation and cooking, 'hall' tests have been used. In these the researcher prepares and cooks the meat and presents it to consumers in a public place – often a hall, hence the name. In hall tests the consumers may come from a restricted group in that only visitors to the particular site will be included whereas greater control over the consumers selected can be exercised if these are chosen by reference to their addresses for example.

Taste panel methods

An excellent general overview of the different types of method available using trained panels is given by Piggott *et al.* (1998) and, as applied to meat, Nute (1996, 1999). There are four main types: difference or discrimination tests, ranking tests, category scaling and sensory profiling.

Difference tests

In difference tests, panellists are asked to make a choice between two or more samples in regard to either which they prefer (non-directional) or which is lesser or greater for some characteristic: for example, which of two samples is tougher (directional). An example of a difference test is the Triangular test (ISO 4120:1983). In this, the assessor is presented with three meat samples simultaneously and must pick the odd one, two of the samples being identical. For two different samples there are therefore six orders of combinations: ABB, AAB, ABA, BAA, BBA and BAB.

Each sample is presented as the odd one out in half of the comparisons and occurring as the 'first', 'second' or 'third' sample equally. Because there are six combinations, the ideal number of assessors is a multiple of six. The probability of selecting the odd sample by chance alone is one in three. The actual number of correct selections is compared with a figure N derived from:

$$N = (\sqrt{n} \times 0.77313) + [(2n + 3)/6]$$

where n is the total number of tests and N is at the 5% level of statistical significance. For example, if there were 12 panellists, n would be 72 (6 × 12).

If the number of correct selections is greater than N then the two samples would be perceived as different at the 5% statistical significance level ($P = 0.05$). A more powerful test is the 'two from five' test since the probability of selecting the two odd samples by chance is only one in ten. The disadvantage of the test is the amount of work required from the assessor and the consequent danger of sensory fatigue influencing the result. Difference tests might be used to see if people could detect a difference between the meat from bulls or steers, or from two different breeds of pig, or to confirm the presence of a suspected taint. Other examples of difference tests are the 'A-Not A' (ISO 8588:1987) and the 'Duo-Trio' (ISO 10399:1991).

Ranking tests

A disadvantage with difference tests is that only two samples can be compared. Ranking tests overcome this. Assessors are presented with a number of samples in random order and must rank them according to some characteristic, for example toughness or flavour intensity. Whether the meat samples differ significantly in the characteristic is tested statistically by the consistency of the rankings between different assessors.

Category scaling

Difference and ranking tests simply tell us whether samples are different from one another. They tell us nothing about how different they are. Category scales, as their name implies, enable samples to be categorized in regard to specified characteristics such as texture, juiciness and flavour. The number of categories can vary but should generally be between five and ten. Fewer than four categories is not a very sensitive scale; more than ten is not necessary (Gacula and Singh, 1984). An example of an eight-point category scale for texture is:

Scale point	Description
8	Extremely tender
7	Very tender
6	Moderately tender
5	Slightly tender
4	Slightly tough
3	Moderately tough
2	Very tough
1	Extremely tough

Panellists assign a category to each meat sample and the average of the panel assessments is taken to define the characteristic for that sample.

Sensory profiling

In category scaling the specified characteristics are defined for the panellists. In sensory profile testing the assessors develop a unique set of descriptors to define characteristics of the sample. This leads to quite subtle descriptions of sensory characteristics such as crumbliness, rubberiness and oiliness. The technique is particularly useful for investigating subtle differences in flavour between samples. The results can often be related to instrumental and chemical measurements (Nute *et al.*, 1987).

The relationship between sensory and instrumental measures of texture

Although one would obviously expect a relationship between the results obtained from instrumental texture measurements and sensory assessment scores from taste panels, the closeness of the correlation varies and may indeed be quite small. For example, a correlation coefficient of about 0.4, which is not unusual, means that using, for example, instrumental shear force values to predict sensory tenderness can account for less than 20% of the variation observed.

There are several potential reasons for the low correlation. The first is that considerably less precision is attached to the results from taste panels because of the nature of the measurement and the fact that different individuals have different perceptions of the tender-to-tough scale. Their scoring may also vary from day to day. Secondly there is the confounding effect of juiciness on texture mentioned previously. This is just a specific example of the complex system that our perception of eating quality is. Thirdly, the relationship may vary depending on cooking method, and particularly cooking temperature. At different temperatures various components making up overall meat texture, such as the myofibrillar and connective tissue elements, will differ in the extent to which they have been broken down or changed. Because it is very likely that the different components contribute differently to overall texture when measured instrumentally or subjectively, cooking method may confound the relationship.

A Strategy for the Assessment of Eating Quality

What therefore should be the strategy for any assessment of meat quality, and particularly eating quality? An ideal is obviously to measure quality in all possible ways to get a complete picture. However, this may be too expensive both in time and sample requirements. Choosing options will then depend on the actual questions to be answered by the study.

Instrumental texture and chemical assessment are objective, reasonably precise ways of detecting actual or potential effects on meat quality. Trained taste panels enable us to put instrumental results into perspective. They will tell us whether statistically significant differences in instrumentally determined texture are detectable by the human taster in practice; in other words, they give us a feel for the size of shear force difference which is important. This may vary in different situations because of the confounding with other sensory characteristics such as juiciness. The consumer panel refines this further. A difference detectable by a trained taste panel under controlled conditions of meat preparation and testing environment may be completely lost when meat is prepared and cooked by a housewife. Taste and consumer panels therefore enable us to evaluate differences in quality in terms of their importance rather than their actual size. However, we still have very poor knowledge of what the minimum reduction in meat quality has to be to influence overall buying patterns. If the tenderness of pork decreased by 5% overall, would this be reflected in a reduction in overall sales and what would the actual relationship be between the size of the quality decrease and the size of the reduction in sales?

References

Aalhus, J.L., Best, D.R., Murray, A.C. and Jones, S.D.M. (1998) A comparison of the quality characteristics of pale, soft and exudative beef and pork. *Journal of Muscle Foods* 9, 267–280.

Adams, C.E. (1990) Use of HACCP in meat and poultry inspection. *Food Technology* 44, 169–170.

Allen, D.M. (1984) Automated grading of beef and pork carcasses. *Proceedings of the 37th Annual Reciprocal Meat Conference of the American Meat Science Association.* American Meat Science Association, Chicago, pp. 94–98.

Allen, W.M. and Smith, L.P. (1974) Deaths during and after transportation of pigs in Great Britain. *Proceedings of the 20th European Meeting of Meat Research Workers,* Dublin, Ireland. An Foras Talúntais, Dublin, p. 45.

Andersen, J.R., Borggaard, C. and Barton-Gade, P. (1989) On-line system for measuring the intrinsic colour of pork. *Proceedings of the 35th International Congress of Meat Science and Technology,* Copenhagen, Denmark. Danish Meat Research Institute, Roskilde, pp. 208–211.

Andersen, J.R., Borggaard, C., Nielsen, T. and Barton-Gade, P. (1993) Early detection of meat quality characteristics: the Danish situation. *Proceedings of the 39th International Congress of Meat Science and Technology,* Calgary, Canada. Agriculture Canada, pp. 153–164.

Anderson, B. and Horder, J.C. (1979) The Australian carcass bruise scoring system. *Australian Agricultural Journal* 105, 281–287.

Anil, M.H. and Sheard, P.R. (1994) Welfare implications of religious slaughter. *Meat Focus International* 3, 404–405.

Annor-Frempong, I.E., Nute, G.R., Wood, J.D., Whittington, F.W. and West, A. (1998) The measurement of the responses to different odour intensities of 'boar taint' using a sensory panel and an electronic nose. *Meat Science* 50, 139–151.

Anon (1965) Table Chickens, Bulletin No. 168, MAFF, HMSO, London, p. 41.

Appleby, M.C. and Hughes, B.O. (eds) (1997) *Animal Welfare.* CAB International, Wallingford.

Arnold, R.N., Arp, S.C., Scheller, K.K., Williams, S.N. and Schaefer, D.M. (1993a) Tissue equilibration and subcellular distribution of vitamin E relative to myoglobin and lipid oxidation in displayed beef. *Journal of Animal Science* 71, 105–118.

Arnold, R.N., Scheller, K.K., Arp, S.C., Williams, S.N., Buege, D.R. and Schaefer, D.M. (1992) Effect of long or short-term feeding of α-tocopheryl acetate to Holstein and crossbred beef steers on performance, carcass characteristics and beef color stability. *Journal of Animal Science* 70, 3055–3065.

Arnold, R.N., Scheller, K.K., Arp, S.C., Williams, S.N. and Schaefer, D.M. (1993b) Dietary α-tocopherol acetate enhances beef quality in Holstein and beef bred steers. *Journal of Food Science* 58, 28–33.

Arthur, P.F. (1995) Double muscling in cattle: a review. *Australian Journal of Agricultural Research* 46, 1493–1515.

Babiker, S.A. and Lawrie, R.A. (1983) Post-mortem electrical stimulation and high temperature ageing of hot-deboned beef. *Meat Science* 8, 1–20.

Bailey, A.J. (1972) The basis of meat texture. *Journal of the Science of Food and Agriculture* 23, 995–1007.

Bailey, C., James, S.J., Kitchell, A.G. and Hudson, W.R. (1974) Air-, water- and vacuum thawing of frozen pork legs. *Journal of the Science of Food and Agriculture* 25, 81–97.

Baldock, N.M. and Sibley, R.M. (1990) Effects of handling and transportation on heart rate and behaviour in sheep. *Applied Animal Behaviour Science* 28, 15–39.

Barbut, S. (1996) Estimates and detection of the PSE problem in young turkey breast meat. *Canadian Journal of Animal Science* 76, 455–457.

Barbut, S., McEwen, S.A. and Julian, R.J. (1990) Turkey downgrading: effect of truck, cage location and unloading. *Poultry Science* 69, 1410–1413.

Bartov, I. and Bornstein, S. (1977) Stability of abdominal fat and meat of broilers: the interrelationships between the effects of dietary fat and vitamin E supplements. *British Poultry Science* 18, 47–57.

Bate-Smith, E.C. and Bendall, J.R. (1956) Changes in muscle after death. *British Medical Bulletin* 12, 230–235.

Bauman, H. (1990) HACCP: Concept, development and application. *Food Technology* 44, 156–158.

Bejerholm, C. (1991) The effect of ageing on the eating quality of normal pork loins. *Proceedings of the 37th International Congress of Meat Science and Technology*, Kulmbach, Germany, Volume I, pp. 48–51.

Bejerholm, C. and Barton-Gade, P. (1986) Effect of intramuscular fat level on eating quality of pig meat. *Proceedings of the 32nd European Meeting of Meat Research Workers*, Ghent, Belgium. Volume II, paper 8:5, pp. 389–391.

Bendall, J.R. (1973) Post mortem changes in muscles. In: Bourne, G.H. (ed.) *The Structure and Function of Muscle*, 2nd edn. Academic Press, New York, Volume II, Part 2, pp. 243–309.

Bendall, J.R. (1976) Electrical stimulation of rabbit and lamb carcasses. *Journal of the Science of Food and Agriculture* 27, 819–826.

Bendall, J.R. and Swatland, H.J. (1988) A review of the relationships of pH with physical aspects of pork quality. *Meat Science* 24, 85–126.

Bennett, M.E., Bramblett, V.D., Aberle, E.D. and Harrington, R.B. (1973) Muscle quality, cooking method and ageing vs. palatibility of pork loin chops. *Journal of Food Science* 38, 536–538.

Bennett, R.M. (1996) Willingness-to-pay measures of public support for farm animal welfare legislation. *Veterinary Record* 139, 320–321.

Berg, R.T. and Walters, L.E. (1983) The meat animal: changes and challenges. *Journal of Animal Science* 57 (suppl. 2), 133–146.

Berry, P.S., Kettlewell, P.J. and Moran, P. (1990) The AFRC Mark 1 Experimental Broiler Harvester. *Journal of Agricultural Engineering Research* 47, 153–163.

Bett, K.L. and Grimm, C.C. (1994) Flavour and aroma – its measurement. In: Pearson, A.M. and Dutson, T.R. (eds) *Quality Attributes and their Measurement in Meat, Poultry and Fish Products.* Blackie Academic and Professional (Chapman and Hall), London, pp. 202–221.

Blackmore, D.K. and Newhook, J.C. (1976) Effects of different slaughter methods on bleeding sheep. *Veterinary Record* 99, 312–216.

Boccard, R., Buchter, L., Casteels, E., Cosentino, E., Dransfield, E., Hood, D.E., Joseph, R.L., MacDougall, D.B., Rhodes, D.N., Schoen, I., Tinbergen, B.J. and Touraille, C. (1981) Procedures for measuring meat quality characteristics in beef production experiments. Report of a working group in the Commission of the European Communities (CEC) Beef production Research Programme. *Livestock Production Science* 8, 385–397.

Boddy, L. and Wimpenny, J.W.T. (1992) Ecological concepts in food microbiology. *Journal of Applied Bacteriology* 73 (Symposium Suppl.), 23S–38S.

Boehm, M.L., Kendall, T.L., Thompson, V.F. and Goll, D.E. (1998) Changes in the calpains and calpastatin during postmortem storage of bovine muscle. *Journal of Animal Science* 76, 2415–2434.

Bonneau, M. (1993) *Measurement and Prevention of Boar Taint in Entire Male Pigs.* Institut National de la Recherche Agronomique, Paris, France.

Boulianne, M. and King, A.J. (1995) Biochemical and colour characteristics of skinless boneless pale chicken breast. *Poultry Science* 74, 1693–1698.

Bouton, P.E., Harris, P.V. and Shorthose, W.R. (1971) Effect of ultimate pH upon the water-holding capacity and tenderness of mutton. *Journal of Food Science* 36, 435–439.

Boyer-Berri, C. and Greaser, M.L. (1998) Effect of postmortem storage on the z-line region of titin in bovine muscle. *Journal of Animal Science* 76, 1034–1044.

Bradley, R. (1993) Transmittable diseases: the lessons from bovine spongiform encephalopathy (BSE). In: Wood, J.D. and Lawrence, T.L.J. (eds) *Safety and Quality of Food from Animals – Occasional Publication No 17.* British Society of Animal Production, Edinburgh, pp. 19–29.

Bratzler, L.J. (1949) Determining the tenderness of meat by use of the Warner–Bratzler method. *Proceedings of the 2nd Reciprocal Meat Conference of the American Meat Science Association.* American Meat Science Association, Chicago, pp. 117–121.

Bray, A.R., Graafhuis, A.E. and Chrystall, B.B. (1989) The cumulative effect of nutritional, shearing and preslaughter washing stresses on the quality of lamb meat. *Meat Science* 25, 59–67.

Bremner, A. and Johnston, M. (1996) *Poultry Meat Hygiene and Inspection.* W.B. Saunders & Co. Ltd, London.

Broom, D.M. (1986) Indicators of poor welfare. *British Veterinary Journal* 142, 524–526.

Broom, D.M. (1994) The effects of production efficiency on animal welfare. In: Huisman, E.A., Osse, J.W.M., van der Heide, D., Tamminga, S., Tolkamp, B.L., Schouten, W.G.P., Hollingsworth, C.E. and van Winkel, G.L. (eds) *Biological Basis of Sustainable Animal Production. Proceedings of the 4th Zodiak Symposium.* EAAP Publication 67, Wageningen, pp. 201–210.

Broom, D.M. (1996) Animal welfare defined in terms of attempts to cope with the environment. *Acta Agriculture Scandinavica, Section A: Animal Science*, Suppl. 27, 22–28.

Bryan, F.J. (1980) Foodborne diseases in the United States associated with meat and poultry. *Journal of Food Production* 43, 140–150.

Buckley, J. and Connolly, J.F. (1980) Influence of alpha tocopherol (vitamin E) on storage stability of raw pork and bacon. *Journal of Food Protection* 43, 265–267.

Butterfield, R.M. and May, N.D.S. (1996) *Muscles of the Ox.* University of Queensland Press, Australia.

Calkins, G.R., Davis, G.W., Cole, A.B. and Hutsell, D.A. (1980) Incidence of bloodsplashed hams from hogs subjected to certain ante-mortem handling methods. *Journal of Animal Science* 50 (Suppl. 1), 15 (Abstract).

Callow, E.H. (1948) Comparative studies of meat II. The changes in the carcass during growth and fattening, and their relation to the chemical composition of the fatty and muscular tissues. *Journal of Agricultural Science (Cambridge)* 38, 174–203.

Campbell-Platt, G. and Cook, P.E. (1995) *Fermented Meats.* Blackie Academic and Professional (Chapman and Hall), London.

Cannon, J.E., Morgan, J.B., McKeith, F.K., Smith, G.C., Sonka, S., Heavner, J. and Meeker, D.L. (1996) Pork chain quality audit survey: quantification of pork quality characteristics. *Journal of Muscle Foods* 7, 29–44.

Cardoso, L.A. and Stock, M.J. (1998) Effect of Clenbuterol on endocrine status and nitrogen and energy balance in food restricted rats. *Journal of Animal Science* 76, 1012–1018.

Carse, W.A. (1973) Meat quality and acceleration of post-mortem glycolysis by electrical stimulation. *Journal of Food Technology* 8, 163–166.

Cassens, R.G., Kauffman, R.G., Scherer, A. and Meeker, D.L. (1992) Variations in pork quality: a 1991 USA survey. *Proceedings of the 38th International Congress of Meat Science and Technology*, Clermont-Ferrand, France, pp. 237–240.

Chan, W., Brown, J., Church, S.M. and Buss, D.H. (1996) *Meat Products and Dishes (Supplement to McCance and Widdowson's 'The Composition of Foods').* The Royal Society of Chemistry, Cambridge and the Ministry of Agriculture Fisheries and Food, London.

Cheah, K.S. Cheah, A.M. and Krausgill, D.I. (1995) Effect of dietary supplementation of vitamin E on pig meat quality. *Meat Science* 39, 255–264.

Cheng, C.S. and Parrish, F.C. (1976) Scanning electron microscopy of bovine muscle: effect of heating on ultrastructure. *Journal of Food Science* 41, 1449–1454.

Chrystall, B.B. (1994) Meat texture measurements. In: Pearson, A.M. and Dutson, T.R. (eds) *Quality Attributes and their Measurement in Meat, Poultry and Fish Products.* Blackie Academic and Professional (Chapman and Hall), London, pp. 316–336.

Chrystall, B.B. and Hagyard, C.J. (1976) Electrical stimulation and lamb tenderness. *New Zealand Journal of Agricultural Research* 19, 7–11.

Cockram, M.S. and Lee, R.A. (1991) Some preslaughter factors affecting the occurrence of bruising in sheep. *British Veterinary Journal* 147, 120–125.

Coleman, M.E., Rhee, K.S. and Cross, H.R. (1988) Sensory and cooking properties of beef steaks and roasts cooked with and without external fat. *Journal of Food Science* 53, 34–36.

Cook, C.J. (1993) A guide to better electrical stunning. *Meat Focus International* 2, 128–131.

Cook, C.J., Devine, C.E., Gilbert, K.V., Smith, D.D. and Maasland, S.A. (1995) The effect of electrical head-only stun duration on electroencephalographic-measured seizure and brain amino acid neurotransmitter release. *Meat Science* 40, 137–147.

Cooper, R.N. and Morris, M.A. (1978) Bobby calf bleeding rates and blood yields. *New Zealand Journal of Agricultural Research* 21, 409–410.

Cornforth, D. (1994) Color – its basis and importance. In: Pearson, A.M. and Dutson, T.R. (eds) *Quality Attributes and their Measurement in Meat, Poultry and Fish Products.* Blackie Academic and Professional (Chapman and Hall), London, pp. 34–78.

Cornforth, D.P., Pearson, A.M. and Merkel, R.A. (1980) Relationship of mitochondria and sarcoplasmic reticulum to cold shortening. *Meat Science* 4, 103–121.

Crouse, D., Koohmaraie, M. and Seideman, S.D. (1991) The relationship of muscle fibre size to tenderness of beef. *Meat Science* 30, 295–302.

Curtis, S.E. and Stricklin, W.R. (1991) The importance of animal cognition in agricultural animal production systems: an overview. *Journal of Animal Science* 69, 5001–5007.

Dainty, R.H. and Mackey, B.M. (1992) The relationship between the phenotypic properties of bacteria from chill-stored meat and spoilage processes. *Journal of Applied Bacteriology* 73 (Symposium Suppl.), 103S–114S.

Davey, C.L., Kuttel, H. and Gilbert, K.V. (1967) Shortening as a factor in meat ageing. *Journal of Food Technology* 2, 53–56.

Davey, C.L., Gilbert, K.V. and Carse, W.A. (1976) Carcass electrical stimulation to prevent cold shortening toughness in beef. *New Zealand Journal of Agricultural Research* 19, 13–18.

Davis, C.E., Townsend, W.E. and McCampbell, H.C. (1978) Early rigor detection in pork carcasses by foreleg position. *Journal of Animal Science* 46, 376–383.

Dawkins, M.S. and Hardie, S. (1989) Space needs of laying hens. *British Poultry Science* 30, 413–416.

Deliza, R., MacFie, H.J.H. and Hedderley, D. (1996) Information affects consumer assessment of sweet and bitter solutions. *Journal of Food Science* 61, 1080–1084.

DeVol, D.L., McKeith, F.K., Bechtel, P.J., Novakofski, J., Shanks, R.D. and Carr, T.R. (1988) Variation in composition and palatability traits and relationships between muscle characteristics and palatability in a random sample of pork carcasses. *Journal of Animal Science* 66, 385–395.

Dorsa, W.J. (1997) New and established carcass decontamination procedures commonly used in the beef-processing industry. *Journal of Food Protection* 60, 1146–1151.

Dransfield, E. (1977) Intramuscular composition and texture of beef muscles. *Journal of the Science of Food and Agriculture* 28, 833–842.

Dransfield, E. (1994a) Optimisation of tenderisation, ageing and tenderness. *Meat Science* 36, 105–121.

Dransfield, E. (1994b) Tenderness of meat, poultry and fish. In: Pearson, A.M. and Dutson, T.R. (eds) *Quality Attributes and their Measurement in Meat, Poultry and Fish Products.* Blackie Academic and Professional (Chapman and Hall), London, pp. 289–315.

Dransfield, E. and MacFie, H.J.M. (1980) Precision in the measurement of meat texture. *Journal of the Science of Food and Agriculture* 31, 62–66.

Dransfield, E., Jones, R.C.D. and MacFie, H.J.H. (1981) Tenderising in m. longissimus dorsi of beef, veal, rabbit, lamb and pork. *Meat Science* 5, 139–147.

Duncan, I.J.H. and Petherick, J.C. (1991) The implications of cognitive processes for animal welfare. *Journal of Animal Science* 69, 5017–5022.

Dutson, T.R. (1983) The measurement of pH in muscle and its importance to meat quality. *Proceedings of the 36th Reciprocal Meat Conference of the American Meat Science Association,* Fargo, North Dakota. 12–15 June. American Meat Science Association, Chicago, pp. 92–97.

Dutson, T.R., Savell, J.W. and Smith, G.C. (1982) Electrical stimulation of antemortem stressed beef. *Meat Science* 6, 159–162.

Edwards, S.A., Armsby, A.W. and Specter, H.H. (1987) Space allowances for growing pigs on fully slatted floors. *Animal Production* 44, 490–491.

Ekstrand, C., Carpenter, T.E., Andersson, I. and Algers, B. (1998) Prevalence and control of foot pad dermatitis in broilers in Sweden. *British Poultry Science* 39, 318–324.

Eldridge, G.A., Barnett, J.L., McCausland, I.P., Millar, H.W.C. and Vowles, W.J. (1984) Bruising and method of marketing cattle. *Proceedings of the Australian Society of Animal Production* 15, 675–680.

Elias, P.S. (1985) Irradiation preservation of meat and meat products. In: Lawrie, R. (ed.) *Developments in Meat Science – 3.* Elsevier Science Publishers, Amsterdam, Chapter 5, pp. 115–153.

Ellis, R.L. (1994) Food analysis and chemical residues in muscle foods. In: Pearson, A.M. and Dutson, T.R. (eds) *Quality Attributes and their Measurement in Meat, Poultry and Fish Products.* Blackie Academic and Professional (Chapman and Hall), London, pp. 441–478.

Enser, M., Hallett, K., Hewitt, B., Fursey, G.A.J. and Wood, J.D. (1996) Fatty acid composition of English beef, lamb and pork at retail. *Meat Science* 42, 443–456.

Enser, M., Hallett, K., Hewitt, B., Fursey, G.A.J., Wood, J.D. and Harrington, G. (1998) Fatty acid content and composition of UK beef and lamb muscle in relation to production system and implications for human nutrition. *Meat Science* 49, 329–341.

Etherington, D.J., Taylor, M.A.J. and Dransfield, E. (1987) Conditioning of meat from different species. Relationship between tenderising and the levels of cathepsin B, cathepsin L, calpain I, calpain II and β-glucuronidase. *Meat Science* 20, 1–18.

Fabiansson, S., Reutersward, A.L. and Libelius, R. (1985) Ultrastructural and biochemical changes in electrically stimulated dark cutting beef. *Meat Science* 12, 177–188.

Farmer, L.J. (1992) Meat flavour. In: Johnston, D.E., Knight, M.K. and Ledward, D.A. (eds) *The Chemistry of Meat-based Foods.* Royal Society of Chemistry, Cambridge, pp. 169–182.

Faustman, C., Cassens, R.G., Schaefer, D.M., Buege, D.R., Williams, S.N. and Scheller, K.K. (1989) Improvement of pigment and lipid stability in Holstein steer beef by dietary supplementation with vitamin E. *Journal of Food Science* 54, 858–862.

Faustman, C., Chan, W.K.M., Schaefer, D.M. and Havens, A. (1998) Beef color update: the role for vitamin E. *Journal of Animal Science* 76, 1019–1026.

FAWC (1993) Second Report on Priorities for Research and Development in Farm Animal Welfare, MAFF, Tolworth, UK.

Finnie, J.W. (1995) Neuropathological changes produced by non-penetrating percussive captive bolt stunning of cattle. *New Zealand Veterinary Journal* 43, 183–185.

Fisher, A.V. (1997) A review of the technique of estimating the composition of livestock using the velocity of ultrasound. *Computers and Electronics in Agriculture* 17, 217–231.

Folch, J., Lees, M. and Sloan-Stanley, G.H. (1957) A simple method for the isolation and purification of total lipids from animal tissues. *Journal of Biological Chemistry* 226, 497–509.

Fortin, A. (1989) Preslaughter management of pigs and its influence on the quality (PSE/DFD) of pork. *Proceedings of the 35th International Congress of Meat Science and Technology.* Danish Meat Research Institute, Roskilde, pp. 981–986.

Fortin, A. and Raymond, D.P. (1988) The use of electrical characteristics of muscle for the objective detection of PSE and DFD in pork carcasses under commercial conditions. *Canadian Institute of Food Science and Technology Journal* 21, 260–265.

Fortin, A., Jones, S.D.M. and Haworth, C.R. (1984) Pork carcass grading: a comparison of the New Zealand Hennessy Grading Probe and the Danish Fat-o-Meater. *Meat Science* 10, 131–144.

Franke, W.C. and Solberg, M. (1971) Quantitative determination of metmyoglobin and total pigment in an intact meat sample using reflectance spectrophotometry. *Journal of Food Science* 36, 515–519.

Freeman, B.M., Kettlewell, P.J., Manning, A.C.C. and Berry, P.S. (1984) Stress of transportation for broilers. *Veterinary Record* 114, 286–287.

Froystein, T., ThornWittussen, H., Røe, M., Bye, M. and Bjørnstad, A. (1993) Entire male pig production in small scale slaughterhouses based on manual analysis of skatole. In: Bonneau, M. (ed.) *Measurement and Prevention of Boar Taint in Entire Male Pigs.* INRA, Paris, pp. 145–149.

Fujii, J., Otsu, K., Zorzato, F., DeLeon, S., Khanna, V.K., Weiler, J.E., O'Brien, P.J. and MacLennan, D.H. (1991) Identification of a mutation in the porcine ryanodine receptor associated with malignant hyperthermia. *Science* 253, 448–451.

Fung, D.Y.C. (1994) Rapid methods for measurement and enumeration of microbial contamination. In: Pearson, A.M. and Dutson, T.R. (eds) *Quality Attributes and their Measurement in Meat, Poultry and Fish Products.* Blackie Academic and Professional (Chapman and Hall), London, pp. 404–440.

Gacula, M.C. and Singh, J. (1984) *Statistical Methods in Food and Consumer Research.* Academic Press, New York.

Garcia-Regueiro, J.A. and Diaz, I. (1989) Evaluation of the contribution of skatole, indole, androstenone and adrostenols to boar taint in back fat of pigs by HPLC and capillary gas chromatography (CGC). *Meat Science* 25, 307–316.

George, M.H., Tatum, J.D., Dolezal, H.G., Morgan, J.B., Wise, J.W., Calkins, C.R., Gordon, T., Reagan, J.O. and Smith, G.C. (1997) Comparison of USDA quality grade with Tendertec for the assessment of beef palatability. *Journal of Animal Science* 75, 1538–1546.

Gerrard, F. (1980) *Macgregor's The Structure of the Meat Animals,* 3rd edn. Oxford Technical Press, Oxford, Chapter 3, pp. 53–84.

Gibney, M.J. (1993) Fat in animal products: facts and perceptions. In: Wood, J.D. and Lawrence, T.L.J. (eds) *Safety and Quality of Food from Animals.* Occasional Publication of the British Society of Animal Production, Edinburgh, pp. 57–61.

Gilbert, K.V., Davey, C.L. and Newton, K.G. (1977) Electrical stimulation and hot boning of beef. *New Zealand Journal of Agricultural Research* 20, 139–143.

Gill, C.O. (1994) The hygienic quality of bruised tissue in red meat carcasses. *Meat Focus International* 3, 369–371.

Gill, C.O. and Harrison, J.C.L. (1982) Microbiological and organoleptic qualities of bruised meats. *Journal of Food Protection* 45, 646–649.

Gill, C.O. and Penney, N. (1988) The effect of the initial gas volume to meat weight ratio on the storage life of chilled beef packaged under CO_2. *Meat Science* 22, 53–63.

GIRA (1997) *World Meat Facts Book.* International Meat Secretariat – GIRA, Geneva, Switzerland, 45pp.

Goll, D.E., Bray, R.W. and Hoeckstra, W.G. (1964) Age-associated changes in bovine muscle connective tissue. III. Rate of solubilisation at 100°C. *Journal of Food Science* 29, 622–628.

Gracey, J.F. (1981) *Thornton's Meat Hygiene,* 7th edn. Baillière Tindall, London.

Gracey, J.F. (1998) *Meat Plant Operations.* Chalcombe Publications, Welton, Lincoln.

Gracey, J.F. and Collins, D.S. (1992) *Meat Hygiene,* 9th edn. Baillière Tindall, London.

Grandin, T. (1980) Mechanical, electrical and anaesthetic stunning methods for livestock. *International Journal for Studies in Animal Problems* 1, 242–263.

Grandin, T. (1991) *Recommended Animal Handling Guidelines for Meat Packers.* American Meat Institute, Washington DC.

Grandin, T. (1993) *Livestock Handling and Transport.* CAB International, Wallingford.

Grandin, T. and Bruning, J. (1992) Boar presence reduces fighting in mixed slaughter-weight pigs. *Applied Animal Behaviour Science* 33, 273–276.

Grandin, T. and Regenstein, J.M. (1994) Religious slaughter and animal welfare: a discussion for meat scientists. *Meat Focus International* 3, 115–123.

Grau, R. and Hamm, R. (1953) Eine einfache Methode zur Bestimmung der Wasserbindung im Muskel. *Naturwissenschaffen* 40, 29–30.

Grau, F.H., Brownlie, L.E. and Roberts, E.A. (1968) Effect of some preslaughter treatments on the *Salmonella* population in the bovine rumen and faeces. *Journal of Applied Bacteriology* 31, 157–163.

Gray, J.I. and Crackel, R.L. (1992) Oxidative flavour changes in meats: their origin and prevention. In: Johnston, D.E., Knight, M.K. and Ledward, D.A. (eds) *The Chemistry of Muscle-based Foods.* Royal Society of Chemistry, Cambridge, pp. 145–168.

Gready, R. (1997) A whole industry approach to farm and quality assurance. *The Pig Journal* 39, 90–96.

Green, B.E., Hsin, I.M. and Zipser, M.Y.W. (1971) Retardation of oxidative color changes in raw ground beef. *Journal of Food Science* 36, 940–942.

Gregory, N.G. (1998) *Animal Welfare and Meat Science.* CABI Publishing, CAB International, Wallingford.

Gregory, N.G. and Wilkins, L.J. (1989a) Effect of stunning current on carcass quality in chickens. *Veterinary Record* 124, 530–532.

Gregory, N.G. and Wilkins, L.J. (1989b) Handling and processing damage in end-of-lay hens. *British Poultry Science* 30, 555–562.

Hadley, P.J., Holder, J.S. and Hinton, M.H. (1997) Effects of fleece soiling and skinning method on the microbiology of sheep carcasses. *Veterinary Record* 140, 570–574.

Hall, S.J.G. and Bradshaw, R.H. (1998) Welfare aspects of the transport by road of sheep and pigs. *Journal of Applied Animal Welfare Science* 1, 235–254.

Hamdy, M.K., Kunkle, L.E. and Deatherage, F.E. (1957) Bruised tissue II. Determination of the age of a bruise. *Journal of Animal Science* 16, 490–501.

Hamm, R. (1986) In: Bechtel, P.J. (ed.) *Muscle as Food.* Academic Press, New York, p. 135.

Hansen, L.J. (1972) Development of the Armour Tenderometer for tenderness evaluation of beef carcasses. *Journal of Texture Studies* 3, 146–164.

Hansen, R., Rogers, R., Emge, S. and Jacobs, N.J. (1964) Incidence of *Salmonella* in the hog colon as affected by handling practices prior to slaughter. *Journal of the American Veterinary Medical Association* 145, 139–140.

Hegarty, P.V.J. (1969) Subjective evaluation of the colour of pig muscle. I. Accuracy of subjective measurement of colour. *Journal of the Science of Food and Agriculture* 20, 685–689.

Heitzman, R.J. (1996) Residues in meat. In: Taylor, S.A., Raimundo, A., Severini, M. and Smulders, F.J.M. (eds) *Meat Quality and Meat Packaging.* ECCEAMST, Utrecht, pp. 155–167.

Hicks, C., Schinckel, A.P., Forrest, J.C., Akridge, J.T., Wagner, J.R. and Chen, W. (1998) Biases associated with genotype and sex in prediction of fat-free lean mass and carcass value in hogs. *Journal of Animal Science* 76, 2221–2234.

Higgs, A.R., Norris, R.T. and Richards, R.B. (1991) Season, age and adiposity influence death rates in sheep exported by sea. *Australian Journal of Agricultural Research* 42, 205–226.

Hileman, S.M., Schillo, K.K., Boling, J.A. and Estienne, M.L. (1990) Effects of age on fasting-induced changes in insulin, glucose, urea nitrogen, and free fatty acids in the sera of sheep. *Proceedings of the Society for Experimental Biology and Medicine* 194, 21–25.

Hofmann, K. (1975) Ein neues Gerät zur Bestimmung der Wasserbindung des Fleisches: Das 'Kapillar-Volumeter'. *Fleischwirtschaft* 55, 25–30.

Honikel, K.O. (1987) How to measure the water-holding capacity of meat? Recommendation of standardised methods. In: Tarrant, P.V., Eikelenboom, G. and Monin, G. (eds) *Evaluation and Control of Meat Quality in Pigs*. Martinus Nijhoff, Dordrecht, pp. 129–142.

Honikel, K.O. and Fischer, C. (1977) A rapid method for the detection of PSE and DFD porcine muscles. *Journal of Food Science* 42, 1633–1636.

Honikel, K.O. and Hamm, R. (1994) Measurement of water-holding capacity and juiciness. In: Pearson, A.M. and Dutson, T.R. (eds) *Quality Attributes and their Measurement in Meat, Poultry and Fish Products*. Blackie Academic and Professional (Chapman and Hall), London, pp. 125–161.

Honkavaara, M. (1993) Effect of a controlled ventilation stock crate on stress and meat quality. *Meat Focus International* 2, 545–547.

Hood, D.E. (1975) Preslaughter injection of sodium ascorbate as a method of inhibiting metmyoglobin formation in fresh beef. *Journal of the Science of Food and Agriculture* 26, 85–90.

Hornsey, H.C. (1956) The colour of cooked cured pork I. Estimation of the nitric oxide-haem pigments. *Journal of the Science of Food and Agriculture* 7, 534–540.

Hostetler, R.L. and Landmann, W.A. (1968) Photomicrographic studies of dynamic changes in muscle fibre fragments. 1. Effect of various heat treatments on length, width and birefringence. *Journal of Food Science* 33, 468–470.

Hostetler, R.L., Carpenter, Z.L., Smith, G.C. and Dutson, T.R. (1975) Comparison of postmortem treatments for improving tenderness of beef. *Journal of Food Science* 40, 223–226.

Hostetler, R.L., Landmann, W.A., Link, B.A. and Fitzhugh, H.A. (1970) Influence of carcass position during rigor mortis on tenderness of beef muscles: comparison of two treatments. *Journal of Animal Science* 31, 47–50.

Hubbard, J.I. (1973) Microphysiology of vertebrate neuromuscular transmission. *Physiological Reviews* 53, 674–723.

Hudson, W.R., Hinton, M.H. and Mead, G.C. (1998) Assessing abattoir hygiene with a marker organism. *Veterinary Record* 142, 545–547.

Humphrey, T.J., Baskerville, A., Whitehead, A., Rowe, B. and Henley, A. (1993) Influence of feeding patterns on the artificial infection of laying hens with *Salmonella enteritidis* phage type 4. *Veterinary Record* 132, 407–409.

Huxley, A.F. and Simmons, R.M. (1971) Proposed mechanisms of force generation in striated muscle. *Nature* 233, 533–538.

Huxley, H.E. (1969) The mechanism of muscular contraction. *Science* 164, 1356–1366.

Huxley, H.E. and Hanson, J. (1954) Changes in the cross-striations of muscle during contraction and stretch and their structural interpretation. *Nature* 173, 973.

Irie, M. and Swatland, H.J. (1993) Prediction of fluid losses from pork using subjective and objective paleness. *Meat Science* 33, 277–292.

Jakobsson, B. and Bengtsson, N.E. (1969a) The influence of high freezing rates on the quality of frozen ground beef and small cuts of beef. *Proceedings of the 15th European Meeting of Meat Research Workers*. p. 482.

Jakobsson, B. and Bengtsson, N. (1969b) Freezing of raw beef: influence of ageing, freezing rate and cooking method on quality and yield. *Journal of Food Science* 38, 560–565.

James, S. (1996) Chilling and freezing of red meat. In: Taylor, S.A., Raimundo, A., Severini, M. and Smulders, F.J.M. (eds) *Meat Quality and Meat Packaging.* ECCEAMST, Utrecht, pp. 45–63.

James, S.J., Creed, P.G. and Roberts, T.A. (1977) Air thawing of beef quarters. *Journal of the Science of Food and Agriculture* 28, 1109–1119.

Jeacocke, R.E. (1977a) Continuous measurements of the pH of beef muscle in intact beef carcasses. *Journal of Food Technology* 12, 375–386.

Jeacocke, R.E. (1977b) The temperature dependence of anaerobic glycolysis in beef muscle held in a linear temperature gradient. *Journal of the Science of Food and Agriculture* 28, 551–556.

Jeacocke, R.E. (1984) The control of post-mortem metabolism and the onset of rigor mortis. In: Bailey, A.J. (ed.) *Recent Advances in the Chemistry of Meat.* Royal Society of Chemistry, London, Chapter 3, pp. 41–57.

Jeacocke, R.E. (1993) The concentration of free magnesium and free calcium ions both increase in skeletal muscle fibres entering rigor mortis. *Meat Science* 35, 27–45.

Jeremiah, L.E. (1984) A note on the influence of inherent muscle quality on cooking losses and palatability attributes of pork loin chops. *Canadian Journal of Animal Science* 64, 773–775.

Jeremiah, L.E., Newman, J.A., Tong, A.K.W. and Gibson, L.L. (1988) The effects of castration, preslaughter stress and zeranol implants on beef: part 2-cooking properties and flavour of loin steaks from bovine males. *Meat Science* 22, 103–121.

Jones, S.D.M. and Tong, A.K.W. (1989) Factors influencing the commercial incidence of dark cutting beef. *Canadian Journal of Animal Science* 69, 649–654.

Jones, S.D.M., Schaefer, A.L., Robertson, W.M. and Vincient, B.C. (1990) The effects of withholding feed and water on carcass shrinkage and meat quality in beef cattle. *Meat Science* 28, 131–139.

Joseph, R.L. (1996) Very fast chilling of beef and tenderness – a report from an EU concerted action. *Meat Science* 43, No. S., S217–S227.

Kauffman, R.G., Wachholz, D., Henderson, D. and Lochner, J.V. (1978) Shrinkage of PSE, normal and DFD hams during transit and processing. *Journal of Animal Science* 46, 1236–1240.

Kauffman, R.G., Eikelenboom, G., van der Wal, P.G., Merkus, G.S.M. and Zaar, M. (1986) The use of filter paper to estimate drip loss of porcine musculature. *Meat Science* 18, 191–200.

Kauffman, R.G., Sybesma, W. and Eikelenboom, G. (1990) In search of quality. *Canadian Institute of Food Science and Technology Journal* 23, 160–164.

Kauffman, R.G., Sybesma, W., Smulders, F.J.M., Eikelenboom, G., Engel, B., Van Laack, R.L.J.M., Hoaving-Bolink, A.H., Sterenburg, P., Nordheim, E.V., Walstra, P. and van der Wal, P.G. (1993) The effectiveness of examining early post-mortem musculature to predict ultimate pork quality. *Meat Science* 34, 283–300.

Kempster, A.J., Cuthbertson, A. and Harrington, G. (1982a) The relationship between conformation and the yield and distribution of lean meat in the carcasses of British pigs, cattle and sheep: a review. *Meat Science* 6, 37–53.

Kempster, A.J., Cuthbertson, A. and Harrington, G. (1982b) *Carcass Evaluation in Livestock Breeding, Production and Marketing.* West View Press, Boulder, Colorado.

Kempster, A.J., Chadwick, J.P. and Jones, D.W. (1985) An evaluation of the Hennessy Grading Probe and the SFK Fat-o-Meater for use in pig carcass classification and grading. *Animal Production* 40, 323–329.

Kempster, A.J., Cook, G.L. and Grantley-Smith, M. (1986) National estimates of body composition of British cattle, sheep and pigs with special reference to trends in fatness. A review. *Meat Science* 17, 107–138.

Kempster, A.J., Cook, G.L. and Southgate, J.R. (1988) Evaluation of British Friesian, Canadian Holstein and Beef breed × British Friesian steers slaughtered over a commercial range of fatness from 16-month and 24-month beef production systems. 2. Carcass characteristics, and rate and efficiency of lean gain. *Animal Production* 46, 365–378.

Kenny, F.J. and Tarrant, P.V. (1987) The behaviour of young Friesian bulls during social regrouping at an abattoir. Influence of an overhead electrified wire grid. *Applied Animal Behavioural Science* 18, 233–246.

Kent, J.E., Molony, V. and Robertson, I.S. (1995) Comparison of the Burdizzo and rubber ring methods for castrating and tail docking lambs. *Veterinary Record* 136, 192–196.

Kerler, J. and Grosch, W. (1996) Odorants contributing to warmed-over flavour (WOF) of refrigerated cooked beef. *Journal of Food Science* 61, 1271–1274.

Kerth, C.R., Miller, M.F. and Ramsey, C.B. (1995) Improvement of beef tenderness and quality traits with calcium chloride injection in beef loins 48 h postmortem. *Journal of Animal Science* 73, 750–756.

Kestin, S.C., Knowles, T.G., Tinch, A.E. and Gregory, N.G. (1992) Prevalence of leg weakness in broiler chickens and its relationship with genotype. *Veterinary Record* 131, 190–194.

Kettlewell, P., Mitchell, M. and Meehan, A. (1993) The distribution of thermal loads within poultry transport vehicles. *Agricultural Engineer* 48, 26–30.

Kirk, R.S. and Sawyer, R. (1991) *Pearson's Composition and Analysis of Foods*, 9th edn. Longman Scientific and Technical, Harlow, Essex.

Kirton, A.H., Bishop, W.H., Mullord, M.M. and Frazerhurst, L.F. (1978) Relationships between time of stunning and time of throat cutting and their effect on blood pressure and blood splash in lambs. *Meat Science* 2, 199–206.

Knapp, R.H., Terry, C.A., Savell, J.W., Cross, H.R., Mies, W.L. and Edwards, J.W. (1989) Characterisation of cattle types to meet specific beef targets. *Journal of Animal Science* 67, 2294–2308.

Knowles, T.G. and Broom, D.M. (1990) The handling and transport of broilers and spent hens. *Applied Animal Behaviour Science* 28, 75–91.

Knowles, T.G., Maunder, D.H.L., Warriss, P.D. and Jones, T.W.H. (1994a) Factors affecting the mortality of lambs in transit to or in lairage at a slaughterhouse, and reasons for carcass condemnations. *Veterinary Record* 135, 109–111.

Knowles, T.G., Maunder, D.H.L. and Warriss, P.D. (1994b) Factors affecting the incidence of bruising in lambs arriving at one slaughterhouse. *Veterinary Record* 134, 44–45.

Knowles, T.G., Warriss, P.D., Brown, S.N. and Kestin, S.C. (1994c) Long distance transport of export lambs. *Veterinary Record* 134, 107–110.

Koh, K.C., Bidner, T.D., McMillan, K.W. and Kim, M.B. (1993) The relationship between ATP and R-values in postmortem bovine longissimus dorsi muscle. *Meat Science* 33, 253–263.

Koh, M.C., Lin, C.H., Chua, S.B., Chew, S.T. and Phang, S.T.W. (1998) Random amplified polymorphic DNA (RAPD) fingerprints for identification of red meat species. *Meat Science* 48, 275–285.

Koohmaraie, M. (1996) Biochemical factors regulating the toughening and tenderization processes of meat. *Meat Science* 43, No. S, S193-S201.

Koohmaraie, M., Babiker, A.S., Schroeder, A.L., Merkel, R.A. and Dutson, T.R. (1988) Acceleration of postmortem tenderization in ovine carcasses through activation of Ca^{2+}-dependent proteases. *Journal of Food Science* 53, 1638–1641.

Koohmaraie, M., Whipple, G. and Crouse, J.D. (1990) Acceleration of post-mortem tenderization in lamb and Brahman-cross beef carcasses through infusion of calcium chloride. *Journal of Animal Science* 68, 1278–1283.

Koohmaraie, M., Shackleford, S.D., Wheeler, T.L., Lonergan, S.M. and Doumit, M.E. (1995) A muscle hypertrophy condition in lamb (callipyge): characterisation of effects on muscle growth and meat quality traits. *Journal of Animal Science* 73, 3596–3607.

Koohmaraie, M., Doumit, M.E. and Wheeler, T.L. (1996) Meat toughening does not occur when rigor shortening is prevented. *Journal of Animal Science* 74, 2935–2942.

Kreikemeier, K.K., Unruh, J.A. and Eck, T.P. (1998) Factors affecting the occurrence of dark-cutting beef and selected carcass traits in finished beef cattle. *Journal of Animal Science* 76, 388–395.

Kropf, D.H. (1993) Colour stability-factors affecting the colour of fresh meat. *Meat Focus International* 2, 269–275.

Kunkel, H.O., Thompson, P.B., Miller, B.A. and Skaggs, C.L. (1998) Use of competing conceptions of risk in animal agriculture. *Journal of Animal Science* 76, 706–713.

Kyle, R. (1994) New species for meat production. *Journal of Agricultural Science, Cambridge* 123, 1–8.

Lautner, B. (1997) Quality assurance in the US. *The Pig Journal* 39, 29–36.

Lavelle, C.L., Hunt, M.C. and Kropf, D.H. (1995) Display life and internal cooked color of ground beef from vitamin E-supplemented steers. *Journal of Food Science* 60, 1175–1178.

Leach, T.M. (1985) Pre-slaughter stunning. In: Lawrie, R. (ed.) *Developments in Meat Science- 3*. Elsevier Applied Science, London, Chapter 3, pp. 51–87.

Ledward, D.A. (1990) Metmyoglobin formation in beef stored in carbon dioxide enriched and oxygen depleted atmospheres. *Journal of Food Science* 25, 33–37.

Lewis, G.J. and Purslow, P.P. (1990) Connective tissue differences in the strength of cooked meat across the muscle fibre direction due to test specimen size. *Meat Science* 28, 183–194.

Light, N., Champion, A.E., Voyle, C. and Bailey, A.J. (1985) The role of epimysial, perimysial and endomysial collagen in determining texture in six bovine muscles. *Meat Science* 13, 137–149.

Lister, D. (1984) *In Vivo Measurement of Body Composition in Meat Animals.* Elsevier Applied Science, London.

Locker, R.H. (1960) Degree of muscular contraction as a factor in tenderness in beef. *Food Research* 25, 304–307.

Locker, R.H. (1985) Cold induced toughness of meat. *Advances in Meat Research* 1, 1–44.

Locker, R.H. and Daines, G.J. (1975) Rigor mortis in beef Sternomandibularis muscle at 37°C. *Journal of the Science of Food and Agriculture* 26, 1721–1733.

Locker, R.H. and Hagyard, C.J. (1963) A cold shortening effect in beef muscles. *Journal of the Science of Food and Agriculture* 14, 787–793.

Locker, R.H. and Wild, D.J.C. (1984) Ageing of cold shortened meat depends on the criterion. *Meat Science* 10, 235–238.

Longdell, G.R. (1996) Recent developments in sheep and beef processing in Australasia. *Meat Science* 43, No. S, S165-S174.

Lopez-Bote, C. and Warriss, P.D. (1988) A note on the relationships between measures of waterholding capacity in the m. longissimus dorsi and total drip loss from butchered pig carcasses during storage. *Meat Science* 23, 227–234.

Lopez-Bote, C., Warriss, P.D. and Brown, S.N. (1989) The use of muscle protein solubility measurements to assess pig lean meat quality. *Meat Science* 26, 167–175.

Lundström, K. and Bonneau, M. (1996) Off flavours in meat with particular emphasis on boar taint. In: Taylor, S.A., Raimundo, A., Severini, M. and Smulders, F.J.M. (eds) *Meat Quality and Meat Packaging.* ECCEAMST, Utrecht, pp. 137–154.

Lundström, K. and Enfält, A-C. (1997) Rapid prediction of RN phenotype in pigs by means of meat juice. *Meat Science* 45, 127–131.

MacDougall, D.B. (1984) Meat Research Institute Light Probe for stressed meat detection. *Analytical Proceedings* 21, 494–495.

MacDougall, D.B. (1994) Colour of meat. In: Pearson, A.M. and Dutson, T.R. (eds) *Quality Attributes and their Measurement in Meat, Poultry and Fish Products.* Blackie Academic and Professional (Chapman and Hall), London, pp. 79–93.

MacDougall, D.B., Cuthbertson, A. and Smith, R.J. (1969) The assessment of pig meat paleness by reflectance photometry. *Animal Production* 11, 243–246.

MacDougall, D.B., Mottram, D.S. and Rhodes, D.N. (1975) Contribution of nitrite and nitrate to the colour and flavour of cured meats. *Journal of the Science of Food and Agriculture* 26, 1743–1754.

Madruga, M.S. and Mottram, D.S. (1995) The effect of pH on the formation of Maillard-derived aroma volatiles using a cooked meat system. *Journal of the Science of Food and Agriculture* 68, 305–310.

Mallikarjunan, P. and Mittal, G.S. (1995) Optimum conditions for beef carcass chilling. *Meat Science* 39, 215–223.

Marsh, B.B. and Leet, N.G. (1966) Studies in meat tenderness III. The effects of cold shortening on tenderness. *Journal of Food Science* 31, 450–459.

Maruyama, K. (1985) Myofibrillar cytoskeleton proteins of vertebrate striated muscle. In: Lawrie, R. (ed.) *Developments in Meat Science – 3.* Elsevier Applied Science, London, Chapter 2, pp. 25–50.

McCance, R.A. and Widdowson, E.M. (1997) *McCance and Widdowson's: The Composition of Foods,* 5th edn. by B. Holland, A.A. Welch, I.D. Unwin, D.H. Buss, A.A. Paul and D.A.T. Southgate. The Royal Society of Chemistry and the Ministry of Agriculture, Fisheries and Food, Cambridge, UK.

McCausland, I.P. and Dougherty, R. (1978) Histological ageing of bruises in lambs and calves. *Australian Veterinary Journal* 54, 525–527.

McFarlane, B.J. and Unruh, J.A. (1996) Effects of blast chilling and postmortem calcium chloride injection on tenderness of pork longissimus muscle. *Journal of Animal Science* 74, 1842–1845.

McGeown, D., Danbury, T.C., Waterman-Pearson, A.E. and Kestin, S.C. (1999) The effect of Carprofen on lameness in broiler chickens. *Veterinary Record* 144, 668–671.

McInerney, J. (1991) Assessing the benefits of animal welfare. In: Carruthers, S.P. (ed.) *Farm Animals: It Pays to be Humane*, CAS paper 22. Centre for Agricultural Strategy, University of Reading, Reading, pp. 15–31.

McLaren, D.G., Novakofski, J., Parrett, D.F., Lo, L.L., Singh, S.D., Neumann, K.R. and McKeith, F.K. (1991) A study of operator effects on ultrasonic measures of fat depth and longissimus muscle area in cattle, sheep and pigs. *Journal of Animal Science* 69, 54–66.

McNally, P.W. and Warriss, P.D. (1996) A study of recent bruising in cattle at abattoirs. *Veterinary Record* 138, 126–128.

McVeigh, J.M. and Tarrant, P.V. (1980) The problem of dark cutting beef. In: Hood, D.E. and Tarrant, P.V. (eds) *The Problem of Dark Cutting Beef.* Martinus Nijhoff, The Hague, pp. 440–453.

Meat Research Institute (1972) Assessment of meat texture by optical diffraction. HMSO, London.

Mikami, M., Sekikawa, M. and Miura, H. (1993) Peptide and free amino acid content of electrically stimulated beef. *Meat Focus International* 2, 537–539.

Miles, C.A. and Fursey, G.A.J. (1974) A note on the velocity of ultrasound in living tissue. *Animal Production* 18, 93–96.

Minton, J.E. (1994) Function of the hypothalamic-pituitary-adrenal axis and the sympathetic nervous system in models of acute stress in domestic farm animals. *Journal of Animal Science* 72, 1891–1898.

Mitchell, A.D., Conway, J.M. and Potts, W.J.E. (1996) Body composition analysis of pigs by dual-energy X-ray absorptiometry. *Journal of Animal Science* 74, 2663–2671.

Mitsumoto, M., Cassens, R.G., Schaefer, D.M., Arnold, R.N. and Scheller, K.K. (1991) Improvement of color and lipid stability in beef longissimus with dietary vitamin E and vitamin C dip treatment. *Journal of Food Science* 56, 1489–1492.

MLC (1985) Concern at ringside damage in pigs. Meat and Marketing Technical Notes No. 4. Meat and Livestock Commission, Milton Keynes, pp. 14–16.

MLC (1989) *Stotfold Pig Development Unit – First Trial Results.* Meat and Livestock Commission, Milton Keynes.

MLC (1992) *Second Stotfold Pig Development Unit Trial Results.* Meat and Livestock Commission, Milton Keynes.

MLC (1993) *Beef Yearbook.* Meat and Livestock Commission, Milton Keynes.

MLC (1995) *Beef Yearbook.* Meat and Livestock Commission, Milton Keynes.

MLC (1997) *A Pocketful of Meat Facts.* Meat and Livestock Commission, Milton Keynes.

Moberg, G.P. (1987) Problems in defining stress and distress in animals. *Journal of the American Veterinary Medical Association* 191, 1207–1211.

Mohan Raj, A.B. (1993) Gas stunning of chickens. *Meat Focus International* 2, 313–317.

Mohan Raj, A.B. (1994a) An investigation into the batch killing of turkeys in their transport containers using mixtures of gases. *Research in Veterinary Science* 56, 325–331.

Mohan Raj, A.B. (1994b) Effect of stunning method, carcase chilling temperature and filleting time on the texture of turkey breast meat. *British Poultry Science* 35, 77–89.

Mohan Raj, A.B. (1999) Behaviour of pigs exposed to mixtures of gases and the time required to stun and kill them: welfare implications. *Veterinary Record* 144, 165–168.

Møller, A.J. and Jensen, P. (1993) Cold induced toughening in excised pork as affected by pH, R value and time at boning. *Meat Science* 34, 1–12.

Moloney, V. and Kent, J.E. (1997) Assessment of acute pain in farm animals using behavioural and physiological measurements. *Journal of Animal Science* 75, 266–272.

Monin, G. and Sellier, P. (1985) Pork of low technological quality with a normal rate of pH fall in the immediate post-mortem period: the case of the Hampshire breed. *Meat Science* 13, 49–63.

Morgan, J.B., Savell, J.W., Hale, D.S., Miller, R.K., Griffen, D.B., Cross, H.R. and Shackelford, S.D. (1991) National beef tenderness survey. *Journal of Animal Science* 69, 3274–3283.

Morgan, J.B., Wheeler, T.L., Koohmaraie, M., Savell, J.W. and Crouse, J.D. (1993) Meat tenderness and the calpain proteolytic system in longissimus muscle of young bulls and steers. *Journal of Animal Science* 71, 1471–1476.

Mortensen, A.B. and Sørensen, S.-E. (1984) Relationship between boar taint and skatole determined with a new analysis method. *Proceedings of the 30th European Meeting of Meat Research Workers,* Bristol. Meat Research Institute, Bristol, pp. 394–396.

Mos, B.W. and Robb, J.D. (1978) The effect of preslaughter lairage on serum thyroxine and cortisol levels at slaughter, and the meat quality of boars, hogs and gilts. *Journal of the Science of Food and Agriculture* 29, 689–696.

Mottram, D.S. (1998) Chemical tainting of foods. *International Journal of Food Science and Technology* 33, 19–29.

Mottram, D.S. (1992) The chemistry of meat flavour. *Meat Focus International* 1, 87–93.

Murray, A.C. and Johnson, C.P. (1990) Evaluation and objective characterisation of the Agriculture Canada Subjective Pork Quality standards. *Canadian Institute of Food Science and Technology Journal* 23, 87–93.

Murray, A.C., Jones, S.D.M. and Tong, A.K.W. (1989) Evaluation of the Colormet Reflectance Meter for the measurement of pork muscle quality. *Proceedings of the 35th International Congress of Meat Science and Technology.* Danish Meat Research Institute, Roskilde, pp. 188–192.

NACMCF (1998) Hazard analysis and critical control point principles and application guidelines. *Journal of Food Protection* 61, 762–775.

Neale, R.J. (1992) Meat iron availability: chemical and nutritional considerations. In: Johnston, D.E., Knight, M.K. and Ledward, D.A. (eds) *The Chemistry of Meat-based Foods.* Royal Society of Chemistry, Cambridge, pp. 183–192.

Newman, P.B. (1980–81) The separation of meat from bone – a review of the mechanics and the problems. *Meat Science* 5, 171–200.

Newsholme, E.A. and Start, C. (1973) *Regulation in Metabolism.* John Wiley & Sons, Chichester.

Newton, K.G. and Gill, C.O. (1981) The microbiology of DFD fresh meats: a review. *Meat Science* 5, 223–232.

Nishimura, T., Liu, A., Hattori, A. and Takahashi, K. (1998) Changes in mechanical strength of intramuscular connective tissue during post-mortem ageing of beef. *Journal of Animal Science* 76, 528–532.

Nour, A.Y.M. and Thonney, M.L. (1994) Technical note: chemical composition of Angus and Holstein carcasses predicted from rib section composition. *Journal of Animal Science* 72, 1239–1241.

Novakofski, J., Park, S., Bechtel, P.J. and McKeith, F.K. (1989) Composition of cooked pork chops: effect of removing subcutaneous fat before cooking. *Journal of Food Science* 54, 15–17.

Nute, G.R. (1996) Assessment by sensory and consumer panelling. In: Taylor, S.A., Raimundo, A., Severini, M. and Smulders, F.J.M. (eds) *Meat Quality and Meat Packaging.* ECCEAMST, Utrecht, pp. 243–255.

Nute, G.R. (1999) Sensory assessment of poultry meat quality. In: Richardson, R.I. and Mead, G.C. (eds) *Poultry Meat Science* CAB International, Wallingford, pp. 349–365.

Nute, G.R., Jones, R.C.D., Dransfield, D. and Whelahan, O.P. (1987) Sensory characteristics of ham and their relationships with composition, visco-elasticity and strength. *International Journal of Food Science and Technology* 22, 461–476.

Offer, G. and Knight, P. (1988a) The structural basis of water-holding in meat. Part 1: General principles and water uptake in meat processing. In: Lawrie, R. (ed.) *Developments in Meat Science – 4.* Elsevier Science, London, Chapter 3, pp. 63–171.

Offer, G. and Knight, P. (1988b) The structural basis of water-holding in meat. Part 2: Drip losses. In: Lawrie, R. (ed.) *Developments in Meat Science – 4.* Elsevier Applied Science, London, Chapter 4, pp. 173–243.

Offer, G. and Trinick, J. (1983) On the mechanism of water-holding in meat: the swelling and shrinkage of myofibrils. *Meat Science* 8, 245–281.

Offer, G., Knight, P., Jeacocke, R., Almond, R., Cousins, T., Elsey, J., Parsons, N., Sharp, A., Starr, R. and Purslow, P. (1989) The structural basis of the water-holding, appearance and toughness of meat and meat products. *Food Microstructure* 8, 151–170.

Okayama, T., Imai, T. and Yamanoue, M. (1987) Effect of ascorbic acid and alpha-tocopherol on storage stability of beef steaks. *Meat Science* 21, 267–273.

Olson, D.G. and Parrish, F.C. (1977) Relationship of myofibril fragmentation index to measurements of beefsteak tenderness. *Journal of Food Science* 42, 506–509.

Pálsson, H. (1955) Conformation and body composition. In: Hammond, J. (ed.) *Progress in the Physiology of Farm Animals.* Butterworths, London, Volume 2, Chapter 10, pp. 430–542.

Park, B., Whittaker, A.D., Miller, R.K. and Hale, D.S. (1994) Predicting intramuscular fat in beef longissimus muscle from speed of sound. *Journal of Animal Science* 72, 109–116.

Parrish, F.C., Olson, D.G., Miner, B.E., Young, R.B. and Snell, R.L. (1973) Relationship of tenderness measurements made by the Armour Tenderometer to certain objective, subjective and organoleptic properties of bovine muscle. *Journal of Food Science* 38, 1214–1219.

Patterson, R.L.S. (1968) 5 α-Androst-16-en-3 one: a compound responsible for taint in boar fat. *Journal of the Science of Food and Agriculture* 19, 31–38.

Patterson, R.L.S. and Jones, S.J. (1990) Review of current techniques for the verification of the species origin of meat. *Analyst* 115, 501–506.

Pearson, A.J., Kilgour, R., de Langen, H. and Payne, E. (1977) Hormonal responses of lambs to trucking, handling and electric stunning. *Proceedings of the New Zealand Society of Animal Production* 37, 243–248.

Pearson, A.M. (1981) Meat and Health. In: Lawrie, R. (ed.) *Developments in Meat Science – 2.* Applied Science, London, Chapter 8, pp. 241–292.

Pearson, A.M. and Dutson, T.R. (eds) (1987) *Advances in Meat Research Volume 3. Restructured Meat and Poultry Products.* Van Nostrand Reinhold, New York.

Petherick, J.C. and Blackshaw, J.K. (1987) A review of the factors influencing the aggressive and agonistic behaviour of the domestic pig. *Australian Journal of Experimental Agriculture* 27, 605–611.

Petrovic, L., Grujic, R. and Petrovic, M. (1993) Definition of the optimal freezing rate – 2. Investigation of the physico-chemical properties of beef m. longissimus dorsi frozen at different freezing rates. *Meat Science* 33, 319–331.

Piggott, J.R., Simpson, S.J. and Williams, S.A.R. (1998) Sensory analysis. *International Journal of Food Science and Technology* 33, 7–18.

Planella, J. and Cook, G.L. (1991) Accuracy and consistency of prediction of pig carcass lean concentration from P_2 fat thickness and sample joint dissection. *Animal Production* 53, 345–352.

Poole, G.H. and Fletcher, D.L. (1995) A comparison of argon, carbon dioxide, and nitrogen in a broiler killing system. *Poultry Science* 74, 1218–1223.

Porter, S.J., Owen, M.G., Page, S.J. and Fisher, A.V. (1990) Comparison of seven ultrasonic techniques for *in vivo* estimation of beef carcass composition with special reference to performance testing. *Animal Production* 51, 489–495.

Proctor, B.E., Davison, S. and Brody, A.L. (1956) A recording strain-gage denture tenderometer for foods. II. Studies on the masticatory force and motion, and the force-penetration relationship. *Food Technology* 10, 327–331.

Proctor, B.E., Davison, S., Malecki, G.J. and Welch, M. (1955) A recording strain-gage denture tenderometer for foods. I. Instrument evaluation and initial tests. *Food Technology* 9, 471–477.

Reece, W.O. (1991) *Physiology of Domestic Animals.* Lea & Febiger, Philadelphia, Chapter 3, pp. 64–80.

Reid, R.L. and Mills, S.C. (1962) Studies on the carbohydrate metabolism of sheep. XIV. The adrenal response to psychological stress. *Australian Journal of Agricultural Research* 13, 282–295.

Renerre, M. (1990) Factors involved in the discolouration of beef meat. *International Journal of Food Science and Technology* 25, 613–630.

Rey, C.R., Kraft, A.A., Topel, D.G., Parrish, F.C. and Hotchkiss, D.K. (1996) Microbiology of pale, dark and normal pork. *Journal of Food Science* 41, 111–116.

Rhodes, D.N., Jones, R.C.D., Chrystall, B.B. and Harries, J.M. (1972) Meat texture II. The relationship between subjective assessments and a compressive test on roast beef. *Journal of Texture Studies* 3, 298–309.

Richardson, R.I. and Mead, G.C. (eds) (1999) *Poultry Meat Science*. Poultry Science Symposium series, Volume 25. CABI Publishing, Wallingford.

Ruusunen, M. and Puolanne, E. (1988) Fiber-type distribution in porcine muscles. *Proceedings of the 34th International Congress of Meat Science and Technology (A)*. Livestock and Meat Authority of Queensland and Meat Research Laboratory. CSIRO Division of Food Processing, Queensland, Australia, pp. 52–54.

Sakata, R., Oshida, T., Morita, H. and Nagata, Y. (1995) Physico-chemical and processing quality of porcine m. longissimus dorsi frozen at different temperatures. *Meat Science* 39, 277–284.

Sandersen, B. (1993) Integrated national research on boar taint in Denmark: causes of boar taint in entire male pigs. In: Bonneau, M. (ed.) *Measurement and Prevention of Boar Taint in Entire Male Pigs*. INRA, Paris, pp. 27–32.

Santos, C., Roseiro, L.C., Gonçalves, H. and Melo, R.S. (1994) Incidence of different pork quality categories in a Portugese slaughterhouse: a survey. *Meat Science* 38, 279–287.

Sañudo, C., Nute, G.R., Campo, M.M., María, G., Baker, A., Sierra, I., Enser, M.E. and Wood, J.D. (1998) Assessment of commercial lamb quality by British and Spanish taste panels. *Meat Science* 48, 91–100.

Sato, K. and Hegarty, G.R. (1971) Warmed-over flavour in cooked meats. *Journal of Food Science* 36, 1098–1102.

Savell, J.W., Dutson, T.R., Smith, G.C. and Carpenter, Z.L. (1978) Structural changes in electrically stimulated beef muscle. *Journal of Food Science* 43, 1606–1609.

Schaefer, A.L., Jones, S.D.M., Tong, A.K.W. and Young, B.A. (1990) Effects of transport and electrolyte supplementation on ion concentrations, carcass yield and quality in bulls. *Canadian Journal of Animal Science* 70, 107–119.

Schaefer, A.L., Jones, S.D.M., Tong, A.K.W., Young, B.A., Murray, N.L. and Lepage, P. (1992) Effects of post-transport electrolyte supplementation on tissue electrolytes, haematology, urine osmolarity and weight loss in beef bulls. *Livestock Production Science* 30, 333–346.

Scott, G.H. (1981) What is animal stress and how is it measured. *Journal of Animal Science* 52, 150–153.

Sebranek, J.G. and Fox, J.B. (1985) A review of nitrite and chloride chemistry: interactions and implications for cured meats. *Journal of the Science of Food and Agriculture* 36, 1169–1182.

Seideman, S.C., Cross, H.R., Oltjen, R.R. and Schanbacher, B.D. (1982) Utilisation of the intact male for red meat production: a review. *Journal of Animal Science* 55, 826–840.

Seidler, D., Nowak, B., Bartnick, E. and Huesmann, M. (1984) PSE-Diagnostik am Schlachtband. Teil 2: Gegenüberstellung der diagnostischen Möglichkeiten mit einem modifizierten MS-Tester und dem FOM-Gerät auf der Basis biochemisch und strukturell orientierter Fleischbeschaffenheitsparameter. *Fleischwirtschaft* 64,1499–1505.

Sellier, P. and Monin, G. (1994) Genetics of pig meat quality: a review. *Journal of Muscle Foods* 5, 187–219.

Sensky, P. (1998) Differences in the calpain enzume system in tough and tender samples of porcine longissimus dorsi. *Proceedings of the British Society of Animal Science*, Scarborough, UK. British Society of Animal Science, Penicuik, Midlothian.

Shackleford, S.D., Koohmaraie, M., Miller, M.F., Crouse, J.D. and Reagan, J.D. (1991) An evaluation of tenderness of the longissimus muscle of Angus by Hereford versus Brahman crossbred haifers. *Journal of Animal Science* 69, 171–177.

Shahidi, F. (1998) Flavor of Meat, Meat Products and Seafoods, 2nd edn. Blackie Academic and Professional (Chapman and Hall), London.

Shahidi, F. and Pegg, R.B. (1991) Encapsulation of the pre-formed cooked cured-meat pigment. *Journal of Food Science* 56, 1500–1504.

Sheard, P.R., Nute, G.R. and Chappell, A.G. (1998a) The effect of cooking on the chemical composition of meat products with special reference to fat loss. *Meat Science* 49, 175–191.

Sheard, P.R., Wood, J.D., Nute, G.R. and Ball, R.C. (1998b) Effects of grilling to 80°C on the chemical composition of pork loin chops and some observations on the UK national food survey estimate of fat composition. *Meat Science* 49, 193–204.

Sheridan, J.J. (1990) The ultra-rapid chilling of lamb carcasses. *Meat Science* 24, 31–50.

Shorthose, W.R. and Wythes, J.R. (1988) Transport of sheep and cattle. *Proceedings of the 34th International Congress of Meat Science and Technology*. Livestock and Meat Authority of Queensland and Meat Research Laboratory. CSIRO Division of Food Processing, Queensland, Australia, p. 122.

Simmons, S.L., Carr, T.R. and McKeith, F.K. (1985) Effects of internal temperature and thickness on palatability of pork loin chops. *Journal of Food Science* 50, 313–315.

Simpson, B.M. (1993) Farm assurance: the Scottish dimension. In: Wood, J.D. and Lawrence, T.L.J. (eds) *Safety and Quality of Food from Animals*. Occasional Publication of the British Society of Animal Production No. 17, British Society of Animal Production, Edinburgh, pp. 69–72.

Simpson, S.P. and Webb, A.J. (1989) Growth and carcass performance of British Landrace pigs heterozygous at the halothane locus. *Animal Production* 49, 503–509.

Sims, T.J. and Bailey, A.J. (1992) Structural aspects of cooked meat. In: Johnston, D.E., Knight, M.K. and Ledward, D.A. (eds) *The Chemistry of Muscle-based Foods*. Royal Society of Chemistry, Cambridge, pp. 106–127.

Skibsted, L.H. (1992) Cured meat products and their oxidative stability. In: Johnston, D.E., Knight, M.K. and Ledward, D.A. (eds) *The Chemistry of Muscle-based Foods*. Royal Society of Chemistry, Cambridge, pp. 266–286.

Smith, G.C. (1985) Effects of electrical stimulation on meat quality, color, grade, heat ring, and palatability. In: Pearson, A.M. and Dutson, T.R. (eds) *Advances in Meat Research: Electrical Stimulation.* AVI, Westport, Connecticut, Volume 1, Chapter 4.

Smith, W.C. and Lesser, D. (1982) An economic assessment of pale, soft, exudative musculature in the fresh and cured pig carcass. *Animal Production* 34, 291–299.

Smulders, F.J.M. (ed.) (1997) *Elimination of Pathogenic Organisms from Meat and Poultry.* Elsevier, Amsterdam.

Smulders, F.J.M., Toldra, F., Flores, J. and Prieto, M. (eds) (1992) *New Technologies for Meat and Meat Products.* ECCEAMST, Utrecht.

Solomon, M.B., Long, J.B. and Eastridge, J.S. (1997) The Hydrodyne: a new process to improve beef tenderness. *Journal of Animal Science* 75, 1534–1537.

Sosniki, A.A. (1993) PSE in turkeys. *Meat Focus International* 2, 75–78.

Sparrey, J.M. and Wotton, S.B. (1997) The design of pig stunning tong electrodes – a review. *Meat Science* 47, 125–133.

Squires, E.J. (1990) Studies on the suitability of a colorimetric test for androst-16-ene steroids in the submaxillary gland and fat of pigs as a simple chemical test for boar taint. *Canadian Journal of Animal Science* 70, 1029–1040.

Squires, E.J., Gullet, E.A., Fisher, K.R.S. and Partlow, G.D. (1991) Comparison of androst-16-ene steroid levels determined by a colorimetric assay with boar taint estimated by a trained sensory panel. *Journal of Animal Science* 69, 1092–1100.

Stevenson, M.H. (1992) Irradiation of meat and poultry. In: Johnston, D.E., Knight, M.K. and Ledward, D.A. (eds) *The Chemistry of Muscle-based Foods.* Royal Society of Chemistry, Cambridge, pp. 308–324.

Strother, J.W. (1975) The commercial preparation of fresh meat at wholesale and retail levels. In: Cole, D.J.A. and Lawrie, R.A. (eds) *Meat.* Butterworth & Co (publishers) Ltd, London, Chapter 9, pp. 183–204.

Sudarmadji, S. and Urbain, W.M. (1972) Flavor sensitivity of selected animal protein foods to gamma radiation. *Journal of Food Science* 37, 671–672.

Swarbrick, O. (1986) The welfare during transport of broilers, old hens and replacement pullets. In: Gibson, T.E. (ed.) *The Welfare of Animals in Transit.* British Veterinary Association, Animal Welfare Foundation, London, pp. 82–97.

Swartz, D.R., Greaser, M.L. and Marsh, B.B. (1993) Structural studies of rigor bovine myofibrils using fluorescence microscopy. II Influence of sarcomere length on the building of myosin subfragment-1, alpha actinin and G-actin to rigor myofibrils. *Meat Science* 33, 157–190.

Swatland, H.J. (1983) Measurement of electrical stunning, rate of exsanguination and reflex activity in pigs in an abattoir. *Journal of the Canadian Institute of Food Science and Technology* 16, 35–38.

Swatland, H.J. (1991) Evaluation of probe designs to measure connective tissue fluorescence in carcasses. *Journal of Animal Science* 69, 1983–1988.

Swatland, H.J. (1994) *Structure and Development of Meat Animals and Poultry.* Technomic, Lancaster, Pennsylvania.

Swatland, H.J., Ananthanarayanan, S.P. and Goldenberg, A.A. (1994) A review of probes and robots: implementing new technologies in meat evaluation. *Journal of Animal Science* 72, 1475–1486.

Swensen, K., Ellis, M., Brewer, M.S., Novakofski, J. and McKeith, F.K. (1998) Pork carcass composition: II Use of indicator cuts for predicting carcass composition. *Journal of Animal Science* 76, 2405–2414.

Sybesma, W. (1966) Die Messung des Unterschiedes im Auftreten des Rigor mortis in Schinken. *Fleischwirtschaft* 46, 637–639.

Tappel, A.L., Brown, W.D., Zalkin, H. and Maier, V.P. (1961) Unsaturated lipide peroxidation catalysed by hematin compounds and its inhibition by vitamin E. *Journal of the American Oil Chemist's Society* 38, 5–9.

Taylor, A.A. and Shaw, B.G. (1977) The effect of meat pH and package permeability on putrefaction and greening in vacuum-packed beef. *Journal of Food Technology* 12, 515–521.

Taylor, A.A., Shaw, B.G. and MacDougall, D.B. (1981) Hot deboning beef with and without electrical stimulation. *Meat Science* 5, 109–123.

Taylor, A.A., Perry, A.M. and Warkup, C.C. (1995) Improving pork quality by electrical stimulation or pelvic suspension of carcasses. *Meat Science* 39, 327–337.

Taylor, D.A. (1993) Dirty cattle. *Veterinary Record* 132, 308 (letter).

Taylor, D.J. (1997) A realistic assessment of the risks of antimicrobial use in animals and its effects on food safety. *The Pig Journal* 40, 46–59.

Taylor, D.M., Fernie, K., McConnell, I., Ferguson, C.E. and Steele, P.J. (1998) Solvent extraction as an adjunct to rendering: the effect on BSE and scrapie agents of hot solvents followed by dry heat and steam. *Veterinary Record* 143, 6–9.

Taylor, S.A. (1996a) Basic considerations in meat packaging. In: Taylor, S.A., Raimundo, A., Severini, M. and Smulders, F.J.M. (eds) *Meat Quality and Meat Packaging*. ECCEAMST, Utrecht, pp. 259–271.

Taylor, S.A. (1996b) Modified atmosphere packaging of meat. In: Taylor, S.A., Raimundo, A., Severini, M. and Smulders, F.J.M. (eds) *Meat Quality and Meat Packaging*. ECCEAMST, Utrecht, pp. 301–311.

Taylor, S.A. (1996c) Improving tenderness by electrical stimulation or hip suspension. In: Taylor, S.A., Raimundo, A., Severini, M. and Smulders, F.J.M. (eds) *Meat Quality and Meat Packaging*. ECCEAMST, Utrecht, pp. 89–105.

Thonney, M.L., Perry, T.C., Armbruster, G., Beermann, D.H. and Fox, D.G. (1991) Comparison of steaks from Holstein and Simmental × Angus steers. *Journal of Animal Science* 69, 4866–4870.

Threlfall, E.J. (1992) Antibiotics and the selection of food-borne pathogens. *Journal of Applied Bacteriology* (Symposium Suppl.) 73, 96S-102S.

Tomkin, R.B. (1990) The use of HACCP in the production of meat and poultry products. *Journal of Food Protection* 53, 795–803.

Topel, D.G., Miller, J.A., Berger, P.J., Rust, R.E., Parrish, F.C. and Ono, K. (1976) Palatability and visual appearance of dark, normal and pale colored porcine m. longissimus. *Journal of Food Science* 41, 628–630.

Tornberg, E. (1996) Biophysical aspects of meat tenderness. *Meat Science* 43, No. S, S175-S191.

Trenkle, A. and Marple, D.N. (1983) Growth and development of meat animals. *Journal of Animal Science* 57 (Suppl. 2), 273–283.

Tribe, D.E. (1964) *Carcase Composition and Appraisal of Meat Animals*. CSIRO, East Melbourne, Victoria, Australia.

Troeger, K. (1989) Plasma adrenaline levels of pigs after different preslaughter handling and stunning methods. *Proceedings of the 35th International Congress of Meat Science and Technology*, Roskilde, Denmark. Danish Meat Research Institute, Roskilde, pp. 975–980.

Tronstad, A. (1997) The Swedish ban on antibiotic growth promoters in animal feeds. *The Pig Journal* 40, 89–98.

Trout, G.R. (1992) Evalution of techniques for monitoring pork quality in Australian pork processing plants. *Proceedings of the 38th International Congress of Meat Science and Technology*, Clermont-Ferrand, France. Station de Recherches sur la Viande, INRA, Theix, France, pp. 983–986.

Tulloh, N.M. (1964) The carcass compositions of sheep, cattle, and pigs as functions of body weight. In: Tribe, D.E. (ed.) *Carcase Composition and Appraisal of Meat Animals*. CSIRO, East Melbourne, Victoria, Australia.

Tuma, H.J., Venable, J.H., Wuthier, P.R. and Henrickson, R.L. (1962) Relation of fibre diameter to tenderness and meatiness as influenced by bovine age. *Journal of Animal Science* 21, 33–38.

Uijtenboogaart, T.G. (1996) Poultry handling, slaughter and primary processing. In: Taylor, S.A., Raimundo, A., Severini, M. and Smulders, F.J.M. (eds) *Meat Quality and Meat Packaging*. ECCEAMST, Utrecht, pp. 125–136.

Van Laack, R.L.J.M. and Smulders, F.J.M. (1989) The effect of electrical stimulation, time of boning and high temperature conditioning on sensory quality traits of porcine longissimus dorsi muscle. *Meat Science* 25, 113–121.

Varnum, A.H. and Sutherland, J.P. (1995) *Meat and Meat Products*. Chapman and Hall, London.

Veerkamp, C.N. (1986) Preslaughter conditions for poultry-good handling gives better yield. *Poultry-Misset* April, 30–33.

Voisey, P.W. (1976) Engineering assessment and critique of instruments used for meat tenderness evaluation. *Journal of Texture Studies* 7, 11–48.

Voyle, C. (1971) *Proceedings of the 17th European Meeting of Meat Research Workers*, Bristol. Meat Research Institute, Bristol, pp. 95–97.

Wabeck, C.J. (1972) Feed and water withdrawal time relationship to processing yield and potential faecal contamination of broilers. *Poultry Science* 51, 1119–1121.

Wachholz, D., Kauffman, R.G., Henderson, D. and Lockner, J.V. (1978) Consumer discrimination of pork color at the market place. *Journal of Food Science* 43, 1150–1152.

Wal, van der, P.G., Bolink, A.H. and Merkus, G.S.M. (1988) Differences in quality characteristics of normal, PSE and DFD pork. *Meat Science* 24, 79–84.

Warkup, C.C. (1993) Improving meat quality: the blueprint approach. In: Wood, J.D. and Lawrence, T.L.J. (eds) *Safety and Quality of Food from Animals*. Occasional Publication of the British Society of Animal Production No. 17, British Society of Animal Production, Edinburgh, pp. 63–67.

Warner, R.D. and Eldridge, G.A. (1988) Preliminary observations of pig meat quality problems in a Victorian abattoir. *Proceedings of the 34th International Congress of Meat Science and Technology*. Livestock and Meat Authority of Queensland and Meat Research Laboratory. CSIRO Division of Food Processing, Queensland, Australia, pp. 573–574.

Warner, R.D., Kauffman, R.G. and Russell, R.L. (1993) Quality attributes of major porcine muscles: a comparison with the longissimus lumborum. *Meat Science* 33, 359–372.

Warriss, P.D. (1984a) Exsanguination of animals at slaughter and the residual blood content of meat. *Veterinary Record* 115, 292–295.

Warriss, P.D. (1984b) The behaviour and blood profile of bulls which produce dark cutting meat. *Journal of the Science of Food and Agriculture* 35, 863–868.

Warriss, P.D. (1984c) The incidence of carcass damage in slaughter pigs. *Proceedings of the 30th European Meeting of Meat Research Workers*, Bristol. Meat Research Institute, Bristol, paper 1:8, pp. 19–20.

Warriss, P.D. (1985) Marketing losses caused by fasting and transport during the pre-slaughter handling of pigs. *Pig News and Information* 6, 155–157.

Warriss, P.D. (1987) The effect of time and conditions of transport and lairage on pig meat quality. In: Tarrant, P.V., Eikelenboom, G. and Monin, G. (eds) *Evaluation and Control of Meat Quality in Pigs.* Martinus Nijhoff, Dordrecht, pp. 245–264.

Warriss, P.D. (1990) The handling of cattle preslaughter and its effects on carcass and meat quality. *Applied Animal Behaviour Science* 28, 171–186.

Warriss, P.D. (1992) Handling animals before slaughter and the consequences for welfare and product quality. *Meat Focus International* 1, 135–138.

Warriss, P.D. (1994) Ante-mortem handling of pigs. In: Cole, D.J.A., Wiseman, J. and Varley, M.A. (eds) *Principles of Pig Science.* University of Nottingham Press, Nottingham, pp. 425–432.

Warriss, P.D. (1995) Ante-mortem factors influencing the yield and quality of meat from farm animals. In: Morgan Jones, S.D. (ed.) *Quality and Grading of Carcasses of Meat Animals.* CRC Press Inc., Boca Raton, Florida, pp. 1–15.

Warriss, P.D. (1996a) Guidelines for the handling of pigs antemortem. *Meat Focus International* 4, 491–494.

Warriss, P.D. (1996b) Instrumental measurement of colour. In: Taylor, S.A., Raimundo, A., Severini, M. and Smulders, F.J.M. (eds) *Meat Quality and Meat Packaging.* ECCEAMST, Utrecht, pp. 221–232.

Warriss, P.D. (1996c) Introduction: what is meat quality? In: Taylor, S.A., Raimundo, A., Severini, M. and Smulders, F.J.M. (eds) *Meat Quality and Meat Packaging.* ECCEAMST, Utrecht, pp. 3–10.

Warriss, P.D. (1996d) The consequences of fighting between mixed groups of unfamiliar pigs before slaughter. *Meat Focus International* 5, 89–92.

Warriss, P.D. (1996e) The welfare of animals during transport. In: Raw, M.E. and Parkinson, T.J. (eds) *The Veterinary Annual.* Blackwell Science Ltd, Oxford, Volume 36, pp. 73–85.

Warriss, P.D. and Brown, S.N. (1983) The influence of pre-slaughter fasting on carcass and liver yield in pigs. *Livestock Production Science* 10, 273–282.

Warriss, P.D. and Brown, S.N. (1987) The relationship between initial pH, reflectance and exudation in pig muscle. *Meat Science* 20, 65–74.

Warriss, P.D. and Brown, S.N. (1993) Relationships between the subjective assessment of pork quality and objective measures of colour. In: Wood, J.D. and Lawrence, T.L.J. (eds) *Safety and Quality of Food from Animals.* Occasional Publication of the British Society of Animal Production No. 17, British Society of Animal Production, Edinburgh, pp. 98–101.

Warriss, P.D. and Brown, S.N. (1994) A survey of mortality in slaughter pigs during transport and lairage. *Veterinary Record* 134, 513–515.

Warriss, P.D. and Wotton, S.B. (1981) Effect of cardiac arrest on exsanguination in pigs. *Research in Veterinary Science* 31, 82–86.

Warriss, P.D., Dudley, C.P. and Brown, S.N. (1983) Reduction of carcass yield in transported pigs. *Journal of the Science of Food and Agriculture* 34, 351–356.

Warriss, P.D., Kestin, S.C., Brown, S.N. and Wilkins, L.J. (1984) The time required for recovery from mixing stress in young bulls and the prevention of dark cutting meat. *Meat Science* 10, 53–68.

Warriss, P.D., Brown, S.N., Bevis, E.A., Kestin, S.C. and Young, C.S. (1987) Influence of food withdrawal at various times pre-slaughter on carcass yield and meat quality in sheep. *Journal of the Science of Food and Agriculture* 39, 325–334.

Warriss, P.D., Kestin, S.C., Brown, S.N. and Bevis, E.A. (1988) Depletion of glycogen reserves in fasting broiler chickens. *British Poultry Science* 29, 149–154.

Warriss, P.D., Bevis, E.A., Brown, S.N. and Ashby, J.G. (1989a) An examination of potential indices of fasting time in commercially-slaughtered sheep. *British Veterinary Journal* 145, 242–248.

Warriss, P.D., Brown, S.N., Lopez-Bote, C., Bevis, E.A. and Adams, S.J.M. (1989b) Evaluation of lean meat quality in pigs using two electronic probes. *Meat Science* 25, 281–291.

Warriss, P.D., Kestin, S.C. and Brown, S.N. (1989c) The effect of β-adrenergic agonists on meat quality in sheep. *Animal Production* 48, 385–392.

Warriss, P.D., Brown, S.N., Franklin, J.G. and Kestin, S.C. (1990a) The thickness and quality of backfat in various pig breeds and their relationship to intramuscular fat and the setting of joints from the carcasses. *Meat Science* 28, 21–29.

Warriss, P.D., Brown, S.N., Rolph, T.P. and Kestin, S.C. (1990b) Interactions between the β-adrenergic agonist Salbutamol and genotype on meat quality in pigs. *Journal of Animal Science* 68, 3669–3676.

Warriss, P.D., Kestin, S.C., Rolph, T.P. and Brown, S.N. (1990c) The effects of the β-adrenergic agonist salbutamol on meat quality in pigs. *Journal of Animal Science* 68, 128–136.

Warriss, P.D., Brown, S.N. and Adams, S.J.M. (1991) Use of the Tecpro pork quality meter for assessing meat quality on the slaughterline. *Meat Science* 30, 147–156.

Warriss, P.D., Bevis, E.A., Brown, S.N. and Edwards, J.E. (1992) Longer journeys to processing plants are associated with higher mortality in broiler chickens. *British Poultry Science* 33, 201–206.

Warriss, P.D., Brown, S.N. and Nute, G.R. (1993a) Differences in meat quality between boars and gilts. In: Wood, J.D. and Lawrence, T.L.J. (eds) *Safety and Quality of Food from Animals.* Occasional Publication of the British Society of Animal Production No. 17, British Society of Animal Production, Edinburgh, pp. 95–97.

Warriss, P.D., Kestin, S.C., Brown, S.N., Knowles, T.G., Wilkins, L.J., Edwards, J.E., Austin, S.D. and Nicol, C.J. (1993b) The depletion of glycogen stores and indices of dehydration in transported broilers. *British Veterinary Journal* 149, 391–398.

Warriss, P.D., Brown, S.N., Adams, S.J.M. and Corlett, I.K. (1994) Relationships between subjective and objective assessments of stress at slaughter and meat quality in pigs. *Meat Science* 38, 329–340.

Warriss, P.D., Brown, S.N., Knowles, T.G., Kestin, S.C., Edwards, J.E., Dolan, S.K. and Phillips, A.J. (1995a) Effects on cattle of transport by road for up to fifteen hours. *Veterinary Record* 136, 319–323.

Warriss, P.D., Brown, S.N., Nute, G.R., Knowles, T.G., Edwards, J.E., Perry, A.M. and Johnson, S.P. (1995b) Potential interactions between the effects of preslaughter stress and post-mortem electrical stimulation of the carcasses on meat quality in pigs. *Meat Science* 41, 55–68.

Warriss, P.D., Kestin, S.C., Brown, S.N. and Nute, G.R. (1996) The quality of pork from traditional pig breeds. *Meat Focus International* 5, 179–182.

Wasserman, A.E. and Gray, N. (1965) Meat flavour. 1. Fractionation of water-soluble flavour precursors of beef. *Journal of Food Science* 30, 801–807.

Webb, J. (1998) MAFF: Role in quality assurance pig assurance scheme (PAS) Farm Assured British Pigs (FABPIGS). *The Pig Journal* 41, 105–109.

Webb, J.E., Brunson, C.C. and Yates, J.D. (1972) Effects of feeding antioxidants on rancidity development in pre-cooked, frozen broiler parts. *Poultry Science* 51, 1601–1605.

Weber, A. and Murray, J.M. (1973) Molecular control mechanisms in muscle contraction. *Physiological Reviews* 53, 612–673.

Webster, A.J.F. (1980) The energetic efficiency of growth. *Livestock Production Science* 7, 243–252.

Webster, A.J.F., Tuddenham, A., Saville, C.A. and Scott, G.B. (1993) Thermal stress on chickens in transit. *British Poultry Science* 34, 267–277.

Webster, J. (1995) *Animal Welfare – A Cool Eye towards Eden.* Blackwell Science, Oxford.

Webster, J. and Saville, C. (1981) Rearing of veal calves. In: *Alternatives to Intensive Husbandry Systems.* Universities Federation for Animal Welfare (UFAW), Potters Bar, pp. 86–94.

Wheeler, T.L. and Koohmaraie, M. (1992) Effects of the β-adrenergic agonist L644, 969 on muscle protein turnover, endogenous proteinase activities, and meat tenderness in steers. *Journal of Animal Science* 70, 3035–3043.

Wheeler, T.L. and Koohmaraie, M. (1994) Prerigor and postrigor changes in tenderness of ovine longissimus muscle. *Journal of Animal Science* 72, 1232–1238.

Wheeler, T.L., Koohmaraie, M. and Shackelford, S.D. (1994) Reducing inconsistent beef tenderness with calcium-activated tenderization. *Proceedings of the Meat Industry Research Conference of the American Meat Science Association.* American Meat Science Association, Chicago, p. 119.

Wheeler, T.L., Koohmaraie, M. and Shackelford, S.D. (1996) Effects of vitamin C concentration and co-injection with calcium chloride on beef retail display color. *Journal of Animal Science* 74, 1846–1853.

Whitfield, F.B. (1998) Microbiology of food taints. *International Journal of Food Science and Technology* 33, 31–51.

Whittaker, J. (1997) The incidence of dark, firm, dry cutting beef in bulls, steers and heifers. MSc Thesis, University of Bristol.

Willis, W.L., Murray, C. and Raczkowski, C.W. (1996) The influence of feed and water withdrawal on *Campylobacter jejuni* detection and yield of broilers. *Journal of Applied Poultry Research* 5, 210–214.

Wilson, A. (1998) *Wilson's Practical Meat Inspection*, 6th edn, revised by Wilson, W. Blackwell Science, Oxford.

Wood, J.D. (1995) The influence of carcass composition on meat quality. In: Morgan Jones, S.D. (ed.) *Quality and Grading of Carcasses of Meat Animals*. CRC Press, Boca Raton, Florida, pp. 131–155.

Wood, J.D. and Butler-Hogg, B.W. (1982) Deposition of fat and its partition between the major fat depots in meat animals. *Journal of the Science of Food and Agriculture* 33, 810–811.

Wood, J.D. and Enser, M. (1997) Factors influencing fatty acids in meat and the role of antioxidants in improving meat quality. *British Journal of Nutrition* 78 (Suppl. 1), S49–S60.

Wood, J.D., Warriss, P.D. and Enser, M.B. (1992) Effects of production factors on meat quality in pigs. In: Johnston, D.E., Knight, M.K. and Ledward, D.A. (eds) *The Chemistry of Muscle-based Foods*. Royal Society of Chemistry, Cambridge, pp. 3–15.

Wood, J.D., Nute, G.R., Fursey, G.A.J. and Cuthbertson, A. (1995) The effect of cooking conditions on the eating quality of pork. *Meat Science* 40, 127–135.

Wood, J.D., Holder, J.S. and Main, D.C. (1998) Quality assurance schemes. *Meat Science* 49 (Suppl. 1), S191-S203.

Wotton, S.B., Anil, M.H., Whittington, P.E. and McKinstry, J.L. (1992) Pig slaughtering procedures: head-to-back stunning. *Meat Science* 32, 245–255.

Wythes, J.R., Round, P.J., Johnston, G.N. and Smith, P.C. (1989) Cattle handling at abattoirs. III. The effects of feeding, and of different feeds, during the resting period before slaughter on liveweight, carcass and muscle properties. *Australian Journal of Agricultural Research* 40, 1099–1109.

Xue, J., Dial, G.D., Holton, E.E., Vicker, Z., Squires, E.J., Lou, Y., Godbout, D. and Morel, N. (1996) Differences in boar taint: relationship between tissue levels of boar taint compounds and sensory analysis of taint. *Journal of Animal Science* 74, 2170–2177.

Yndgaard, C.F. (1973) Technical note: a routine procedure for pH measurements in pig carcasses. *Journal of Food Technology* 8, 485–488.

Zalick, N. (1993) The Welsh lamb premium scheme in practice. In: Wood, J.D. and Lawrence, T.L.J. (eds) *Safety and Quality of Food from Animals*. Occasional Publication of the British Society of Animal Production No. 17, British Society of Animal Production, Edinburgh, pp. 73–76.

Index